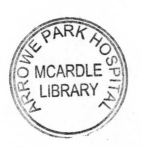

Synopsis of
Otolaryngology

Fifth edition

Synopsis of
Otolaryngology

Roger F. Gray FRCS
Consultant ENT Surgeon, Addenbrooke's Hospital, Cambridge

Maurice Hawthorne FRCS
Consultant ENT Surgeon, Midlesborough

Fifth edition

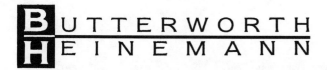

Butterworth-Heinemann Ltd
Linacre House, Jordan Hill, Oxford OX2 8DP

 PART OF REED INTERNATIONAL BOOKS

OXFORD   LONDON   BOSTON
MUNICH   NEW DELHI   SINGAPORE   SYDNEY
TOKYO   TORONTO   WELLINGTON

First published 1957
Second edition 1967
Third edition 1978
Reprinted 1982 1983
Fourth edition 1985
Fifth edition 1992

British Library Cataloguing in Publication Data
Gray, Roger F.
  Synopsis of otolaryngology. – 5th ed.
  – (Synopsis series)
  I. Title II. Hawthorne, Maurice III. Series
  617.5

ISBN 0 7506 1358 0

Library of Congress Cataloguing in Publication Data
Gray, Roger F., 1946–
  Synopsis of otolaryngology. – 5th ed./Roger F. Gray, Maurice Hawthorne.
    p. cm.
  Rev. ed. of: A synopsis of otolaryngology/John Groves, Roger F. Gray.
  4th ed. 1985.
  Includes bibliographical references and index.
  ISBN 0 7506 1358 0
  1. Otolaryngology—Handbooks, manuals, etc. I. Hawthorne, Maurice.
  II. Groves, John. Synopsis of otolaryngology. III. Title.
  [DNLM: 1. Otorhinolaryngologic Diseases. WV 100 G781s]
  RF56.G73   1992
  617.5'1–dc20
  DNLM/DC
  For Library of Congress   91-23288
                                                                    CIP

Composition by Scribe Design, Gillingham, Kent
Printed in Great Britain at the University Press, Cambridge

Preface to the fifth edition

New ways of treating old diseases and the appearance of new ones have necessitated extensive revision of 'Synopsis'. These changes may not be obvious because the publishers have urged that we keep to the successful format of the 4th edition.

Sections on the salivary glands, rhinoplasty, aesthetic facial surgery, aspiration and ENT aspects of systemic disease, particularly AIDS, have been added, together with 15 new illustrations. Inspiration for these has come from several excellent texts and we owe the authors a debt of gratitude where we have adapted their style to fill our needs. The beautiful and anatomically precise images of the CT scanner now grace our pages.

We say goodbye to John Groves, a leading architect of the the first four editions, and wish him well in his retirement. His contribution will be appreciated by those who have obtained higher specialist qualifications in otolaryngology studying with 'Synopsis'. Always an enthusiastic teacher, this book has made the English speaking world his classroom for three decades. It was during a visit to Madras in 1987 that I became aware of the extensive use made of 'Synopsis' by young surgeons in India preparing for a career in otolaryngology, and this has been a source of great encouragement.

Maurice Hawthorne is my new co-editor, the last Royal Free Hospital registrar to train under both John Groves and John Ballantyne; we benefit from his polished style and his experience in Bristol and particularly Zurich where he has held an otological fellowship.

Thanks go to Dr Nathanial Blau, Consultant Neurologist, whose excellent pages on neurology for otolaryngologists remains largely unchanged, also to Mr David Baguley, Audiological Scientist, for his advice on paediatric tests and hearing aids. I wish to thank Dr Geoffrey Smaldon for his gentle but persistent encouragement and to both our wives for their patience and endurance during the hours of preparation of this edition.

Roger F. Gray

Preface to the first edition

We hope that this book will prove to be a useful addition to the 'Synopsis' series. It is intended for quick reference and revision, especially by those who are studying for postgraduate examinations in the specialty.

Much material has inevitably been drawn from the current standard textooks and journals dealing with the subject. In this respect we wish particularly to acknowledge the liberal help we have obtained from the book by the late Sir StClair Thomson and Sir Victor Negus, and from those edited by Mr Maxwell Ellis, Mr W. G. Scott-Brown, and Mr F. W. Watkyn-Thomas. Many other sources have been consulted, including original articles in the *Journal of Laryngology and Otology*, the *Archives of Otolaryngology* of the American Medical Association, and the *Annals of Otology, Rhinology and Laryngology*.

The principles of operative procedures are stated but the details of technique are not considered to lie within the compass of such a book. So rapidly have chemotherapy and the antibiotics developed in the past few years that we have thought it wise, in many instances, to use a generic term – Systemic Disinfection – when such drugs are indicated.

We feel that the association between neurology and diseases of the ear, nose, and throat deserves special attention, and for this reason a section on the subject has been incorporated. We thank Dr Charles Harold Edwards for his valued collaboration in writing this section. Conversely, we have reduced the chapters on the trachea and bronchi to a minimum, as this subject is being increasingly absorbed by the rapidly-expanding specialty of Thoracic Surgery.

We are much indebted to Mrs Murray Laing, who has produced many of the illustrations and whose skill and advice in this respect have been much appreciated. Mr John Groves, Senior Registrar to the Ear, Nose and Throat Department of St Mary's Hospital, has rendered great assistance by reading the early drafts, and we have gladly taken advantage of his many pertinent criticisms and suggestions. He has also drawn a considerable number of the illustrations. He has our most sincere thanks.

We wish to thank Mr Henry J. Shaw, Assistant Director to the Professorial Unit at the Institute of Laryngology and Otology, London, W.C.l, for cheerfully undertaking the labour of correcting the final proofs.

Finally, we should like to record the friendly co-operation and help that we have received from Mr L. G. Owens, BSc, Director of the firm of John Wright & Sons Ltd, throughout the preparation of this volume.

JFS IGR JCB

Contents

Chapter 23 **Diseases of the nervous system in relation to otolaryngology 545**

Part I
The ear

Chapter 1

Surgical anatomy

DEVELOPMENT OF THE EAR

Visceral arches and clefts

During the third week of fetal development, a series of six *visceral arches* appears on the lateral aspect of the head. These mesenchymal arches form ridges in the overlying ectoderm and corresponding projections in the ento-derm of the pharynx. The ridges become separated from one another by a series of furrows where ectoderm and entoderm come into contact with one another. The ectodermal furrows form the visceral clefts. The entodermal furrows form the *pharyngeal* pouches (Figure 1.1).

Each arch has its own nerve supply and arch artery. In man the arch nerves have branches which pass into the territory of the preceding arches.

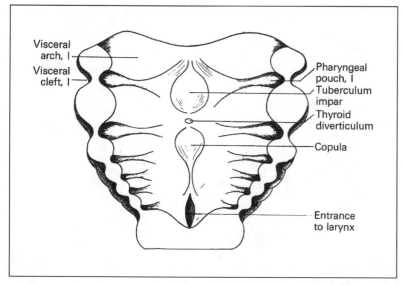

Figure 1.1 Visceral arches and clefts, and pharyngeal pouches

The vagus nerve (arches 4 and 6) has an auricular branch which supplies part of the pinna, external auditory meatus and tympanic membrane.

Auricle

Develops from a series of six tubercles which form round the margins of the first visceral cleft.

External auditory canal

This is formed from the ectoderm of the first visceral cleft.

Tympanic membrane

This has three layers:

1. An outer *epithelial* layer, from the ectoderm of the cleft.
2. A middle *fibrous* layer, from the mesoderm between the first visceral cleft and the tubotympanic recess.
3. An inner *'mucosal'* layer, from entoderm of part of the tubotympanic recess.

Eustachian tube and tympanic cavity

The dorsal recesses of the first and second entodermal pouches fuse to form the tubotympanic recess. The recess expands around the ossicles and chorda tympani clothing them in entoderm and so forms the eustachian tube and tympanic cavity. A cartilaginous process grows from the lateral part of the capsule to form the *tegmen tympani* and the lateral wall of the eustachian tube. In this way the tympanic cavity and proximal part of the tube are included in the petrous temporal bone. During the sixth or seventh month the mastoid antrum appears as a dorsal expansion of the middle ear cavity.

Malleus and incus

These are derived from the mesoderm of the first visceral arch (Figure 1.2).

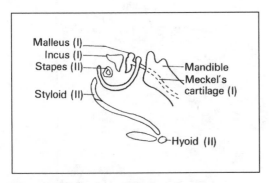

Figure 1.2 Derivatives of the visceral arches

Stapes

The head, neck and crura are derived from the mesoderm of the second visceral arch; the footplate comes from the otic capsule which develops in the mesoderm surrounding the membranous labyrinth (Figure 1.2).

Inner ear

Bilaterally, an ectodermal placode sinks below the surface to form the auditory vesicle — the primordium of the membranous labyrinth. The mesoderm surrounding it becomes the cartilaginous ear capsule, which finally ossifies to form the bony labyrinth. The otic vesicle contributes to the acousticofacial complex of neural crest material. After separation of the geniculate ganglion the otic vesicle becomes subdivided into vestibular and cochlear parts. The peripheral process of the bipolar neuroblasts of the vestibular and spiral ganglia grows into the membranous labyrinth while the central process grows proximally to synapse with the vestibulocochlear complex in the floor of the IV ventricle. The inner ear has reached its full adult size and form by the end of the fourth fetal month.

DEVELOPMENT OF THE TEMPORAL BONE

Morphological elements

There are four distinct elements which become fused together (Figure 1.3). 1. *Tympanic ring* is formed in membrane and is an incomplete circle deficient above. Its concavity is grooved by the *tympanic sulcus* for the attachment of the greater part of the circumference of the tympanic membrane. This circumference is thickened into a definite rim which allows the surgeon to dislocate the membrane out of the sulcus without tearing. The ring grows

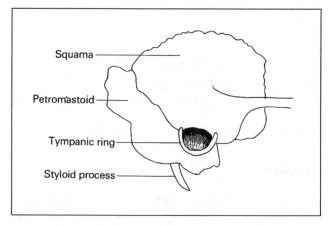

Figure 1.3 Parts of the temporal bone

laterally and slightly backwards to form the tympanic plate, but the anterior and posterior portions grow more rapidly than the rest. This leaves a foramen in the floor of the canal (the foramen of Huschke). This may persist through life.

2. *Squama* is also ossified in membrane and is developed to help in the protection of the brain. The postero-inferior portion of the squama grows downwards behind the tympanic ring to form the lateral wall of the mastoid antrum.

3. *Styloid process* is developed from the cranial end of the cartilage of the second visceral arch.

4. *Petromastoid* is preformed in cartilage as a protecting capsule for the membranous labyrinth.

The bony capsule has three layers:

- A thin outer or *periosteal* layer.
- A thick middle or *enchondral* layer.
- A thin inner or *endosteal* layer.

Ossification may be defective in the middle layer, particularly in the region of the *fissula ante fenestram*. This is at the junction of cochlea and vestibule, just in front of the oval window, and is the site of election for a focus of otosclerotic bone.

Development of mastoid process

The mastoid portion of the temporal bone is flat at birth and the stylomastoid foramen, through which the *facial nerve* emerges, lies immediately behind the tympanic ring. As air cells develop, the lateral part of the mastoid portion grows downwards and forwards to form the *mastoid process*. Hence the stylomastoid foramen comes to lie on the under-surface of the bone. This descent is accompanied by an increase in length of the facial nerve canal. The mastoid process does not form a definite elevation until the end of the second year of life. The mastoid antrum lies *above* the tympanic cavity in the infant, about 2 mm deep to the bony surface.

Mastoid types

There are three types of definitive mastoid process (Figure 1.4):

1. *Cellular,* where air cells are large and numerous.
2. *Diploic,* where cells are small and less numerous. Marrow spaces are present.
3. *Sclerotic* (or 'ivory'), where cells and marrow spaces are absent.

Pneumatization of mastoid

Eighty per cent of mastoids are pneumatized, 20% diploic or sclerotic. The pneumatized mastoid can therefore be regarded as normal. The individual type is usually, but not necessarily, the same on both sides.

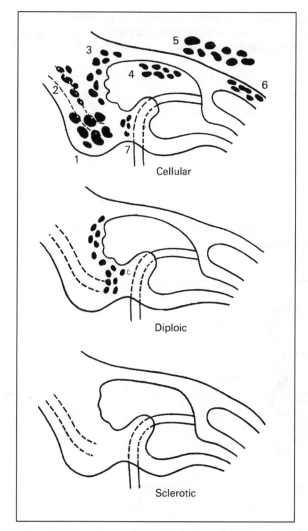

Figure 1.4 Threes types of mastoid. In the cellular type the following groups of cells may be present: 1, tip; 2, perisinus; 3, sinodural angle or petrosal; 4 perilabyrinthine; 5, superficial to dura; 6, zygomatic; 7, perifacial

Theories of deficient pneumatization

There are three main theories:
1. *Tumarkin* believes that 'frustration of pneumatization' results from failure of aeration of the middle ear cleft, from blockage of the eustachian tube. This occurs particularly in upper respiratory 'catarrh'.

This view has been confirmed by Lindeman by further radiological studies in children with middle ear effusions.
2. *Diamant and Dahlberg* believed that dense bone is congenital and that all sizes of air-cell system may be normal variants.

3. Wittmaack believed that the dense mastoid resulted from infantile otitis media, which interfered with the normal absorption of diploe and hence with pneumatization. This is not supported by evidence.

ANATOMY OF THE EAR

External ear

The external ear consists of two parts:

1. Auricle (Figure 1.5)

The auricle has a framework of cartilage except in the lobule. The skin is closely adherent to the perichondrium.

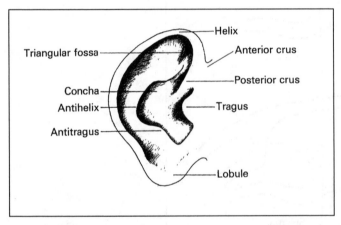

Figure 1.5 Right ear (auricle)

2. External auditory canal

The adult external auditory canal is about 2.5 cm in length from the concha to the tympanic membrane. It is subdivided into:

- A *cartilaginous* portion, in its outer third which is directed medially and slightly upwards and backwards. The cartilage, deficient superiorly, is continuous with that of the auricle. The deficiency is continuous with the space between the tragus and the crus of the helix. The skin is vibrissae bearing and produces wax from pilosebaceous and ceruminous glands which binds with desquamated keratin.
- A *bony* portion, in its inner two-thirds. The posterosuperior portion is formed by the squama, the remainder by the tympanic plate. The thin hairless and gland-free skin is closely adherent to the sutures between the tympanic plate and the squama. Prominent anterior and posterior bony

meatal spines may project from the free outer border of the tympanic plate at the squamotympanic and tympanomastoid sutures (Figure 1.6). These *endomeatal sutures and spines* add to the difficulty of separating an intact flap of skin from the bony canal.

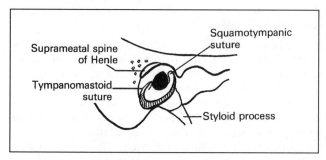

Figure 1.6 Endomeatal spines and sutures (right ear)

Relations of external auditory meatus

1. Temporomandibular joint, in front.
2. Mastoid air cells, behind.
3. Middle cranial fossa, above.
4. Mastoid antrum, posteromedial and superomedial to the sloping squamous portion of the deep bony canal.
5. Parotid gland, in front and below.

Sensory nerve supply of external ear (See Figure 1.18)

Vascular supply of external ear

1. Auriculotemporal branch of superficial temporal artery, anteriorly.
2. Branches of postauricular division of external carotid artery, posteriorly.

Lymphatic drainage of auricle

1. Parotid lymph nodes, in front (preauricular).
2. Posterior lymph nodes, behind (postauricular).
3. External jugular lymph nodes, below.

Constrictions and anterior recess of meatus

There are two constrictions in the external auditory canal:

1. At the medial end of the cartilaginous portion.
2. About 5 mm from the tympanic membrane, in the bony portion (*isthmus*). From the isthmus, the floor of the canal dips steeply downwards and forwards to form the anterior recess. It is often difficult to remove debris from this recess.

Middle ear cleft

The eustachian tube and antero-inferior part of tympanic cavity are lined with respiratory epithelium (columnar ciliated). Elsewhere the epithelium is cuboidal. The cleft consists of:

1. Eustachian (pharyngotympanic) tube

The lower orifice lies in the lateral wall of the nasopharynx on a level with the posterior end of the inferior turbinate. In the adult this 3.7 cm tube runs laterally and posterosuperiorly, to open in the anterior wall of the tympanic cavity. The lateral third is bony, while the lower superior and medial parts are cartilaginous and the remainder membranous. The tube is closed at rest, but is opened on yawning or swallowing by the combined actions of the sphincter of the nasopharyngeal isthmus and the tensor palati muscle, which is attached to the cartilaginous medial wall of the tube. The tube is more horizontal and relatively wider and shorter in the infant than in the adult.

2. Tympanic cavity

This biconcave disc-shaped cavity measures about 13 mm anterior to posterior, 15 mm in height and 2 mm at its narrowest point in the centre. The *lateral wall* is formed mainly by the tympanic membrane and its surrounding bone. The cavity is artificially divided into three parts:

- Mesotympanum, lying medial to the membrane.
- Epitympanum (attic), lying medial to the bone of the horizontal part of the squama (outer attic wall), above the membrane.
- Hypotympanum, below the drumhead, medial to the tympanic plate.

Tympanic membrane (drumhead) consists of three layers:

- An outer *epithelial* layer, continuous with the epithelium of the external auditory canal.
- A middle *fibrous* layer, containing (inner) circular and (outer) radial fibres, and the handle of the malleus.
- An inner *'mucosal'* layer.

The *pars tensa* (see Figure 1.19) is thickened peripherally into a fibrocartilaginous *annulus*, which fits into the grooved tympanic sulcus of the temporal bone.

The fibrous layer is absent above the malleolar folds and this portion of the membrane is called the *membrana flaccida*.

The drumhead is set obliquely, the anterior and inferior aspect being the most medial. It is convex towards the tympanic cavity.

The *medial wall* (Figure 1.7) has several obvious features which are:

- The *promontory*, the bony projection covering the basal turn of the cochlea.
- The *fenestra ovale*, occupied by the footplate of the stapes and the annular ligament, closes the middle ear from the scala vestibuli.
- The *facial nerve*. The horizontal portion of the nerve in its bony canal lies just above the oval window.

- The ampullary end of the *horizontal semicircular canal*, which lies just above the second genu of the facial nerve.
- The *fenestra rotunda*, closed by the round window membrane separates the middle ear from the scala tympani. It lies postero-inferior to the promontory.

Anterior wall has four openings, from above downwards:

- Canal of Huguier, through which the chorda tympani escapes from the middle ear.
- Canal for tensor tympani muscle.
- Tympanic orifice of eustachian tube.
- The petrotympanic suture, containing the tympanic artery and the anterior ligament of the malleus.

Posterior wall presents an opening (*aditus ad antrum*) which leads backwards from the epitympanum into the mastoid antrum. Below this is the *pyramid*. Through it passes the tendon of the stapedius muscle, which is inserted into the neck of the stapes. Deep to the pyramid and the vertical portion of the facial canal (Figures 1.7, 1.23) between the windows and a little behind them, lies the *sinus tympani;* superficial to the pyramid and facial canal, and deep to the posterosuperior part of the tympanic annulus, lies the *facial recess.*

Floor is a thin plate of bone separating the cavity from the jugular bulb. A dehiscence may be present. It is in this portion of the bulb that the *glomus jugulare* (jugular body) is situated.

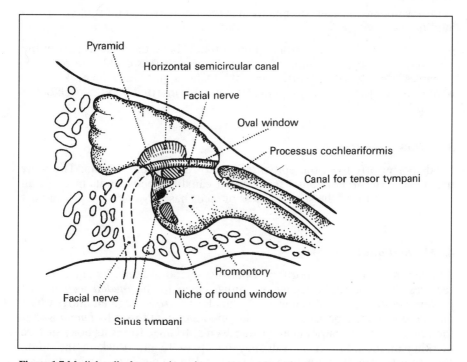

Figure 1.7 Medial wall of tympanic cavity

Roof (tegmen tympani) separates the cavity from the middle cranial fossa and is continuous with the tegmen antri. This thin plate of bone passes laterally from petrous to join the squama. The petrosquamous suture may be deficient, so providing a preformed pathway for infection.

Ossicles transmit sound energy from the surface of the tympanic membrane to the oval window and thence to the cochlear fluids.

- *Malleus* has a head, neck, anterior and lateral processes, and a handle. The head lies in the epitympanum; the handle, directed downwards and backwards, is firmly attached to the fibrous layer of the tympanic membrane. A short process projects laterally from the neck.
- *Incus* has a body (articulating with head of malleus) and a short process (both in epitympanum); also a long process which descends behind the handle of malleus and parallel to it. This bends medially at its lower end (lenticular process) to articulate with the head of stapes.
- *Stapes* has a head, neck, anterior and posterior crura (the anterior being the thinner), and a footplate which is held in the oval window by the annular ligament.

Chorda tympani nerve, a branch of the facial, arises in the Fallopian canal above the stylomastoid foramen. It enters the middle ear cavity through the posterior wall, lateral to the pyramid; thence it passes forwards, lateral to the incus and medial to the malleus, to escape from the cavity through the canal of Huguier and squamotympanic fissure.

Tympanic plexus of nerves lies on the promontory, deep to the mucous membrane.

Intratympanic muscles are mainly striated but may contain some non-striated fibres.

- *Tensor tympani.* Arising from a bony tunnel above the osseous part of the eustachian tube, its tendon turns round the processus cochleariformis and passes laterally to its insertion into the malleus, just below its neck.
- *Stapedius.* Occupies the pyramid. Its tendon is inserted into the neck of the stapes.

3. Aditus ad antrum

Leads posteriorly from the epitympanum to the mastoid antrum. The bony prominence of the horizontal semicircular canal lies between its medial wall and floor. The tip of the short process of incus has a ligamentous attachment to its floor.

4. Mastoid antrum

Situated in the posterior portion of petrous temporal bone. Its anterior wall receives the posterior opening of aditus. Deep to the *medial wall* lie the posterior and horizontal semicircular canals. The *roof* (tegmen antri) which may be deficient, separates it from the middle cranial fossa. Its *lateral wall* is the squama, and the suprameatal (Macewen's) triangle forms its bony surface marking in the adult. This wall may be up to 15 mm thick in the adult. *Postero-inferiorly* it communicates by several openings with the mastoid air cells. Although the mastoid air cells can vary considerably in size, number and distribution the antrum is always present.

5. Compartments and mucosal folds of the tympanic cavity

The attic or epitympanum is almost completely separated from the mesotympanum by the ossicles and their folds (Figure 1.8). The mucosal folds may limit infection to one or several of these compartments of the middle ear.

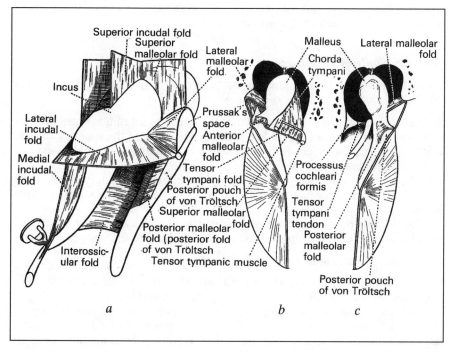

Figure 1.8 The compartments and folds of the middle ear (after Proctor). a, Posterosuperior and lateral view of the right middle ear; b, Prussak's space; c, posterior pouch of von Tröltsch

Relations of middle ear cleft

Complications of inflammatory and neoplastic disease of the middle ear cleft result from direct spread to surrounding structures. Its relations are therefore of the utmost importance.

External auditory canal is separated from the middle ear cleft by the tympanic membrane.

Temporal lobe of brain is separated from the tympanic cavity, aditus ad antrum by the tegmen tympani et antri.

Labyrinth is related to the medial walls of the tympanic cavity, aditus ad antrum. Infection spreads through the windows, by erosion of the bony semicircular canal, or directly from the perilabyrinthine air cells of the petrous.

Facial nerve. In its horizontal and vertical portions is closely related to the tympanic cavity. In the horizontal portion its bony covering may be deficient.

Lateral sinus (sigmoid portion) is related posteromedially to the mastoid process.

Jugular bulb is closely related to the bony floor of the tympanic cavity. Rarely, if the floor is deficient, the bulb may be seen as a dark blue mass medial to the lower part of the tympanic membrane.

Cerebellum lies posteromedial to the lateral sinus, in the posterior cranial fossa.

Vth and VIth cranial nerves are closely related to the apex of the petrous pyramid (Figure 1.9) and may be involved in the spread of inflammation to the apex in well pneumatized temporal bones.

Vascular supply of middle ear

Derived from numerous branches of both external and internal carotid arteries.

1. Superior petrosal and superior tympanic arteries and ramus nutricia incudomallei (all branches of the middle meningeal artery) to the superior region.
2. Inferior tympanic artery (a branch of the ascending pharyngeal artery) to the inferior region.
3. Anterior tympanic artery (a branch of the internal maxillary artery) and ramus tympanici (a branch of the internal carotid artery) to the anterior region.
4. Posterior tympanic artery (a branch of the mastoid branch of the stylomastoid artery, derived from the postauricular artery) to the posterior region.

The *ossicles* are supplied by the following vessels:

1. *Anterior tympanic artery,* which sends branches to malleus and incus.
2. *Ramus nutricia incudomallei,* supplying malleus and incus.
3. Branches of the *anterior, posterior and inferior tympanic arteries* supply the stapes, incudostapedial joint and lenticular process of incus. The vessels pass down the incus, up the stapedial crura and along the stapedius tendon.

Nerve supply of middle ear

1. *Sensory.* From the IXth cranial nerve, through the *tympanic plexus,* which receives a twig from the VIIth nerve.
2. *Motor*
   - From the mandibular branch of the Vth cranial nerve to the *tensor tympani* muscle.
   - From the stapedial branch of the VIIth cranial nerve, to the *stapedius* muscle.

Inner ear

The inner ear lies in the temporal bone. It is called the labyrinth (from its complexity) and consists of:

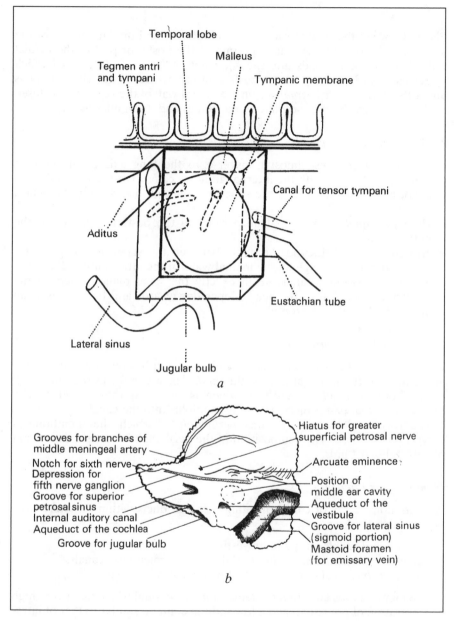

Temporal lobe

Malleus

Tegmen antri
and tympani

Tympanic membrane

Canal for tensor tympani

Aditus

Eustachian tube

Lateral sinus

Jugular bulb

a

Grooves for branches of
middle meningeal artery

Notch for sixth nerve
Depression for
fifth nerve ganglion
Groove for superior
petrosal sinus
Internal auditory canal
Aqueduct of the cochlea

Groove for jugular bulb

Hiatus for greater
superficial petrosal nerve

Arcuate eminence

Position of
middle ear cavity
Aqueduct of the
vestibule
Groove for lateral sinus
(sigmoid portion)
Mastoid foramen
(for emissary vein)

b

Figure 1.9 a, Diagram of relations of middle ear; b, Relation of middle ear. Medial and superior aspect of temporal bone

Osseous labyrinth

A series of cavities in the petrous part of the bone. There are three main parts:

1. Vestibule

Placed between the medial wall of the middle ear and the lateral end of the internal auditory canal. A small aperture in the posterior part of the medial wall of the vestibule leads into the *aqueduct of the vestibule,* a canal which passes backwards to the posterior surface of the petrous bone, where it opens under the dura. The *fenestra ovale,* in the lateral wall of the vestibule, is closed to the middle ear by the footplate of the stapes and its annular ligament.

2. Bony semicircular canals

* *Superior canal.* Lies almost transverse to the long axis of the petrous making a 60° angle with the internal auditory canal. The arcuate eminence is not a surface marking of the superior canal but lies close to its highest point.
* *Posterior canal.* Lies in a plane parallel to the posterior surface of the petrous.
* *Horizontal canal.* Lies in the angle between the superior and posterior canals. It makes a bulge on the medial walls of the attic, aditus ad antrum. The two horizontal canals lie in exactly the same plane, which, in the anatomical position of the head, slopes downwards and backwards at an angle of 30° to the horizontal.

3. Bony cochlea (Figure 1.10)

Lies in front of the vestibule. Snail shell in shape, it has two and a half turns in the human. It has a central axis, the *modiolus,* which forms the inner wall of the bony canal of the cochlea, which is wound spirally round it. The *osseous spiral lamina* projects from the modiolus into the canal.

The osseous labyrinth contains *perilymph* in which the membranous labyrinth is situated. The composition of the perilymph is very similar to that of extracellular fluids.

Membranous labyrinth

A continuous series of communicating sacs and ducts within the bony cavities. It consists of:

1. *Saccule and utricle,* in the bony vestibule.
2. *Membranous semicircular ducts,* in the bony semicircular canals.
3. *Cochlear duct* (scala media) in the bony cochlea.

The membranous labyrinth contains *endolymph* fluid which has a very high concentration of potassium and a low sodium content, similar to that of intracellular fluids.

The *basilar membrane* stretches from the free border of the osseous spiral lamina to the outer wall of the bony canal of the cochlea.

Reissner's membrane extends diagonally from the osseous spiral lamina to the outer wall of the bony cochlea.

Sensory cells concerned with hearing are contained in the cochlear duct *(scala media),* a portion of the membranous labyrinth which ends blindly at the *helicotrema.*

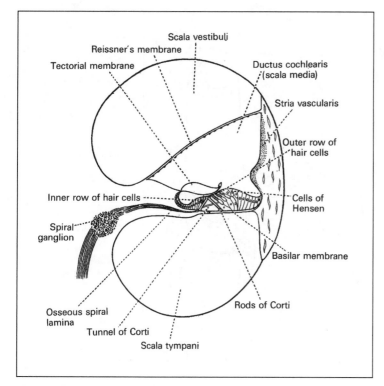

Figure 1.10 Cochlea with organ of Corti

The *scala vestibuli* and *scala tympani* lie above and below the scala media respectively and both contain perilymph. They communicate with each other at the helicotrema in the apex of the cochlea. The scala vestibuli communicates functionally with the middle ear through the oval window, the scala tympani through the round window. The scala tympani is connected with the subarachnoid space through the bony *aqueduct of the cochlea*.

Organ of Corti

Consists of a series of neuroepithelial structures arranged along the inner edge of the basilar membrane. A tunnel, composed of two rows of *rods of Corti*, and forming a triangle with the basilar membrane, divides the organ into inner and outer portions. On the inner side of the inner rod there is a single row of hair cells (IHCs). These inner hair cells are bulbous in shape. The 'hairs' of each cell consist of 120 *stereocilia* arranged in two rows in the form of a double V, with their apices directed away from the modiolus (Figure 1.11a). On the outer side of the outer rod there are three or four rows of hair cells. These outer hair cells (OHCs) are columnar in shape, with 46–148 *stereocilia* arranged in three rows in the form of a wide triple W, with their apices also directed away from the modiolus (Figure 1.11b). The OHC cilia are 2 μm long in the basal turn and increase in length to 6 μm at the

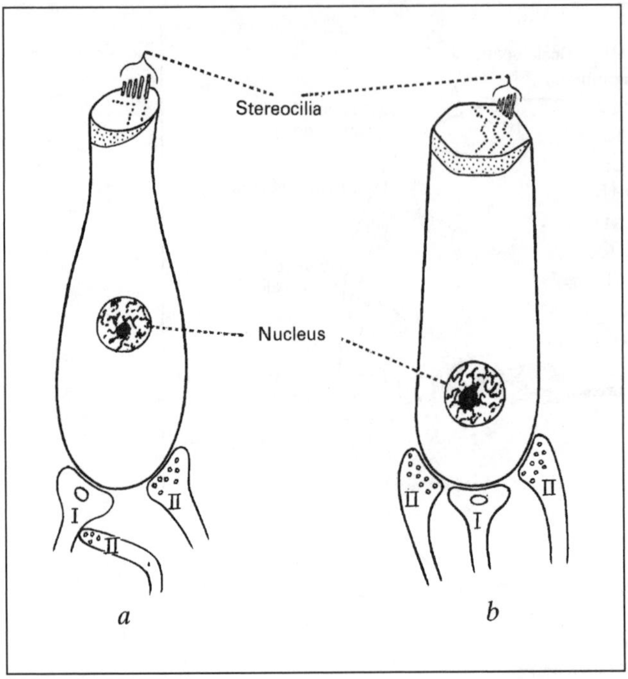

Figure 1.11 Structure of cochlear hair cells: a, inner hair cell; b, outer hair cell

apex. The *kinocilia* of the vestibular hair cells (q.v.) are represented in the cochlear hair cells by a simple *basal body*. The free surface of each hair cell is the cuticular plate, and the hair cells are separated by supporting cells. There are about 4 500 IHCs and 12 500 OHCs in each ear.

The *tectorial membrane* overhangs the organ of Corti. Outside the outer hair cells are the *cells of Hensen*. Lining the outer side of the scala media is the stria vascularis which is important in regulating Na and K ions. Thickened endosteum lining the outer wall of the bony canal of the cochlea is called the *spiral ligament*.

Cochlear division of VIIIth cranial nerve

The terminal fibres end in contact with the hair cells. These fibres are of two types: Type I fibres, sparsely granulated and probably afferent; and Type II fibres, richly granulated and probably efferent (Figure 1.11a and b). The fibres pass in the *spiral lamina* to the spiral ganglion in the modiolus, to become the auditory branch of the VIIIth cranial nerve.

Central connections

After leaving the internal auditory canal, the cochlear nerve (Figure 1.12) enters the brainstem at the upper border of the medulla, just below the pons and close to the inferior cerebellar peduncle. It enters the brainstem lateral and inferior to the entrance of the vestibular nerve.

The nerve bifurcates immediately after entering the brainstem, and terminates in the dorsal and ventral cochlear nuclei. Thence most of the fibres decussate, via the striae acousticae and corpus trapezoideum, to the lateral lemniscus of the opposite side and then pass to the medial geniculate body and inferior corpus quadrigeminum (primary auditory centres). Other fibres reach the homolateral centre.

Thence they pass to the higher auditory centres in the superior temporal gyrus of the cerebral cortex. The fibres of this last relay are not myelinated at birth, when only 'reflex' subcortical hearing is present. Gradual myelination in the first ten, and especially in the first three, years of life is responsible for a child's ability to learn the pattern of integrated sounds such as language (comprehensive hearing).

Apart from the 23 000–40 000 afferent fibres (Figure 1.12a) most of which are distributed to the IHCs, there have been found some 500–600 centrifugal fibres coursing from the brainstem to the hair cells. Most of these efferent fibres are distributed near the base of the cochlea. They originate in the superior olivary nucleus, about one fifth being homolateral, the remainder

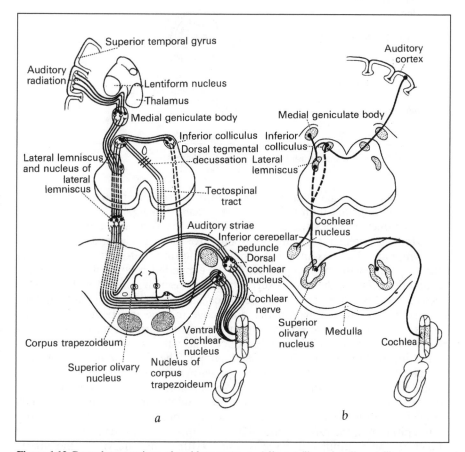

Figure 1.12 Central connections of cochlear nerve. a, Afferent fibres; b, efferent fibres

contralateral, in origin. These efferent fibres appear to be linked, at brain-stem level, with the cochlear nuclei and to be under control from cortical levels by descending fibres (Figure 1.12b). The significance of these efferent fibres is not yet fully understood.

Anatomy of the vestibular labyrinth

The vestibular labyrinth is situated behind the cochlea within the petrous bone. It consists of a system of membranous sacs and ducts within the bony vestibule and semicircular canals (Figure 1.13). The three *semicircular ducts* open into the *utricle* by five separate openings and are set at right angles to one another. Hence they represent the three planes of space.

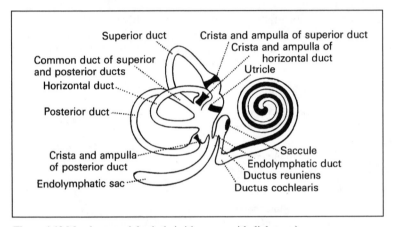

Figure 1.13 Membranous labyrinth (with neuroepithelial areas)

Membranous semicircular ducts open into the posterior part of the *utricle,* which communicates indirectly with the saccule through the *endolymphatic duct.* This duct occupies the bony aqueduct of the vestibule and divides into two branches, which separate to open into the saccule and utricle. The endolymphatic duct has an initial dilatation, the *sinus* before it narrows at the isthmus, to enter the bony aqueduct. In the expanded portion of the aqueduct beyond the *isthmus,* the duct is surrounded by vascular connective tissue. The smooth distal portion of the duct becomes expanded into the endolymphatic sac which is contained within the dura covering the cerebellum. The duct curves at an acute angle on leaving the utricle to form an *utriculoendolym-phatic valve* over the orifice of the duct. The valve is so constructed as to permit inflow but not overflow of endolymph. The *ductus reuniens* connects the saccule with the ductus cochlearis (scala media). The utricle and semicir-cular ducts are the organs of balance. The function of the saccule is uncertain. At one end, each of the semicircular ducts dilates into an *ampulla,* which completely fills a corresponding dilatation of its bony canal. A special sensory neuroepithelium, the *crista,* is found in each ampulla and each is supplied by a branch of the vestibular division of the VIIIth cranial nerve. In the utricle (and saccule) there is also a patch of specialized epithelium, the *macula,* which is a receptor organ (Figure 1.14). The macula of the utricle is in a horizontal plane, that of the saccule in a vertical plane.

Vestibular receptor organs. These are the ampullary cristae and the utricular maculae (otolith organ). Their epithelium is formed of cells surmounted by long hairlets. The vestibular cells are of two types: the Type 1 cell (Figure 1.15a), which is rounded and flask-shaped and surrounded by a nerve chalice; and the Type 2 cell (Figure 1.15b), which is cylindrical and has no

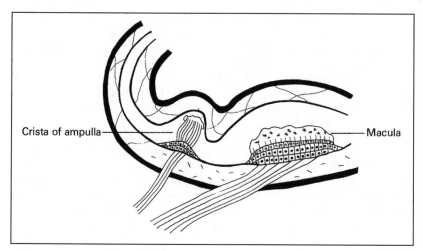

Crista of ampulla ———————————— Macula

Figure 1.14 Vestibular receptor organs

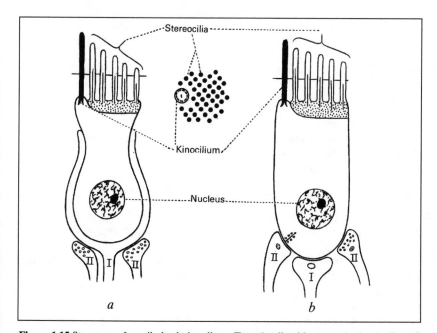

Figure 1.15 Structure of vestibular hair cells. a, Type 1 cell, with nerve chalice; b, Type 2 cell

nerve chalice. Hence the Type 1 cell bears a morphological resemblance to the inner hair cells, and the Type 2 cell resembles the outer hair cell of the cochlea (q.v.). In the ampullary crista there are relatively more Type 1 cells on the summit of the crista, relatively more Type 2 cells on its sides. The hairs do not jut freely into the endolymph but into a mucus-like substance, dome-shaped in the ampullae (*cupola*), cylindrical in the utricle, where there are a number of calcareous particles (*otoliths*) embedded in it.

The bundle of sensory hairs protruding from the free surface of each sensory cell is composed of one kinocilium and 50–110 stereocilia, the latter being anchored in the cuticular plate. The kinocilium is the longest of the sensory hairs and in each bundle the stereocilia diminish in length with increase in distance from the kinocilium. Hence, there is morphological (and functional) *polarization* of the vestibular sensory cells, a displacement of the sensory hairs towards the kinocilium being accompanied by depolarization of the cell and an increased rate of discharge in the afferent nerve, with a decreased discharge rate when the hairs are displaced in the opposite direction.

Innervation and central connections (Figure 1.16). The axis cylinders of the nerve fibres ramify round the hair cells of the receptor organs. As in the cochlea, these fibres are of two types: Type I fibres, which are probably afferent, and Type II fibres, which are richly granular and probably efferent. The fibres are gathered together to form the vestibular nerve, which passes through the internal auditory canal. The neurones pass, in the two main subdivisions of the vestibular nerve, through the internal auditory canal, to the large bipolar cells of the vestibular (Scarpa's) ganglion. The superior branch (which has anastomotic connections, the nerve of Oort, with the facial nerve) innervates the cristae of the superior and lateral semicircular canals, and the macula of the utricle; the inferior branch innervates the posterior canal and most of the macula of the saccule. The nerve then enters the lower border of the pons, where it separates from the cochlear nerve. The vestibular nerve passes backwards into the medulla, to reach the vestibular nuclei in the pons and medulla, close to the floor of the fourth ventricle.

Vestibular nuclei. The four main nuclei are

1. Lateral. In the lateral portion of the medulla.
2. Superior. Above the lateral and in the angle of the fourth ventricle.
3. Medial. Lying medial to (1) and (2).
4. Inferior.

Secondary central pathways. Arise from the nuclei and pass to:

1. Vestibulospinal tract, and thence to the spinal cord, from the lateral nucleus. The nucleus is responsible for myotactic reflexes and reflex muscle tone.
2. Medial longitudinal bundle, which receives ascending fibres from the superior, and a few from the medial nucleus. This nucleus exerts its influence on the extrinsic muscles of the eye, through the nuclei of the IIIrd, IVth and VIth cranial nerves.
3. Cerebellum, from the inferior nucleus. There are both crossed and uncrossed fibres in the central vestibular pathways.

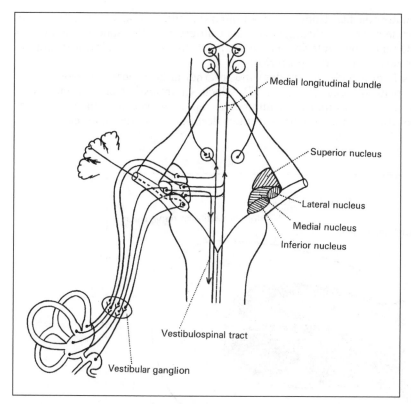

Figure 1.16 Central connections of vestibular nerves

Blood supply of the labyrinth

The blood supply of the labyrinth is derived principally from the internal auditory artery, which arises usually from the anterior inferior cerebellar artery, sometimes directly from the basilar artery.

The internal auditory artery travels down the internal auditory canal and divides into two branches: anterior vestibular and common cochlear, the latter soon subdividing into the vestibulocochlear and cochlear branches. After running a spiral course around the modiolus, the cochlear branch of the vestibulocochlear artery anastomoses with the cochlear branch of the common cochlear artery.

In the cochlea, the cochlear artery runs a serpentine course around the modiolus, as the spiral modiolar artery, from which arterioles run centrifugally to radiate over the scala vestibuli and the osseous spiral lamina. They end in spiral capillary systems both in the external wall of the cochlea where they form the *stria vascularis* and in the lamina.

Internal auditory canal

Nearly 1 cm in length and passes into the petrous bone in a lateral direction. It transmits the VIIth and VIIIth cranial nerves and the internal auditory artery and vein.

When approached from above, through the middle cranial fossa, the facial nerve is seen to run through the canal anterior to the superior vestibular nerve. On a deeper (inferior) plane lie the cochlear nerve, anteriorly, and the inferior vestibular nerve, posteriorly.

At its lateral end (the fundus) the internal auditory canal is closed by a vertical plate of bone (Figure 1.17), which separates it from the inner ear. This plate is perforated by a number of openings which transmit the filaments of the two cranial nerves to their destinations in the inner ear.

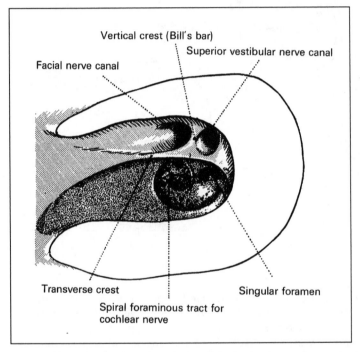

Figure 1.17 Right internal auditory bony canal – fundus as seen from posterior cranial fossa

Referred otalgia

Pain is commonly referred to the ear from lesions of remote or related structures whose nerve supply also sends branches to the ear.

Sensory nerve supply of the ear

Can be summarized diagrammatically (Figure 1.18).

Causes of referred otalgia

Are best considered on an anatomical basis. Pain may be referred:

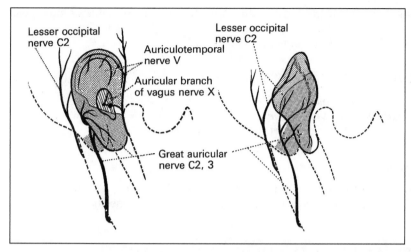

Figure 1.18 Sensory nerve supply of ear. a, Lateral aspect; b, medial aspect The IXth cranial supplies the medial wall of the tympanic cavity through the tympanic plexus (not illustrated)

Via the Vth cranial nerve

Referred pain from inflammation, infection or neoplasm in the territories supplied by the ophthalmic and maxillary divisions is uncommon with the exception of lesions of the nasopharynx.

1. *Lesions of the teeth and jaws*
   - Impaction of the molar teeth, particularly in the lower jaw.
   - Dental caries.
   - Apical abscess.
   - Malocclusion, including overclosure of the jaws and temporo-mandibular joint strain.
   - Temporomandibular arthritis (rare).
2. *Lesions of the salivary glands and ducts*
   - Acute infection.
   - Calculus.
3. *Sphenopalatine neuralgia*
4. *Lesions of the tongue*

Via the IXth and Xth cranial nerves

1. *Lesions of the oro– and laryngopharynx*
   - Acute pharyngitis and tonsillitis.
   - Peritonsillar abscess (quinsy).
   - Parapharyngeal and retropharyngeal abscesses.
   - Tonsillectomy. Almost universally.
   - Tuberculous ulceration.
   - Neoplasms.
2. *Lesions of the tongue*
   - Ulceration.
   - Neoplasms.
   - Infection.

3. *Elongated styloid process* causing stretching of the glossopharyngeal nerve, as it winds round the process.
4. *Glossopharyngeal neuralgia.*

Via the IInd and IIIrd cervical spinal nerves

1. *Cervical disc lesions.*
2. *Arthritis of the cervical spine.*
3. *'Fibrositis'* of the upper part of the sternomastoid muscle.

Relative incidence

The commonest causes of referred otalgia are impaction of a lower molar tooth; infection or removal of the tonsils; and dental malocclusion.

PHYSICAL EXAMINATION OF THE EAR

Only four parts of the ear are accessible to visual inspection:

1. Auricle

2. External auditory meatus

3. Tympanic membrane

- Posterior malleolar fold.
- Pars flaccida.
- Anterior malleolar fold.
- Long process of incus.
- Lateral (short) process.
- Handle of malleus.
- Pars tensa.
- Light reflex.

As seen through an aural speculum, this is shown in Figure 1.19, the membrane is grey, lustrous and translucent. The *handle of the malleus,* normally yellowish in colour, passes downwards and slightly backwards from the lateral (short) process. The *light reflex* passes downwards and slightly forwards from the umbo, the lowest point of the malleus. The light reflex is a reflection of light from that point of the malleus. The light reflex is a reflection of light from that small part of the membrane which lies at right angles to the beam of light. The *long process of the incus* may sometimes be seen behind the handle of the malleus, parallel to it and midway between it and the posterior bony wall of the canal. The *anterior* and *posterior malleolar* folds mark the upper end of the fibrous layer and separate it into:

- *Pars tensa* below.
- *Pars flaccida* above. A perforation in this portion is usually described as an 'attic' perforation – incorrectly, as the 'attic' is that part of the tympanic

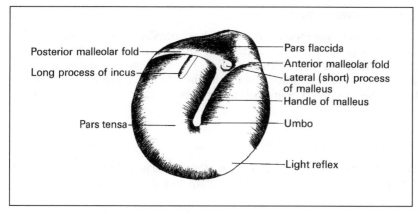

Figure 1.19 Right tympanic membrane

cavity lying above the membrane. Such a perforation does, however, usually indicate disease in the 'attic' and the term is retained for clinical convenience. Changes in the middle ear cleft are deduced clinically from changes seen in the tympanic membrane.

Siegle's pneumatic speculum allows magnification through an obliquely-set lens and mobility of the drumhead can be determined by alternate compression and release of the bulb.

Very fine details of the drumhead are best observed with the binocular operating microscope.

4. Eustachian tube

- Can be inspected at its lower end:
- Indirectly, by postnasal mirror.
- Directly by fibrescope or Yankauer's nasopharyngeal speculum.

Patency of Eustachian tube

Can be determined in five ways:

1. *Valsalva's method*

While the examiner views the tympanic membrane, the patient is instructed to close the mouth, hold the nose and exhale forcibly into it. The membrane moves outwards on inflation if the tube is patent and the membrane intact. Not everyone can do this.

2. *Politzerization*

The nozzle of a Politzer bag is inserted into one nostril. Both nostrils are compressed and the bag is squeezed as the patient swallows. Air entering the ears can be felt if the tubes open.

3. *Eustachian catheterization*

The catheter, beak downwards, is passed horizontally along the floor of the nose until it slips over the posterior end of the palate. It is then turned outwards to lie in the orifice of the tube. The test ear is connected to the examiner's by an auscultation tube, the nozzle of a rubber bulb being attached to the catheter. Compression of the bulb results in a soft, dry sound if the tube is patent.

4. *Indirect measurement of middle ear pressure*

By acoustic impedance meter. This method replaces Politzerization and catheterization where the equipment (a tympanometer) is available.

5. *By the release of positive meatal air pressures*

On swallowing, in the presence of a perforation.

RADIOGRAPHIC EXAMINATION OF THE TEMPORAL BONE

Radiological examination is particularly valuable in assessing the anatomical features of the mastoid, i.e. whether:

1. Cellular, diploic or sclerotic.
2. Sigmoid sinus backwardly or forwardly placed.

Pathological changes may be demonstrable as in opacity and blurring of cell outlines in inflammatory conditions arising in a cellular mastoid; bony erosion in inflammatory and neoplastic conditions; widening of internal auditory meatus in tumours of the VIIIth cranial nerve; evidence of basal skull fractures involving the petrous.

Views

Five standard projections are recommended:

1. 25–35° Fronto-occipital (Towne's) view

Both sides are demonstrated on one film and can be directly compared. This view shows:

- Internal auditory canals.
- Mastoid antrum and air cells.
- Superior and lateral semicircular canals.

2. Submentovertical (axial) view

Again both sides are demonstrated on one film, and this view shows:

- Internal and external auditory canals.
- Tympanic cavity and ossicles.
- Mastoid air cells.
- Bony eustachian tube.
- Petrous apices.
- Foramina spinosum and ovale.
- Stylomastoid foramen.
- Foramen lacerum and carotid canal.

3. 30–35° Lateral oblique (Stockholm B) view

The two sides are taken separately. The following structures are demonstrated:

- The groove and plate of the sigmoid sinus.
- Aditus ad antrum.

4. Posteroanterior oblique (Stenvers and Stockholm C) view

Each side is examined separately. Structures seen include:

- Superior semicircular canal.
- Cochlea.
- Internal auditory canal.

5. Owen's view

The malleus and incus are projected into the middle ear cavity. The aditus and antrum are clearly seen.

Tomography

Provides a better method of demonstrating the extent of destructive processes in the temporal bone, or of assessing the degree of congenital malformation in the ear. It is often the only reliable way of showing the facial canal and labyrinth. A number of projections are used: anteroposterior; anteroposterior oblique; axial; and lateral.

A hypocycloidal or spiral movement of the tube and plate is used to give a thin 'slice' of the bone radiographically in focus. Thus the detail is improved. Routinely, coronal cuts are performed and then lateral or obliques if further information is required. Bony detail is well shown but soft tissue shadowing is poor.

On coronal tomography the loss of the scutum (outer attic wall) is an early sign of cholesteatoma. Widening of the internal auditory canal is highly suspicious of an acoustic neuroma. However, lateral tomography should be performed to demonstrate that the cross sectional area of the canal is greater than normal. Tomography in two planes is required to demonstrate the course of the facial nerve and is therefore recommended in facial palsy as the result of trauma. The vestibular aqueduct can be demonstrated on lateral or 10° oblique tomography. Failure to visualize the aqueduct or type 3 periaqueductal pneumatization as described by Stahle and Wilbrand is associated with Menière's syndrome. Otosclerotic foci or Paget's disease can be identified. Congenital abnormalities can also be elucidated.

High definition CT scan

This gives very precise imaging of the temporal bone and its contents, including the ossicular chain, middle ear contents and internal auditory meatus. Some soft-tissue detail is identifiable. Further information can be obtained by using intravenous, intrathecal, or intraductal contrast. Transverse sections are normally obtained; lateral or coronal sections can be difficult or impossible to obtain directly. Consequently, computer generated reconstructions are made to view in other planes. These have poor detail.

Magnetic resonance imaging

This technique is capable of generating high resolution images with excellent soft tissue contrast in all planes of the human body without ionizing radiation. MRI is contraindicated in patients with cardiac pacemakers, aneurysm clips and cochlear implants. Following research, Applebaum and Valvasorri conclude that there is no apparent danger of stapedectomy prostheses being displaced when subjected to the electromagnetic fields of MRI units.

The technique is particularly useful in detecting small acoustic neuromas especially when combined with gadolinium contrast. It can differentiate between a petrous apex dermoid and a cholesterol granuloma.

Angiography

Angiography is of value in demonstrating vascular tumours and their blood supply. Carotid arteriography and retrograde internal jugular venography may be needed to identify anatomical anomalies of the internal carotid and of the jugular bulb. The introduction of digitalized angiography has increased the safety and usefulness of vascular radiographic investigations.

Selective catheterization of the external carotid arterial system has led to the introduction of therapeutic embolization to facilitate surgical removal of highly vascular lesions such as temporal paragangliomas (glomus jugulare tumours). This technique is not without risk of stroke due to reflux of embolic material into the internal carotid system. In major resections of the petrous bone requiring ligation of the carotid artery, detachable balloons can be placed in the carotid syphon under EEG control prior to the actual start of surgery. This technique reduces the risk of stroke compared to a ligation of the internal carotid artery in the neck.

Ultrasound

In the vertiginous patient or the sufferer from tinnitus information on arterial blood flow in the neck can be obtained by Doppler ultrasound studies.

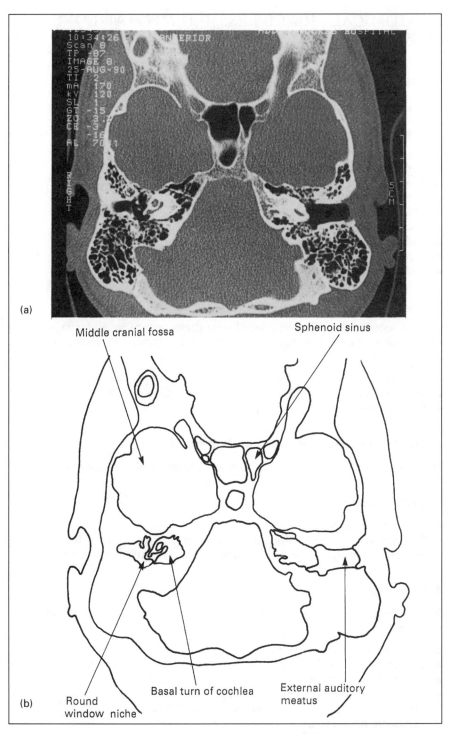

Figure 1.20 (a) Axial CT at the level of the temporal bones; (b) diagrammatic representation

ANATOMICAL PRINCIPLES OF TEMPORAL BONE SURGERY

Incisions

1. Postaural

This is preferred in operations on the highly pneumatized mastoid. It is used for:

- Cortical mastoidectomy for acute mastoiditis.
- Re-opening of old mastoid cavity or mastoid reconstruction.
- Tympanoplasty.
- Exploration of facial nerve.
- Cochlear implants.
- Endolymphatic sac decompression.
- Translabyrinthine route to the internal meatus.
- Osseous labyrinthectomy.

2. Endaural

Can be successfully employed in all operations on the acellular mastoid or where the procedure is directed mainly to the tympanic cavity, aditus ad antrum. It is used for:

- Radical and subradical operations, in chronic suppurative disease.
- Membranous labyrinthectomy for Menière's disease.
- Myringoplasty.

3. Combined postaural and endaural (in continuity)

When wide exposure is required, as in certain cases of tympanoplasty.

4. Extensions 1 and 2

- Horizontally, towards occiput.
- Superiorly, as an extension to a postaural incision, shaped like a lazy S over the temporalis muscle and parietal bone in skull base surgery.

5. Permeatal

Tympanotomy or atticotomy through a permeatal approach is of particular value in:

- All forms of stapes surgery.
- Congenital lesions limited to the contents of the tympanic cavity.
- Ossiculoplasty for chronic or traumatic ear disease.
- Limited infective or neoplastic disease in meso- and epitympanum, e.g. an epithelial attic 'pearl' or glomus tympanicum tumour.
- Tympanic neurectomy.
- Membranous labyrinthectomy.

6. Preauricular

A straight preauricular incision extending superiorly over the root of the zygoma as high as the parietal bone for middle fossa surgery.

Surgical approach to mastoid antrum (Figure 1.12)

- Using the postaural incision, the antrum is approached through Macewen's triangle. Using the endaural incision, the antrum is approached directly through the sloping posterosuperior part of the bony external meatus.

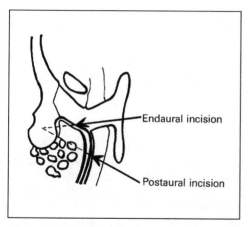

Figure 1.21 Surgical approach to mastoid antrum. Schematic horizontal section through external auditory meatus and middle ear cleft, as seen from above

Subsequent procedures

The following operations are commonly employed:

1. Cortical mastoidectomy

This is the operation for acute mastoiditis, sometimes referred to as 'Schwartze mastoidectomy'.

It aims at wide exenteration of the entire cellular system of the mastoid.

After exposure of the antrum, cells are exenterated from the antral region, root of zygoma, mastoid tip and sinodural angle (the angle between the sigmoid venous sinus and the dura mater of the middle cranial fossa which are both commonly seen during the operation). The bony canal wall is left intact.

2. Exposure of the endolymphatic sac

The sac lies in front of the lateral sinus, on the posterior surface of the temporal bone. A tangent drawn to the floor of the bony external auditory meatus passes through the position of the sac just below the posterior semicircular canal (Figure 1.22).

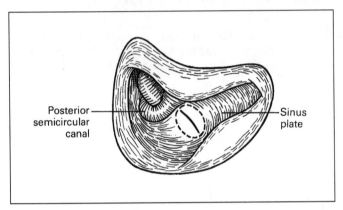

Figure 1.22 Position of endolymphatic sac (by transmastoid approach)

3. Posterior tympanotomy

The mesotympanum can be exposed, without removing the posterior bony canal wall, through a posterior tympanotomy, by drilling between the chorda tympani laterally, the descending facial nerve medially, and the fossa incudis above in the antrum threshold angle (Figure 1.23a). This gives access to the facial nerve (Figure 1.23b), and the round window for placement of a cochlear electrode. When added to a permeatal incision a posterior tympanotomy becomes a combined approach tympanoplasty (often abbreviated to CAT). This allows small cholesteatomas and cholesterol granulomas to be removed and is known as the 'canal wall up' technique.

4. Radical mastoidectomy

Used for some chronic suppurations of the middle ear cleft, usually with cholesteatoma.

After exposure of the antrum, the outer wall of the 'attic' is taken down and the posterior canal wall is reduced to create the so-called 'facial ridge' overlying the nerve. Finally the 'bridge' formed by the outer wall of the aditus is removed. Sometimes this is referred to as the 'canal wall down' technique.

Any remains of ossicles and/or tympanic membrane are picked out. All diseased tissue must be removed, with absolute respect for the facial nerve and oval window contents.

A kidney-shaped cavity results which is then partially lined by a flap of skin derived from the external auditory meatus supplemented by temporalis fascia grafts.

5. Subradical mastoidectomy

There are many modifications of the radical operation designed to preserve hearing.

The outer 'attic' wall and facial ridge are removed, but any healthy remains of ossicles or tympanic membrane are retained.

The commonest of these is the 'attico-antrostomy' in which the incus and head of malleus are removed, together with the 'bridge'.

The extent of surgery required, i.e. whether radical or subradical, can be determined only at the time of operation, but subradical operations can later be converted to radical if they fail. Lifelong cavity cleaning is usually required and a deliberately enlarged meatus (meatoplasty) is essential. In favourable cases restoration of some hearing is attempted, see Figure 2.4).

6. Mastoid obliteration

Obliteration of the cavity behind a new canal wall immediately after mastoidectomy is a time-consuming option which, however, avoids the need for a meatoplasty. Fresh bone paté collected from an area well away from the cholesteatoma may be used to fill the cavity. The bone chips to make the paté are collected on a filter interposed between the sucker and its tubing.

The new canal wall may be cartilage taken from the concha of the ear or preformed in synthetic hydroxylapatite. The wall is wedged between the facial ridge below and the roof of the cavity where the antrum used to be and covered with grafts of fascia (Figure 1.24).

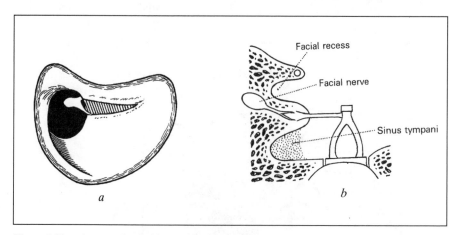

Figure 1.23 a, Antrum threshold angle; b, the sinus tympani

7. Fenestration of horizontal semicircular canal

This is practically never used now in otosclerosis, but the same approach may be used in tympanoplastic procedures (of the so-called 'Type 5').

The principles of the various tympanoplastic procedures are discussed briefly under 'Physiology of Hearing'.

Stapedectomy

Usually performed through a permeatal tympanotomy.

The skin of the posterior deep meatus is elevated from the bone until the attachment of the tympanic membrane is reached. The fibrous annulus is lifted out of its bony sulcus and the middle ear is thus exposed.

The crura of the stapes are removed after separation of the incudostapedial joint and division of the stapedius tendon. The footplate is removed or perforated and a prosthesis is applied between the oval window and the lower end of the long process of the incus.

Labyrinthectomy

The labyrinth can be effectively destroyed by avulsion of the saccule (through the oval window) by permeatal tympanotomy. By a postaural transmastoid approach the membranous semicircular canals can be drilled out and a more radical destruction achieved.

Labyrinthectomy removes all prospect of a cochlear implant.

Exploration of facial nerve

Vertical (mastoid) segment

Through a postauricular incision the mastoid air cells are cleared to expose the lateral sinus, posterior end of horizontal canal, and digastric ridge.

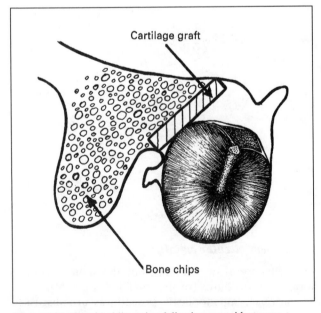

Figure 1.24 Mastoid obliteration following mastoidectomy

(Posterior meatal wall and cortical shell of mastoid tip are left intact.) The stylomastoid foramen is found at the anterior end of the digastric ridge by following medially and upwards the periosteum through a window cut in the cortex of the deep surface of the mastoid process. The Fallopian canal runs vertically up from the foramen to a point just below the semicircular canal, and is exposed and opened by drill strokes parallel to the nerve.

Horizontal (tympanic) segment

May be followed forward (below incus) from the vertical segment exposure (see above). Alternatively, it may be approached by permeatal tympanotomy and atticotomy.

Petrous segment

Can be followed from the geniculate ganglion medially, by drilling down through the floor of cranium exposed by middle fossa craniotomy (Figure 1.25). Alternatively, if the inner ear is expendable, by postauricular and translabyrinthine approach to internal auditory meatus.

Intracranial segment

Exposed by classic posterior fossa craniectomy.

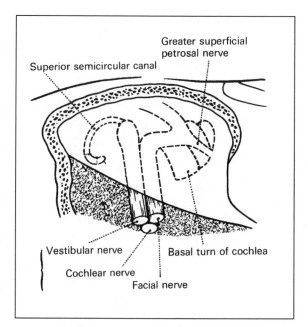

Figure 1.25 Middle cranial fossa approach showing disposition of internal auditory canal, labyrinth and labyrinthine portion of facial nerve

Exposure of internal auditory canal

Can be effected by the routes given above for the intracranial and petrous parts of the facial nerve, i.e. by approaching it through the posterior or middle cranial fossae, or by a translabyrinthine approach.

Chapter 2

Audiology

Audiology is the science of hearing. It includes all aspects, i.e. acoustics, physiology of hearing, disorders of hearing, functional examination of hearing, medical and surgical problems of deafness, education and rehabilitation of deaf and hard-of-hearing, hearing aids and cochlear implants.

PHYSICAL PROPERTIES OF SOUND

Sound waves

Sound travels from its source (voice, tuning fork, piano, etc.) to the ear by waves consisting of alternating compression and rarefaction of molecules in the air, water or other medium through which it is transmitted. Sound travels in air at 340 metres per second (760 m.p.h.) at 20° temperature and atmospheric pressure. Sound has certain objective physical properties which are related to subjective sensations perceived by the hearer.

1. Frequency

Subjective *pitch* is determined by the frequency of vibration of the sound source. If a tuning fork vibrates 256 times to and fro in 1 second, i.e. has a frequency of 256 cycles (double vibrations) per second (Hz), the hearer perceives the note of middle C in the musical scale. Doubling the frequency, i.e. to 512 Hz, produces a note one octave higher.

2. Intensity

The sensation of *loudness* is related to intensity of applied sound energy.

The *decibel* is a logarithmic unit and indicates the ratio between two different intensities. If the two intensities are I_1 and I_2 then the ratio of the intensities in dB equals 10 times the logarithm of the simple ratio to the base 10, or:

n dB = $10 \log_{10} I_1/I_2$

For example, if one intensity is twice as great as another, then the difference in the intensities in dB is

$$10 \times log_{10} \, 2 = 10 \times 0.3010 = 3.01 \text{ dB}.$$

Again, a tenfold increase in intensity is equivalent to a change of 10 dB, a hundredfold increase to a change of 20 dB. A hearing loss of 60 dB means that the patient can only hear sounds above an intensity of one million times the normal threshold, since 60 dB = $10 \times log_{10}$ 1 000 000. The levels used in clinical audiometry are related to a reference intensity pressure of 0.00024 dyne cm^{-2} at 1000 Hz.

By chance it happens that one decibel is roughly equal to the least perceptible difference of loudness detectable by the human ear in the frequencies concerned with speech.

In clinical work the threshold of normal hearing is defined as 0 dB. From a distance of 1 m, a whisper has an intensity of 30 dB; normal conversation 60 dB; a shout 90 dB. Discomfort is felt at 120 dB.

It is important to understand the difference between dBHL and dBSPL. dBHL is a biological scale whereas dBSPL is based on absolute sound pressure levels.

The sensitivity of the human ear to sound varies with frequency. A normal hearing person should have a threshold of 0 db at all frequencies; a new scale (ISO standard R389) or reference has been defined and the units are dBHL. They differ on average about 3–11 dB from dBSPL. Examples of conversion are given in Figure 2.1.

Hz	250	500	1k	2k	4k
dB (HL)	80	90	100	105	100
+ Factor	25	11	7	9	9
dB (SPL)	105	101	107	114	109

Figure 2.1 Conversion table

The reader should be aware that free field measurements such as are made for children too small to wear headphones, and the output of hearing aids are in dBSPL and are not therefore directly comparable with audiograms which are usually measured in dBHL.

3. Overtones

Quality (*timbre*) is determined by overtones or harmonics inherent in the instrument producing sound, whether voice, musical instrument or other source. Overtones are simple multiples of the frequency of the lowest note (fundamental).

PHYSIOLOGY OF HEARING

For physiological purposes, the ear is divided into two parts—*conducting apparatus,* consisting of external ear, tympanic membrane, chain of ossicles, eustachian tube and labyrinthine fluids; and *perceiving (sensorineural) apparatus,* consisting of end-organ (organ of Corti), auditory division of VIIIth cranial nerve, and central connections.

Conduction of sound

Sound can be transmitted to the inner ear in one of three ways:

1. *By way of the ossicular chain,* from the vibrating tympanic membrane to the oval window. This is the most important route.
2. *Directly across the middle ear,* when waves fall on the round window membrane. This may occur when there is a large perforation of the drumhead.
3. *By bone conduction,* sound energy is taken up and transmitted to the inner ear through the bones of the skull.

Function of ossicles

The malleus handle is firmly attached to the tympanic membrane. As the membrane moves in and out, the malleus and incus move in and out by rotating about an axis through the anterior ligament of the malleus and the tip of the short process of the incus. The stapes rocks around an axis passing vertically through the posterior border of the footplate (Figure 2.2).

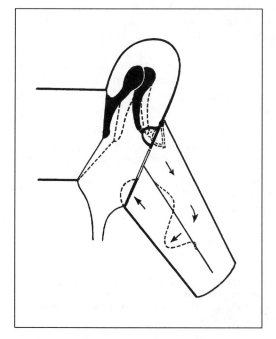

Figure 2.2 Function of ossicles

Vibration of the incompressible fluid (endolymph and perilymph) in the rigid bony labyrinth is made possible by the movement in opposite phase of the structures sealing the round and oval windows. This is achieved by the preferential distribution of sound energy to the oval window through the ossicular chain from the tympanic membrane.

The transformer mechanism of the middle ear

Acoustic energy collected by the large area of the tympanic membrane is applied through the ossicles to the small area of the stapes footplate. The effective ratio of these areas is about 14:1. The ossicles themselves constitute a lever mechanism (acting through the rotational axis of malleus and incus) which has a mechanical advantage of 1.3:1. The product of these area and lever ratios (14 and 1.3) is about 18:1, which represents the *transformer ratio* of the whole mechanism. By its effect the *amplitude* of vibration at the stapes is reduced as compared with that of the membrane, while the *force* exerted by the stapes upon the labyrinthine fluids is increased in the same proportion. By the interposition of this middle ear transformer device the widely differing acoustic impedances* of the external air and the labyrinthine fluids are matched, an arrangement necessary for the maximum transference of acoustic energy from the one medium to the other.

Pathological states causing conductive deafness

1. Non-marginal perforation of the tympanic membrane with intact ossicular chain. (Hearing loss approximately 10–30 dB.) (Figure 2.3a.)
2. Posterosuperior marginal perforation of the tympanic membrane with disruption of the ossicular chain. (Hearing loss 40–60 dB.)
3. Total or subtotal perforation of the tympanic membrane with loss of malleus and incus, the stapes remaining mobile (Figure 2.3b). (Hearing loss 60–80 dB.)

This state is approximated by a radical mastoidectomy. Such hearing as remains is probably due to a difference in acoustical loading upon the fluids of the scala vestibuli and scala tympani respectively. A possible explanation is that the expression of blood through veins leaving the labyrinth allows a

---

*Any medium (e.g. air, water) has *specific acoustic resistance* (unit: acoustical ohm) indicative of its resistance to the passage of sound energy. The value depends upon density *(d)* and elasticity (stiffness—*s*) of the medium. ($R = \sqrt{d} \times s$.)

In a complex vibrating system such as the ear frictional resistance also requires attention and the *impedance* is calculated from the formula:

Impedance $= \sqrt{(r^2 + [\mathrm{m}f - \mathrm{s}/f]^2)}$, where f = frequency and

r = frictional resistance
m = mass
s = stiffness
of the vibrating parts.

The middle ear serves to match approximately the acoustic resistance of air to that of the labyrinth. Lesions affecting the mass or stiffness of its parts reduce its efficiency (producing deafness) in a frequency-selective manner, as the formula shows. Lesions affecting friction alone would impair conduction equally for all frequencies.

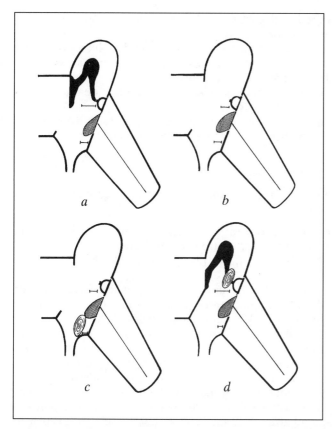

Figure 2.3 Pathological conditions causing conductive deafness. a, Non-marginal perforation of the tympanic membrane with intact ossicular chain. The sound energy transmitted to the oval window is reduced but remains greater than that at the round window; b, total or subtotal perforation of the tympanic membrane with loss of malleus and incus, the stapes remaining mobile. The sound energy transmitted to the oval window is so reduced as to be equalled by that at the round window; c, shielding of the round window by granulation. The sound energy transmitted to each window is reduced, but that at the oval window is greater than that at the round window. A 'differential' therefore exists, again in favour of the oval window; d, epitympanic disease with 'attic' perforation and disruption of the ossicular chain between incus and stapes. The resuting gap is bridged by a cholesteatoma

greater yielding to sound pressures on the vestibular side than on the tympanic side of the cochlear partition.

Hearing can be partially restored if the round window is shielded by granulations or the introduction of a disc of silicone rubber moistened with paraffin (Figure 2.3c).

4. Epitympanic disease, usually with 'attic' perforation and often with granulations and/or cholesteatoma. (Hearing loss 10–60 dB, according to the condition of the ossicular chain.)

The ossicular chain is often disrupted but occasionally the resulting gap may be bridged by the cholesteatoma itself, so allowing transmission (Figure 2.3d).

5. Increased stiffness (reduced compliance) due to chronic adhesive otitis media, tympanosclerosis, or bony ankylosis (otosclerosis).
6. Traumatic disconnection of the ossicular chain, behind an intact tympanic membrane. Results from head injury, blast injury or surgical accident. (Hearing loss 40–60 dB.) (Increased compliance.)
7. Middle ear fluid, the mass effect of which may produce deafness more marked in the higher frequencies. (Reduced compliance.)
8. Pressure changes in the middle ear, as in eustachian tube dysfunction. These probably act by increasing the stiffness of the vibrating parts.

Principles in restoration of sound conduction

Attempts can be made to restore the 'differential' between the two labyrinthine windows by:

1. *Myringoplasty.* Closure of a central perforation by an 'underlaid' fascia graft applied to raw edges of the perforation (Figure 2.4a).
2. *Tympanoplasty with columella effect (*Figure 2.4b*).* The graft is placed upon the stapes head.
3. *Ossiculoplasty.* Restoration of ossicular continuity by incus transposition or by use of incus or malleus homograft, autogenous cartilage or bone graft or inert prosthesis, made of ceramic, plastic or metal (Figure 2.4c, d, e).

Such procedures are most applicable in ears with 'safe' central tympanic defects, free from cholesteatoma. In the presence of cholesteatomatous attico-antral disease they may only be safely used when it is certain that all epithelial disease has been eradicated. If the latter demands a modified radical mastoidectomy residual hearing may still be conserved or improved by a flap or a fascia graft placed so as to rest upon the stapes head. If only the stapes footplate remains a baffle of 'drum' remnant, or a fascia graft is placed so as to shield the round window. It is essential that the stapes be mobile. A vein or fascia graft is applied to the bared promontory and to the lower half of the circumference of the deep external auditory meatus. The essential air space between the upper orifice of the eustachian tube and the round window is preserved initially by absorbable gelfoam packing.

Tympanic muscle reflexes

Contraction of the intratympanic muscles increases the stiffness of the middle ear conducting apparatus. Their action is a reflex one, the stimulus being sound at levels of 90 dB and above. By attenuating loud sounds, especially in the lower frequency range, the reflex probably protects the inner ear against acoustic trauma. Impact or explosive noise reaches the cochlea before the reflex is activated hence it is more damaging than steady state noise.

Hearing by bone conduction

Occurs when the skull is set in vibration as by the subject's own voice, by sound waves in the surrounding atmosphere or by a tuning fork applied to the head. Acoustic vibrations of the cochlear fluids and basilar membrane result from the following mechanisms:

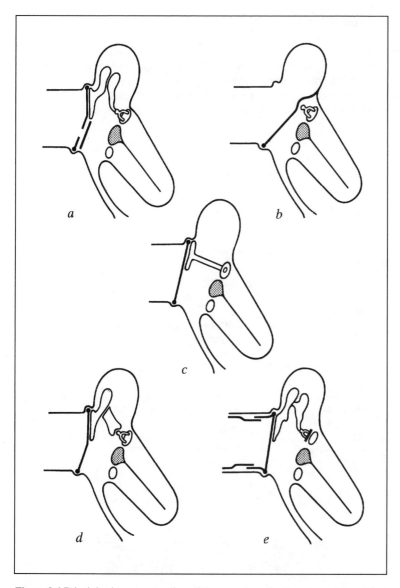

Figure 2.4 Principles in reconstruction of the sound conducting apparatus. a, Myringoplasty; b, tympanoplasty with columellar effect; c, total ossicular replacement: homograft or prosthesis; d, partial ossicular replacement: an incus is often reshaped for this purpose; e, homograft replacement of membrane and ossicles

1. Inertia of the ossicular chain.
2. Compressional effects on the labyrinth due to deformation of the skull.
3. Inertia of the mandible, which causes acoustic vibration in the external auditory meatus.

Perception of sound

Within the cochlea the vibrations of the cochlear fluids are processed and analysed in such a way that data representing frequency, intensity and phase relationships may be transmitted along the auditory nerve (Figure 2.5). In order that the necessary hydrodynamic, electrical and metabolic processes may occur special biological conditions are present in the cochlea.

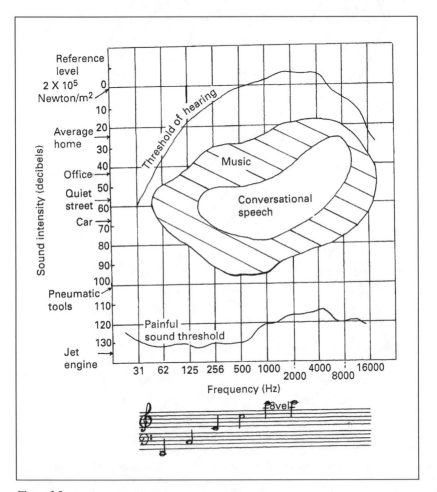

Figure 2.5

Resting conditions

Perilymph has a chemical composition generally similar to that of other extracellular fluids and to CSF. There are minor differences, however, despite the apparent connection between perilymph and CSF through the aqueduct of the cochlea. It is most probable that perilymph is formed as a blood filtrate within the labyrinth but the precise mechanism is uncertain.

Endolymph has a different chemical composition with high potassium and low sodium levels (like intracellular fluids). It is probably secreted and reabsorbed by specialized epithelium in the stria vascularis. An alternative theory suggests that it diffuses across Reissner's membrane and is selectively reabsorbed by the stria. Endolymph is the sole source of *oxygen supply* for the organ of Corti, which itself has no blood vessels.

Circulation of endolymph is probably radial, across not along the scala media. The ductus and saccus endolymphaticus have a debatable part in endolymph production and absorption.

'*Cortilymph*', the fluid in the tunnel of Corti, cannot be endolymph, since high potassium concentration would prevent neuronal activity. Its exact nature and origin require further study.

Resting electrical potentials

As shown by microelectrode studies in animals these are:

Scala media +80 millivolts
Outer hair cells –70 millivolts
Inner hair cells +45 millivolts
Scala vestibuli +5 millivolts

all with reference to scala tympani. The origin and purpose of these electrical potentials are not completely understood.

Dynamic conditions

Events within the cochlea in response to sound vibrations are as follows:

1. Hydrodynamic

Vibration of the stapes at very low speeds (subsonic frequency) will produce a flow of perilymph up the scala vestibuli, through the helicotrema, and down the scala tympani to the round window membrane, which bulges

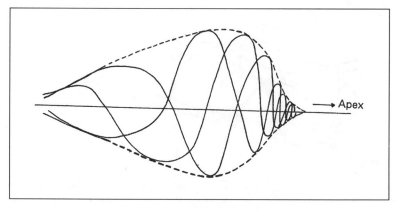

Figure 2.6 Basilar membrane movement in response to acoustic energy

outwards in opposite phase to the footplate. With the rapid vibrations of audio frequencies, however, the acoustic impedance of the inner ear opposes the simple hydraulic effect described, and acoustic energy displaces the cochlear partition to and fro between the upper and lower scalae. If the actual vibrations of the basilar membrane are observed, a *travelling wave* (Békésy) (Figure 2.6) is seen to start from the base of the cochlea and progress towards the helicotrema with increasing amplitude to a sharply defined region of maximum displacement, the position of which depends upon the frequency. Beyond this the wave is rapidly dissipated and disappears. For high frequencies maximum displacement of basilar membrane is confined to the basal turn. Low frequencies cause a longer travelling wave with maximum amplitude near the apex of the cochlea.

2. Mechanical excitation of the hair cells

Vibration of the basilar membrane results in a sliding, or shearing, movement between the tectorial membrane and the reticular lamina. The hairs of the hair cells are thus displaced relative to their cell bodies (Figure 2.7). It is this motion which produces the cochlear microphonic (CM) and is probably the final mechanical event preceding neuronal stimulation.

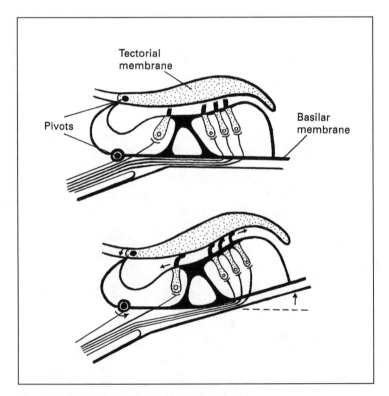

Figure 2.7 Generation of the cochlear microphonic

Transduction, the conversion of acoustical energy into nerve-fibre activity, is not understood. Possibly CM stimulates the nerve endings. Alternatively, chemical mediation may play a part.

Electrical activity in response to acoustic stimulation

Wever and Bray first described 'microphonic potentials' in the cochlea when acoustic stimulation occurs. These microphonics, aptly named, reproduce electrically the wave form of the sound signal. They can be analysed into:

- *Cochlear microphonic potentials* (CM), arising in the vicinity of the hair cells being stimulated. CM 1 is oxygen dependent whereas the smaller component, CM 2, persists for a short while after the death of the animal. CM is absent in any part of the cochlea where the hair cells are damaged or destroyed.
- *Summating potentials* (SP), special variants of microphonic, occur with very high intensity stimuli, probably arising from the inner hair cells; SP is a rectified derivative of the sound signal, unlike CM whose wave-form is a direct electrical equivalent of the original sound.
- *Auditory nerve action potentials* (AP), the algebraic sum of the neural discharges in the whole of the cochlear nerve. Each auditory nerve fibre has an optimum stimulus frequency for which the threshold is lowest. Its rate of firing increases to a maximum about 25 dB above threshold. The fibres responding to the higher frequencies are arranged around the outside of the nerve trunk, consistently with their origin from the basal turns of the cochlea.

Theories of hearing attempt to explain the conversion of all the dimensions of sound into a representative pattern of auditory nerve-fibre activity. The possible variations in the nerve action pattern depend upon:

1. Which particular nerve fibres are being activated.
2. The total number of fibres being activated.
3. The rate of firing in individual fibres (below 1000 Hz).
4. The temporal relationships of neural discharges between individual fibres and groups of fibres.

'Place' theories of cochlear action (e.g. that of Helmholtz) postulate that perception of pitch relies upon the selective vibratory action of the basilar membrane. The hair cells and the particular nerve fibres activated by them correspond to the point of maximum displacement of the membrane by the travelling wave. This has recently been confirmed by re-examining von Békésy's travelling wave at fixed observation points in the living cochlea. Mechanical tuning thus measured is sufficiently precise to permit accurate identification of pitch by this resonance mechanism alone (Figure 2.8).

Rutherford's *telephone* theory suggested that pitch perception is based upon the rate of firing in individual nerve fibres. The latent period of nervous action limits this theory to the perception only of frequencies below 1000 Hz, if the relation between sound-wave frequency and nerve impulse has a simple 1:1 ratio.

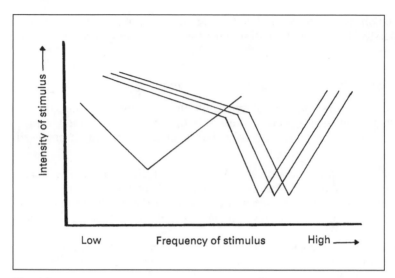

Figure 2.8

Wever's *volley* theory combines both place and telephone principles, postulating that:

1. High frequencies are perceived by place alone (in the basal turn).
2. Low frequencies (below 1000 Hz) stimulate nerve action potentials at a rate equal to the stimulus frequency.
3. Intermediate frequencies are represented in the auditory nerve by asynchronous discharges in groups of neurones, whose *combined* activity represents the frequency of the stimulus.

Loudness perception must be encoded in the variations of possible nerve activity patterns (*see above*) which are not pre-empted by the mechanisms employed in pitch perception. It is known that 95% of nerve fibres innervate inner hair cells, also that the majority of nerve fibres have thresholds of 10–15 dB, only a few of 80 dB. Loudness probably grows by arithmetic sum of fibres active as intensity rises. The outer hair cells are innervated by the efferent cochlear bundle of Rasmussen and contain actin and myosin. They may 'focus' mechanical energy upon a single inner hair cell to enhance its threshold.

Localization of sound

The direction from which a sound comes is perceived by correlation within the CNS of differences between the sound patterns on the two sides of the head. The clues are:

1. Loudness difference (important for high frequencies).
2. Difference in time of reception the two ears (important for complex sounds and transients.
3. Phase difference (important for low frequencies).

FUNCTIONAL EXAMINATION OF HEARING

Live voice and whisper tests

These are applied as single words or short sentences. They are of limited value since standardization is impossible. Even with the same examiner, intensities will vary from test to test and under different acoustic conditions.

Tuning fork tests

Forks of 256 Hz and 512 Hz are the more commonly used.

Rinne test

The patient is usually asked to say whether the vibrating fork seems louder by air conduction (AC) close to the meatus, or by bone conduction (BC) with the base of the fork on the mastoid bone. More correctly the test is done by requiring the subject to indicate as soon as the fork becomes inaudible by AC and then quickly transferring it to the mastoid. If it is then audible again, the duration of its continuing audibility is noted in seconds. If it is not heard by BC in this sequence the order is reversed, beginning with audible BC and transferring the fork to AC at the meatus as soon as the sound disappears. Again, the difference is noted in seconds.

In modern practice the precision of the formal, classic method is seldom required, because pure-tone audiometry usually gives the same, or better reliability. Nevertheless, the test is a valuable double check on the correctness of the audiograph.

Normal subjects. AC better than BC (Rinne positive).

Conductive deafness. BC better than AC (Rinne negative).

Sensorineural deafness. AC better than BC (Rinne positive). Often the BC is not heard.

False negative Rinne

In severe unilateral sensorineural deafness, BC may be heard apparently better than AC as the sound is transmitted through the skull to the better hearing ear. This may cause considerable confusion, if not suspected in all cases of unilateral deafness and if masking (e.g. with a Bàràny box) is not applied to the good ear.

Weber test

A bone conduction test, useful only in cases of unilateral deafness or where a marked difference exists between the two ears. The base of the vibrating tuning fork is placed on the middle of the skull (usually the forehead).

Normal subjects and patients with bilateral equal deafness, the sound is heard in the midline, in both ears equally or in the head generally.

Conductive deafness. The sound is heard in or towards the deafened ear.

Sensorineural deafness. The sound is usually heard in or towards the better hearing ear. Occasionally it is not lateralized, especially in longstanding cases.

Absolute bone conduction (ABC) test

Bone conduction is made 'absolute' for clinical purposes by excluding airborne sound. This is done by pressing the tragus inwards and so occluding the external acoustic meatus. The ABC of the patient is compared with that of the examiner (assuming the examiner to have normal hearing).

Conductive deafness. ABC is normal (i.e. the same as that of the examiner).

Sensorineural deafness. ABC is reduced (i.e. less than that of the examiner).

Stenger test

A test for non-organic hearing loss. If two identical tuning forks are used and one is presented to each ear of a normal subject, he can only perceive the nearer of the two forks. If the examiner holds the two forks behind the blindfolded patient and places one fork about 25 cm from the good ear, the patient will say he hears the sound. Next the other fork is brought to about 8 cm from the ear under test. A patient with true deafness will still hear the fork placed 25 cm from his good ear, but the patient with non-organic deafness will deny that he hears any sound at all.

Chimani–Moos test

A modification of the Weber test, to detect non-organic hearing loss. If a tuning fork is placed on the forehead, the malingerer states that he hears the sound in his good ear (simulating a sensorineural deafness). If the meatus of the good ear is occluded, the truly deaf patient still hears the sound in the occluded ear, but the malingerer may deny that he hears the tuning fork at all.

Audiometry

Hearing requires far more than just an intact ear, auditory nerve and brainstem. Hearing is a perceptive process. It is the ability to detect sounds and then to associate those sounds with a specific memory within the brain so that they become meaningful. Only subjective audiometry can show that the entire system functions. Objective tests can identify responses to sound stimuli at lower neurological and peripheral levels.

Subjective audiometry

Methods of measuring hearing which rely upon the subject responding voluntarily.

1. Pure-tone audiometry

The most generally useful technique which determines the subject's threshold of hearing for pure tones of several seconds' duration. Pure tones are delivered to the ear under test through a suitable earphone (AC) or by a vibrator applied to the mastoid (BC). The frequencies tested usually range from 125 Hz to 8 000 Hz, in octave or half–octave steps, at intensities from –10 dB to 120 dB, in 5 dB steps. Calibration is adjusted so that at each frequency 0 dB is the average threshold of a sample of normally-hearing, healthy ears. The accepted standard in general clinical use conforms with the ISO recommendation (R. 389, international Reference Zero for the calibration of pure-tone audiometers). The threshold curves may take various forms and useful comparisons may be made before and after treatment or from one attendance to another (Figure 2.9 a,b,c,d,e).

Masking in pure-tone audiometry. Is vital:

● To obtain true thresholds when there is a difference in AC sensitivity between the two ears of more than 45 dB.
● In all bone-conduction measurements. The masking is applied to the non–test ear to prevent any noticeable sensation arising from the vibration being transmitted through or around the skull. Narrow–band filtered white noise centred on the test frequency is the most useful masking noise. BC levels are not valid unless correct masking is used and this is difficult to do in a busy clinic. Such a test should be reserved for cases in which exact BC measurements are required, e.g. in the pre– and postoperative assessment of otosclerotic patients.

Recruitment. The loudness recruitment phenomenon is an aspect of certain forms of deafness wherein the growth of loudness of sound of increasing intensity is greater than in normal ears. At least two mechanisms of recruitment have been suggested:

● The sensation of loudness is determined partly by the number of cochlear nerve fibres that are activated by a stimulating sound. Recruitment is thought to depend on the fact that each cochlear nerve fibre makes contact not only with one hair cell, but with several. The inner hair cells receive many times more fibres than the outer hair cells.

If a sound of weak intensity is applied to the deafened ear, the stimulation of the remaining outer hair cells is only sufficient to activate a few of the nerve fibres which innervate them. Therefore the sensation of loudness experienced by the deafened ear is less than normal.

If a sound of strong intensity is applied, the stimulation of the inner hair cells is able to 'saturate' a large number of nerve fibres. The sensation of loudness experienced by the deafened ear will now equal that of the normal ear.

● At very high intensities, the deafened ear may hear the sound louder than the normal ear (over–recruitment). A neural feedback circuit exists whereby the output of the outer hair cells inhibits the output of the inner hair cells. Loss of the outer hair cells damages this mechanism and results in the output of the inner hair cells being unchecked.

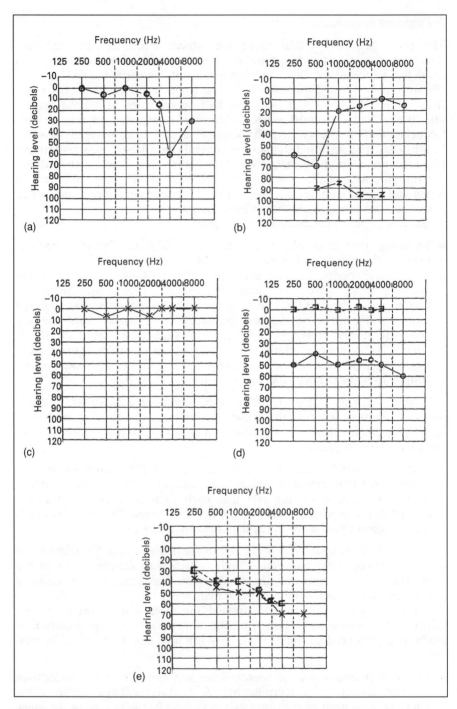

Figure 2.9 Typical audiograms. (a) Noise-induced hearing loss; (b) Menière's disease; (c) normal hearing; (d) ossicular discontinuity; (e) presbyacusis

Recruitment is almost diagnostic of a cochlear (sensory) hearing disorder. Approximately 10% of acoustic neuromas, however, exhibit recruitment and this figure is higher in cases of multiple neurofibromatosis. Patients with brainstem lesions may also show recruitment.

Clinical tests for recruitment, based on investigating changes in the sensation of loudness with change of intensity, are as follows:

- *Alternate binaural loudness balance test (Fowler).* This compares the stimulus intensities which give equal loudness in the normal and the deafened ear in patients with unilateral deafness. A frequency of 1000 Hz is the commonest used and the loudness is compared at threshold and then at 10–dB steps above.

Complete recruitment occurs when the sensation of loudness in the deafened ear grows to equal that in the other ear.

Incomplete recruitment occurs when the sensation of loudness in the deafened ear grows towards, but does not equal, that in the other ear.

Over-recruitment occurs when the sensation of loudness in the deafened ear becomes greater than that in the other ear.

Absence of recruitment is noted when the sensation of loudness in the deafened ear grows equally (in parallel) with the other ear. This occurs in either conductive or neural (retrocochlear) forms of deafness.

Loudness reversal occurs when the sensation of loudness in the deafened ear grows more slowly than that in the other ear. This is almost pathognomonic of a neural type of deafness.

- *Monaural loudness balance test (Reger).* Compares two sensations of loudness, as in the binaural test, but uses sounds of different frequency in the same ear. This test can only be applied to the more astute patient.
- *Difference limen test.* Measures the change in intensity of a sound just sufficient to produce a perceptible alteration of loudness (difference limen of loudness, or DL). If DL remains unchanged or increases with increasing intensity, recruitment is absent. If DL decreases with increasing intensity, recruitment is present.
- *Short increment sensitivity index (SISI).* A continuous pure tone at 20 dB above threshold is increased in intensity by 1 dB for 0.3 s every 5 s. This cycle occurs 20 times. Results are recorded as the number of increments heard, expressed as a percentage.

A score under 20% is typical of normal subjects, conductive and neural deafness.

A score over 60% is typical of severe cochlear deafness (e.g. Meniere's disease).

The test is probably more valid if the procedure is performed with higher intensities (90 dB ISO or 20 dB above threshold, whichever is the greater).

Tone decay. A phenomenon where a pure tone of constant intensity is perceived to grow faint (temporary threshold drift, TTD). It is found in nerve fibre deafness (e.g. acoustic neuroma) and where central auditory connections are impaired.

A small amount of tone decay, especially at higher frequencies, is very common in sensory disorders. The more useful test frequencies appear to be 1000 Hz and 4000 Hz.

In Carhart's test, a tone is presented continuously at 5 dB above the subjective threshold for 60 sec. If the subject ceases to hear the tone, the intensity is increased without break by 5 dB. The test is continued until the patient is able to hear the tone for 30 sec, or until a maximum of 3 min has elapsed from the start.

A decay of 0–14 dB occurs in normal subjects and conductive hearing losses.

A decay of 0–20 dB occurs in sensory deafness. Over 30 dB occurs in neural deafness.

2. Békésy self–recording audiometry

Sweep frequency testing. Signal frequency is swept from low to high, the traverse requiring about 10 minutes. Intensity is switched, so as to increase or diminish, by the patient himself. He is instructed to reduce the volume as soon as he can hear the tone and to increase the volume whenever the tone becomes inaudible. Interrupted (pulsed) or continuous tones are used. The intensity, as determined by the patient, is automatically plotted on a graph against the frequency. The resulting curve indicates the pure–tone threshold. The amplitude of the intensity variations represents the DL (difference limen) for pure tones. Small amplitudes indicate recruitment. It is principally used in the evaluation of hearing in industry.

3. Speech audiometry

Used to analyse graphically the percentage of words heard correctly by the subject. Standardized pre–recorded word lists are used to analyse the percentage of words heard correctly by the subject. Usually groups of 25 words are used at each intensity. Every correctly repeated word scores 1 and close attempts score 1/2, and the total score when multiplied by a factor of 4 is the percentage. Another system of scoring uses words of one syllable each containing three sound components or phonemes. A point is given for each correctly repeated phoneme. In this way each reply that the patient makes can be scored between 0 and 3. Earphones are used to obtain monaural information (providing the other ear is correctly masked). Free field testing is also possible, even when the subject is using a hearing aid.

Normal ears. 100% discrimination score is usually achieved by 60 dB intensity levels.

Conductive deafness. 100% discrimination or near is usually reached, but at higher intensity levels.

Sensory deafness. Often patients are unable to reach high scores (e.g. 50–70% max.) before discrimination deteriorates.

Neural deafness. Classically very poor discrimination scores are achieved.

Objective audiometry

Methods of measuring auditory function which do not require the active cooperation of the subject.

1. Impedance audiometry

A low frequency signal or probe tone (e.g. 220 Hz) is introduced into the sealed external acoustic meatus. If the tympanic membrane is stiff, more of the sound is impeded than when the tympanic membrane is mobile and absorbant (compliant). The amount of sound reflected is monitored by a sound pressure level meter. (Figure 2.10)

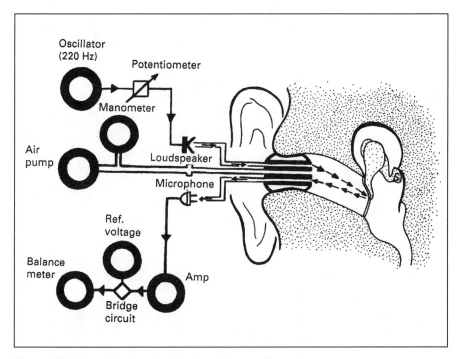

Figure 2.10 Schematic representation of impedance audiometry

- *Tympanometry.* The tympanic membrane may be made artificially stiffer by changing the pressure in the external acoustic meatus from –400 mm H_2O to +200 mm H_2O by using a small air pump attached to a manometer. Changes of acoustic impedance are shown by the meter needle, or automatically plotted as a graph against the pressure changes. The compliance is maximal when the air pressure in the external meatus equals that within the middle ear cavity, and diminishes as the pressure increases or diminishes, thus causing the tympanic membrane to be stretched. The graph shows characteristic changes in different conditions of the middle ear.

(*a*) Normal ears (Figure 2.11a). A symmetrical graph with maximum compliance to 0 mm H_2O. A compliance range of approximately 0.6 ml is average.

(*b*) Seromucinous otitis media (Figure 2.11b). The graph usually shows a negative middle ear pressure (e.g. –300 mm H_2O) and a flat curve indicating a marked decrease in compliance.

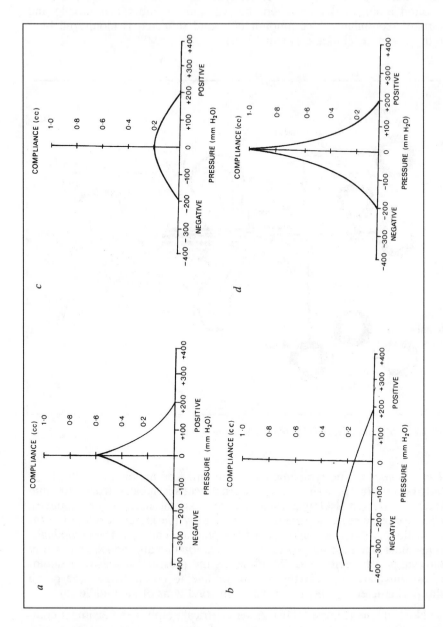

Figure 2.11 Tympanometry. a, Normal; b, eustachian obstruction; c, otosclerosis; d, ossicular disconnection

(*c*) Otosclerosis (Figure 2.11c). Often a normally shaped graph is obtained, with decreased compliance. If the maximum compliance is less than 0.3 ml, usually a type 3 or type 4 footplate is found at surgery.

(*d*) Ossicular disconnection (Figure 2.11d). Increased compliance is usual. If a 800 Hz probe tone is used, the graph may be double peaked.

(*e*) Eustachian tube function. May be assessed:

In patulous Eustachian tube, the needle of the meter will often move with respiration.

In blocked Eustachian tube, if the drumhead is intact, there is a negative pressure within the middle ear. The function can be estimated by inducing a negative or a positive pressure within the external acoustic meatus and then asking the patient to swallow or to carry out Valsalva's or Toynbee's manoeuvres.

In perforation of the tympanic membrane, if the Eustachian tube is patent, it is impossible to obtain an airtight seal. If the tube is blocked, a flat graph is obtained with a compliance of 2.0–2.5 ml.

These methods can be used to assess grommet patency and Eustachian tube function in such cases.

- *Intra–aural reflex measurements.* Contraction of the intra–aural muscles causes a stiffening of the tympanic membrane. The resulting change in drum compliance may be recorded by using acoustic impedance measurements.

(*a*) Non-acoustic reflex. In man, a puff of air directed across the cornea or into the meatus causes the tensor tympani muscle (probably alone) to contract bilaterally. Measurement of this reflex is used to assess the integrity of the neural pathway concerned.

(*b*) Stapedius reflex. In man, sounds of more than 70 dB intensity probably cause the stapedius muscle (alone) to contract bilaterally, unless the sound is of sufficient intensity to cause a general startle reaction. Frequencies between 500 Hz and 4000 Hz are best used clinically. The minimum intensity required to evoke the reflex is termed the stapedius reflex threshold (SRT).

In *normal ears,* the SRT for pure tones (500–4000 Hz) occurs with sound between 70 and 100 dB above the subjective pure tone threshold. The SRT for noise stimuli lies at lower intensities.

In *conductive deafness,* the reflex may be unobtainable owing to the middle ear pathology (e.g. fixation of the stapes in otosclerosis). The SRT, if obtainable, lies at 70–110 dB above the subjective threshold.

In *recruiting deafness,* the SRT often occurs at levels less than 70 dB above the subjective threshold.

In *neural deafness,* usually the SRT occurs at levels in excess of 70 dB above the subjective threshold, providing that the neural pathway is intact.

In *facial paralysis,* if the facial nerve is damaged proximally to the branch to the stapedius muscle, the reflex is unobtainable. It is therefore of value in conditions such as traumatic facial paralysis. In idiopathic paralysis (Bell's palsy), it may be used to verify the completeness of the palsy.

SRT for pure tones cannot be used alone to predict the hearing acuity, since the SRT is obtained at levels relatively closer to the threshold in patients with recruiting pathologies. If wide-band noise is used in addition to pure tones, hearing can be predicted with acceptable accuracy.

$$PTT = SRT_1 - 2.5 \times (SRT_1 - SRT_2)$$

where PTT is the average pure-tone threshold (500–4000 Hz); SRT_1 is the average stapedius reflex threshold (500–4000 Hz); SRT_2 is the stapedius reflex threshold for wide-band noise.

This test has considerable value in screening young children and suspected cases of non-organic hearing loss.

Stapedius reflex decay can be detected by presenting the tone continuously and noting any loss of amplitude of contraction. In normal subjects, there is no decay of the reflex at 500 Hz or 1000 Hz. Patients with neural deafness often show reflex decay and the contraction amplitude is halved in about 3 s.

In *multiple sclerosis*, interesting abnormalities of the stapedius reflex are sometimes found. The reflex may be absent in one or both ears. The reflex rise-time may be prolonged.

2. Evoked (electric) response audiometry (ERA)

The measurement of the tiny physiological electric events occurring in response to sound stimulation. Clinically, ERA involves the use of averaging equipment which can add together individual responses so that the sum becomes visible and background 'noise' is diminished.

- *Electrocochleography (ECochG).* Measurement of the electrical output of the cochlea. The nearer the active electrode is placed to the round window, the larger the responses obtained.

Transtympanic ECochG. A thin needle electrode is placed through the tympanic membrane to lie on the promontory, just anterior to the round window niche. Adults are tested under local anaesthesia and children under general anaesthesia. No masking is required and anaesthesia does not affect the results. Action potentials from the VIIIth nerve, cochlear microphonics and summating potentials are encountered. The action potentials are synchronized by using clicks so that the 'whole nerve action potential' is recorded (Figure 2.12). This gives a clear indication of the cochlear threshold which is a good measure of the hearing threshold. Most of the information comes from the basal coil of the cochlea and is therefore only related to the higher frequencies.

There are two main clinical uses of ECochG:

(i) Prediction of hearing thresholds. ECochG is a robust test for predicting the hearing status of young children. The accuracy is within 15 dB.

(ii) Otoneurological diagnosis. ECochG has great potential in the diagnosis of various conditions that affect the ear. A clear measure of recruitment can be made. Neural lesions (e.g. acoustic neuroma) yield a broad action potential while often the cochlear microphonics are relatively normal. Brainstem lesions may yield a normal ECochG while brainstem and cortical responses are absent.

- *Brainstem responses*

Electrodes are placed on the ear lobe or mastoid, and the vertex. Using acoustic clicks an interesting series of waves is obtained (Figure 2.13). The

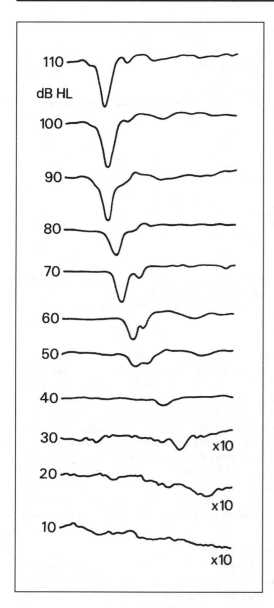

110
dB HL
100
90
80
70
60
50
40
30   x10
20
      x10
10
      x10

Figure 2.12 Electrocochleograph. The large downward deflection is the whole nerve action potential in response to acoustic clicks. In this normal ear the response is visible to within 10 dB of threshold

the cochlear nucleus, the third in the superior olivary nucleus, the fourth and fifth in the inferior colliculus. The last two waves may be used to measure auditory acuity to within 10 dB of threshold. Delay between I and V occurs with acoustic neuroma.

● *Cortical ERA (CERA)*
Records, by the use of electrodes placed on the vertex, and on the ear lobe or mastoid, a tiny cortical auditory response buried in the on-going EEG rhythms. Pure tones are used at 0.5–2 s intervals, and a train of 30–60 pulses

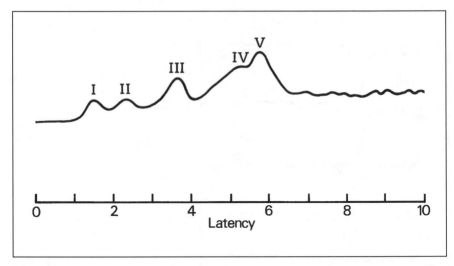

Figure 2.13 Brainstem acoustic response. Five waves are seen when the response to acoustic clicks are averaged to exclude muscle potentials. Each probably corresponds to a synapse in the brainstem and has a characteristic time appearance. Scale shows time after stimulus in milliseconds

is necessary. A typical adult response consists of a small inconsistent positive peak (P1) at 50–60 ms, a large negative peak (M1) at about 100 ms, and a large positive peak (P2) at about 175 ms. This is usually followed by a low second negative peak (N2) at 200–250 ms which is often very prominent in young children. The usefulness of CERA is severely limited by the marked influence on the responses of level of consciousness or awareness.

CERA gives an accurate objective measure of the pure tone audiogram in adults and older children, and it causes no discomfort to the patient. Passive cooperation is essential, as movements blur the response. It takes about 1 hour to perform the test. Young children do not give such accurate results and, unfortunately, sedation makes interpretation of the responses hazardous. There are no definite criteria for using CERA data for otoneurological diagnosis.

● *Postauricular myogenic responses (PAM)*
These are found in the vestigial muscles of the pinna in response to loud clicks. They are subject to variation in muscle tone and give the least accurate thresholds. However, the test is quick and simple to apply and active children untestable by other means without sedation often give clear responses. It is possible to use this test as a screening procedure during actual clinics before deciding on more intensive testing. It may also be used to test the integrity of the neural pathways involved.

Hearing tests in children

The earlier an auditory defect is diagnosed, the better the chances of helping a child to overcome its handicap and to integrate into normal society. If a

'Can your baby hear you?'

Here is a checklist of some of the general signs you can look for in your baby's first year:–

Shortly after birth   YES/NO
Your baby should be startled by a sudden loud noise such
as a hand clap or a door slamming and should blink or
open his eyes widely to such sounds

By 1 month
Your baby should be beginning to notice sudden
prolonged sounds like the noise of a vacuum cleaner and
he should pause and listen to them when they begin.

By 4 months
He should quieten or smile to the sound of your voice
even when he cannot see you. He may also turn his head
or eyes towards you if you come up from behind and
speak to him from the side.

By 7 months
He should turn immediately to your voice across the room
or to very quiet noises made on each side if he is not too
occupied with other things.

By 9 months
He should listen attentively to familiar everyday sounds
and search for very quiet sounds made out of sight. He
should also show pleasure in babbling loudly and
tunefully.

By 12 months
He should show some response to his own name and to
other familiar words. He may also respond when you say
'no' and 'bye bye' even when he cannot see any
accompanying gesture.

> Your health visitor will perform a routine hearing screening test on your
> baby between seven and nine months of age. She will be able to help and
> advise you at any time before or after this test if you are concerned about
> your baby and his development. If you suspect that your baby is not hearing
> normally, either because you cannot answer yes to the items above or for
> some other reason, then seek advice from your health visitor.

Figure 2.14 Checklist for general signs of childs hearing in the first year. (By kind permission of Dr Barry McCormick)

parent suspects a child to be deaf, that child is deaf until proved otherwise. The health visitor may administer a questionnaire to aid in identifying children with a hearing problem (Figure 2.14). Auditory testing of children depends on mental rather than chronological age, and allowances must be made for other handicaps (e.g. mental retardation or blindness).

Reflex tests

1. At birth. Moro or startle reflex. Aureo-palpebral reflex. Onset of crying.
2. At 3 months. Stilling, when the child quietens in response to a sound. Blinking and frowning.
3. At 5 months. Eyes turn towards a sound source.
4. At 6 months. The head turns towards a sound source.

Behavioural tests

The behaviour of a small child to a sound stimulus depends in part upon its mental ability. These tests are beautifully described in the STYCAR (Screening Tests for Young Children and Retardates) manual. Sounds of interest for a child are a high frequency rattle (8 kHz), low humming (500 Hz), a whispered 'S' (2–4 kHz) and a xylophone (500–2 kHz). The intensity is estimated using a sound level meter and tests are performed in a sound-treated room.

1. At 7–18 months. Distraction tests are used. The child seated on his mother's lap is distracted by an assistant. This is usually done with a toy. When the child is absorbed in playing with the toy, the assistant takes it away. At this point the child is in a state of heightened awareness so the examiner presents a test sound from behind or from the side.
2. At 18 months–2.5 years. Cooperation is sought. The child performs a simple task in response to the sounds.

Performance tests

Between 2 and 5 years, the child may be asked verbally to perform tasks (e.g. 'Place the doll on the chair').

Alternatively, the child is seated at a small table and a series of graduated cups fitting into one another may be placed upon it. He is taught to pick out one cup each time he hears the word 'Go' (a very loud word). When the reflex is firmly established, it is possible to measure the distance at which this word is just heard. This is recorded as 'Hears "Go" at X feet'. The response forms an excellent basis for audiometry as soon as the child learns to respond to pure tones.

In an older child who has acquired a knowledge of, or familiarity with, certain common objects, pictures may be used instead of cups. He is requested to 'show me the man' and 'show me the van'. By using carefully graded words, in picture form, it is possible to measure the distances at which the child can distinguish:

1. Vowels (relatively loud).
2. Consonants (relatively soft).

If there is no hearing for speech, musical instruments (such as a drum or xylophone) may be substituted. High-frequency loss may sometimes be determined in this way. If this fails, further attempts are made with a hearing aid.

These tests give information exceeding that of simple audiometry.

Subjective tests

It is vital that pure-tone subjective audiometry be achieved as early as possible in all children with suspect hearing. Techniques are varied to entice the child to cooperate.

1. *Visual reinforced audiometry.* The young child is conditioned to press a button when a sound is heard. This switches on a light which illuminates a series of pictures as a reward.
2. *Conditioned audiometry.* The child is taught to build a tower of bricks or to put bricks into a basket each time he hears the test sound.

Objective tests

ECochG and BSER are performed under intravenous general anaesthetic as day cases in those infants in which a threshold cannot be established. Ketamine produces a brief period in which it is possible to insert the transtympanic electrode and run a series of tests at various loudness levels. Middle ear fluid is sometimes found and a grommet inserted. Levels within 10 dB of the true threshold are found. The tests do not show that the child is capable of understanding sounds.

Fraser's test for labyrinthine fistula

The hearing by pure tones or speech audiometry is tested in two postures, one calculated to minimize a leak of perilymph and the other to maximize it. Twenty minutes separates the two audiograms and the results are contrasted. A marked difference implies a leak of perilymph.

Psychogenic deafness

There are three varieties:

Feigned deafness, or malingering

In which the person deliberately pretends to be deaf to gain a definite advantage for himself. This is most commonly seen in compensation cases.

Hysterical deafness

In which the subject's motive is unconscious although it is connected with personal gain. The hysterical personality is emotionally unstable, immature and suggestible. Often the deafness is bilateral and severe.

Psychosomatic deafness

It is thought that, in certain subjects, stress produces emotional tensions which result in objective changes. It is possible that the effect is mediated by vascular changes.

Tests for psychogenic deafness

1. *Tuning fork tests.* As previously described in the present chapter (Stenger and Chimani–Moos tests, p. 52).
2. *Pure-tone audiometry.* The pure tone audiometric thresholds often vary from one test to another. Often shadow curves are not admitted, even in the absence of masking of the good ear.
   The Stenger test may be employed using pure tones.
3. *Békésy audiometry.* A type V is typical of feigned deafness or hysteria.
4. *Delayed speech feedback.* The patient reads aloud and receives intermittently through earphones his own recorded and amplified speech a few milliseconds after it has been spoken. The test works best in the more literate subject. If he hears his delayed speech, his speech monitoring mechanisms are deceived and his articulation falls away into unintelligibility.
5. *Objective tests.* These are of great value, but transtympanic ECochG is rarely justifiable. The best tests are SRT and BSER.

HEARING AIDS

Aims

To help a person with a hearing impairment to identify desired sounds, including speech (and especially his own), by selective amplification.

Limitations

Due to:

1. Characteristics inherent in the aid (see later).
2. Difficulties in dealing with:
(a) Different speech components: vowels are composed of low frequencies which give power to make speech audible, and consonants of high frequencies which make speech intelligible. By the use of adjustable tone controls, amplification provided throughout the range can be attenuated for high or low frequencies or both to suit individual need.
(b) Competing noise and reverberation in places with hard walls.
(c) Different types of deafness. Conductive loss is restored by simple amplification; sensorineural losses require amplification with strict attention to the details of frequency and growth of loudness. If these are underestimated the patient experiences increase in loudness with no increase in discrimination. Distortion increases with gain and loudness discomfort with the degree of recruitment.

Non-electrical types

Include auricles, trumpets and speaking tubes. These are light in weight but obvious and cumbersome, and have a limited range of usefulness. A gain of intensity up to 29 dB is obtainable with the speaker 75 cm from the aid.

They cause no distortion and may therefore be useful for persons with marked recruitment who cannot tolerate an electrical aid. They may also be used by the aged, whose sensitivity of touch may be diminished and whose only requirement may be to hear one voice at a time or the radio.

Electrical types

Components

1. *Microphone.* Electret condensor type, may be forward facing, unidirectional or omnidirectional.
2. *Amplifier.* A series of transistors, at the centre of an integrated circuit in up-to-date aids. The aid size is dictated by battery requirements and the finger controls.
3. *Receiver (loudspeaker).* Of three types:
(a) *Air conduction* either in 'button' attached to an ear mould, or built in to the case of the aid in ear-level models.
(b) *Bone conduction,* indicated (in less than 2% of patients) because of meatal discharge or stenosis, or of marked subjective preference for bone conduction reception. Used with headband on body-worn aids, or built into spectacle-type aids. Overall amplification is limited to a smaller band of frequencies and battery consumption is greater.
(c) *Bone anchored.* A 20 dB gain is available if the aid is directly anchored to the skull by a percutaneous titanium implant. This is driven by an ear level aid with a button battery. A bone anchored magnet beneath scalp driven by an external electromagnet also has advantages but the gain is not so great, and a body worn driver with large batteries may be required.

Characteristics

1. Amplification

Is the 'acoustic gain' or amount of increase of sound available.
It must be over 25 dB for weak sounds to be heard. Owing to average low 'sensitivity' (ability to amplify weak sounds) of microphone and receiver, the electrical gain of an amplifier must be 85 dB to obtain an acoustic gain of 50 dB.

2. Output

The maximum intensity which the most powerful aid is made to deliver is 148 dB. An aid with this very high output should be used with caution and for limited periods.
Limitation of output. The severely deaf person requires high acoustic gain over a wide frequency range. Selective limitation of unduly loud sounds, which would otherwise cause loss of intelligibility or discomfort, is effected by one of two methods:
(a) Peak clipping (PC): the output voltage is limited to give each sine wave a 'square' waveform. The strong vowel sounds are clipped more than the weak consonant sounds, and some distortion occurs.

(b) Automatic gain control (AGC): retains crests of sine waves and also reproduces their rising characteristic, but the amplitude increases more slowly at the beginning than with PC. Control is exercised over practically the entire dynamic range of speech. There is no perceptible time lag. It may be thought of as an 'auto pilot' on the gain control. AGC on the input is quicker to act but less precise, AGC on the output is slower in onset but more appropriate.

3. Frequency range

The average requirement is 500–4000 Hz. Many variations are required and can be provided.

4. Frequency response

For selective amplification the best response curve is one rising gradually from 500 Hz by 6 dB per octave. Modifications of responses are effected by:

● Changing the receivers.
● Continuously adjustable tone controls.
● Varying the length and diameter of polythene tube to the earpiece.
● Design of ear mould.
● Filters placed in ear mould or tubing.

Types of model available in the British NHS

1. Body-worn

These incorporate a flex to receiver in ear.
   Advantages are:

● Great power available.
● Maximum amplification with minimum feed-back.
● Ability to incorporate induction coil and provide variable settings of input, gain, output, frequency response, peak clipping and AGC.
● Space to have many transistors to give better sensitivity or higher fidelity.
● Ideal for patients without manual dexterity to manipulate the miniature controls of an ear-level aid.

   Disadvantages are physical awkwardness, psychological disfavour, inconvenience of flex, clothes-rub, and inability to produce stereophonic effect.
   NHS current types:
Body-worn BW61 – with a pick-up coil, peak clipping facility and tone control. It is powerful enough to take a bone conduction receiver (max. gain 60–76 dB).
Body-worn BW81 – facilities as above but with a maximum gain of 88–93 dB and uses two alkaline manganese batteries. Both models have a switch for use of pick-up coil and microphone, allowing patients to monitor their own voices.

2. Behind-the-ear ('ear-level')

These have a receiver incorporated in the aid or separate in a 'button' with ear mould. Available in forms 'behind the ear', 'all in ear', 'hair-slide', and in spectacle frames. The position of the microphone opening usually makes less difference than expected.

Advantages are smallness of size, inconspicuousness, freedom from flex and clothes-rub, modification of sound patterns only by diffraction effects of head rather than body, and the stereophonic effect when binaural reception used.

NHS current types:

BE1O series are medium gain (45–47 dB).

BE16, BE17, BE18 and BE19 aids all have forward facing microphones and telecoil pick-ups. The BE18 has a peak clipping facility.

BE30 series – higher gain instruments (53–57 dB).

The 34 and 35 both have pick-up coils, tone control and peak clipping facilities. An audio input facility is available on the 35.

BE5O series – The 51,52 and 53 aids are power post aurals (63–64 dB gain) with front facing microphone, tone control, peak clipping facilities, pick-up coil and selector switch for off, coil, and microphone functions. The 51 and 52 aids allow inputs from both microphone and telecoil to be presented simultaneously (MT switch).

Special adaptations

1. Induction coil

Incorporated in the aid to pick up sound from a wire loop placed round rooms, halls, or classrooms. Can also be used with telephones and television. Provides better sound quality and also allows other listeners to have sound at a comfortable level.

2. Auditory training unit

A powerful portable amplifier with wide frequency range. Helpful for corrective speech training.

3. Group aid

A powerful unit with a number of head-set receivers attached to classroom desks.

4. Radio aid

VHF, radio microphones and receivers for school use. Uses radio transmission of sound from a teachers microphone to childrens hearing aids, thereby avoiding poor classroom acoustics.

5. Amplifying adaptors

Available for telephone, radio and television receivers.

Binaural hearing

An aid for each ear is extremely helpful if useful hearing is present in both ears, especially for children and in quiet surroundings. The chief difficulty is to produce accurate matching for intensity and phase. Two head-worn aids may be carefully adjusted, or one body-worn aid may be used with a Y lead.

Fitting hearing aids

An aid should be tried when deafness becomes a handicap. This is usual when there is an overall loss for pure tones of more than 30–35 dB in the speech range, and in the better ear. Losses up to 100 dB can be helped with a behind-the-ear aid and up to 120 dB with a body-worn aid. Unilateral deafness generally does not call for a hearing aid. However, if needed, the solution may be to use a CROS (contralateral routing of signals) aid, in which a microphone on the deaf side is connected via the sides and front of a pair of spectacles to an amplifier housed in the arm of the spectacles on the good side. This does not interfere with the natural reception of sound in the good ear.

A well-fitting ear mould is an essential part of the amplification system, but is not usually recommended in the presence of a discharge or in otitis externa. In such cases a bone conductor should be fitted if possible. Patients need instruction in the wearing and use of an aid to ensure the best results. Rehabilitation may take months.

Patients must face up to the embarrassment of wearing an aid. They can be assured that if the correct aid fits well and does not cause too marked distortion of speech, it cannot by itself lead to increase of deafness. A good, well-designed hearing aid will give low distortion even under overloading conditions. Rehabilitation into suitable employment is advised. Children (and sometimes adults) with aids need special auditory training. Lip-reading should be practised in combination with the improved hearing.

Acoustic feedback

The whistling sound due to loudspeaker output reaching microphone. This is the factor limiting amplification and is minimized by a well fitting ear mould. Feedback developing around a hitherto good mould means a new development in the canal or middle ear. Wax or otitis media with effusion is usually to blame and should be promptly rectified.

Quality control using a test box

The hearing aid test box will answer two vital questions. First is this aid performing to manufacturer's specifications? Second, given an input of 60 dB, is the output in the speech frequencies sufficient for the patient's needs? Remember that hearing loss is measured in dB HL, a biological scale and aid output measured in dB SPL, a physical scale. A correction must be made before the two can be compared (see Figure 2.1).

Cochlear implants

Electrical stimulation of residual fibres of the cochlear nerve restores hearing when all hair cell function is lost and there is no discrimination of speech with a powerful hearing aid.

Single channel implant

Single active electrode, usually platinum rests against the round window (extracochlear) or is passed into the scala tympani (intracochlear). Circuit completed through indifferent electrode nearby. Restores rhythm of sounds and speech, enhances lip-reading. Minimal discrimination of speech without vision.

Multichannel implant (Figure 2.15)

Four to 22 electrodes on a silicone rubber 'finger' are passed deep into the scala tympani to reach vicinity of all remaining dendrites of cochlear nerve at hibenula perforata. Circuit completed through adjacent electrode (bipolar stimulation) or through remote indifferent electrode (unipolar stimulation). Provides samples of speech at fixed frequencies dictated by effectiveness of nerve electrode interface at fixed sites beneath the basilar membrane. Enhances lip-reading. In 60% of cases allows discrimination of speech without vision. Patients with an excellent result can use the telephone.

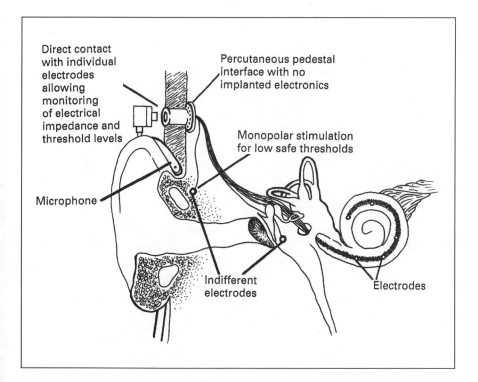

Figure 2.15 Cochlear implant

Speech processor

Body worn box containing amplifiers and frequency selective filters linked to implanted part of device by plug or inductive coupling. Drives the electrode at or within the cochlea. Requires tuning for each individual.

Selection of patients

Acquired deafness beyond the reach of a hearing aid. No active CSOM. Well motivated, no debilitating disease. Meningitis causes bony obliteration of scala tympani in 14% of cases, not a contraindication but much drilling into the scala tympani is required to insert a long electrode array.

Congenitally deaf signing teenagers make no use of implants if fitted. Prospects for 2–3 year old child unknown, doubts are certainty of loss and size of mastoid to support hardware, difficulties should not be insurmountable.

Chapter 3

Equilibrium

PHYSIOLOGY OF THE VESTIBULAR SYSTEM

The vestibular system has two major functions:

1. Maintenance of our equilibrium and hence prevention of injury.
2. Maintenance of the position of the eyes in order to obtain maximum resolution of any object that is being observed.

The detailed anatomy and physiology of the vestibular system is complex but can simply be divided into interconnecting component parts. The sensory side of the system consists of the vestibular labyrinth, eyes and the somatosensors in muscle, joints and skin. These sensory organs connect directly with the brainstem. They also connect with the cerebellum and cerebrum.

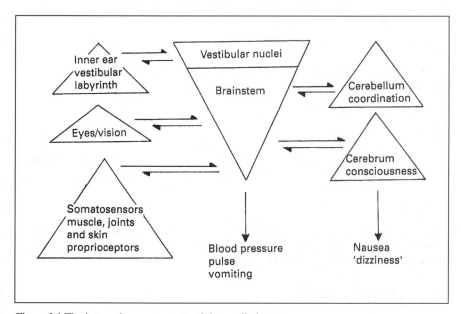

Figure 3.1 The interacting components of the vestibular system

Cerebral interpretation of visual clues such as the horizon, floors, walls, and the effects of gravity gives valuable information about the body's orientation. The brainstem and cerebellum coordinate the sensory information and send out a reflex response to the muscles that maintain posture and eye position.

Labyrinthine function

The receptor organs in the membranous vestibular labyrinth are concerned with the reflex adjustments of posture as well as with subjective sensations.

Utricle

Utricular maculae, situated in the horizontal plane, are quiescent as long as the head is horizontal and stationary. They respond (by gravity) to the slightest tilt and to linear acceleration. Such a movement also results in compensatory ocular reflexes whereby the visual axis is fixed when the head is deviated slightly from its previous position.

Semicircular ducts

Respond to angular acceleration of the head, the horizontal pair to rotations about a vertical axis, the posterior and superior pairs to tipping displacements of the head about a horizontal axis. Each duct shows sensitivity to rotation in its own plane. Movements of endolymph within the ducts stimulate the cristae. Stimulation causes reflex nystagmus, in which the eyes rotate slowly in one direction and then, by a sudden flick, in the opposite direction. The slow component is labyrinthine, the quick one cerebral. In clinical practice, nystagmus is named after the direction of the quick component.

Saccule

The macula of the saccule is at right angles to the macula of the utricle. It may sense linear acceleration.

Posture

The labyrinthine reflexes are normally concerned, with others, in the maintenance of posture. There are two main types of postural reflexes:

Static reflexes

These are the postural reactions of the body when at rest. Together with reflexes arising in the muscles, joints and other structures, they include the following labyrinthine (utricular) reflexes:

1. Tonic labyrinthine reflexes

With effects on the limbs, neck, trunk and eyes.

2. *Labyrinthine righting reflexes*

Which restore the body to its normal position when it is brought to rest in an abnormal position.

Kinetic reflexes

The postural reactions of the body when in movement. They are produced by actual movement with acceleration which is either:

1. *Angular,* as in movements of rotation in any plane.
2. *Progressive,* as in movements in a straight line.

When a part of the body is moved, reflex adjustment of pose is often necessitated to maintain balance. In general, the kinetic reflexes bring the body into its normal stance, while pose is maintained by activation of the various static reflexes.

Vestibular nerve activity

Animal experiments show that there is a steady resting neural discharge equal on both sides. Stimulation of end-organs, e.g. cristae or maculae, has an inhibitory effect in one direction, or a stimulatory effect in the other. Either change is complemented by opposite changes on the other side, a correlation which reflects the anatomical polarization of the hair cells of the cristae. Acute deprivation (for example by nerve section) leaves the brainstem swamped by unbalanced unilateral neural impulses. Vertigo and nystagmus result.

FUNCTIONAL EXAMINATION OF THE LABYRINTH

The function of the vestibular labyrinth can be assessed by stimulating it artificially to produce nystagmus. Congenital nystagmus and squint should be recognized and labyrinthine sedatives withdrawn 3 days before tests.

Nystagmography can be used to record and measure frequency, amplitude, eye speed and duration of nystagmus, either photographically (less commonly) or electrically (the more usual method).

In *electronystagmography* (ENG) electrodes are attached to the skin close to each eye. Changes in the corneoretinal potentials *as recorded at the electrode sites* are proportional to angle of rotation of the eyes from the straight-ahead position. These changes of electrical potential therefore follow faithfully the nystagmus and, after amplification, are recorded permanently on a moving paper strip.

Caloric tests

If water at 30° or 44°C (i.e. 7° below or above normal body temperature) is run into the ear under certain standard conditions, nystagmus is produced in

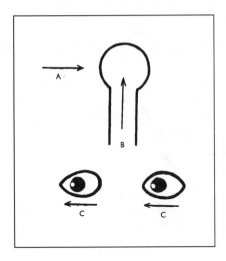

Figure 3.2 Physiology of caloric stimulation. A, Hot water syringed into right ear. Horizontal canal made vertical; B, flow of endolymph towards ampulla; C, nystagmus is to the right

the normal person with a healthy labyrinth. Hot and cold air stimulation is replacing water. There is less risk of electrocution and none of infection with the pseudomonas that colonizes caloric water baths.

Physiology of caloric stimulation

The caloric response is usually ascribed to simple physical changes (Figure 3.2). In a recumbent subject, with the head inclined forwards at 30°, the horizontal semicircular canal is vertical. Hot water heats the fluid in the duct, the specific gravity of the fluid falls and the fluid rises, i.e. moves towards the ampulla. This causes nystagmus with quick component to the stimulated side. When cold water or air is used, the endolymph moves away from the ampulla and produces nystagmus in the opposite direction. The responses are abolished in space (weightlessness).

1. Hallpike caloric test

The patient lies on a couch with the head-rest tilted upwards at 30° to the horizontal. This brings the horizontal semicircular duct into the vertical plane. Water at the desired temperature is run into the ear from a douche-can placed 61 cm above the patient's head. A continuous stream is directed against the tympanic membrane for 40 s. Nystagmus usually results if the labyrinth is normal and commonly lasts for about 2 minutes from the beginning of stimulation. Each ear is tested separately by hot and by cold stimulation, an interval of 5 minutes being allowed between each separate stimulation. The duration of the nystagmus in each case is recorded graphically (Figure 3.3a).

Canal paresis is present if the duration of nystagmus is reduced equally for both 'hot' and 'cold' tests (Figure 3.3b). The condition may be unilateral or bilateral.

Directional preponderance is present if the nystagmoid responses towards one side are of shorter duration than those towards the other (Figure 3.3c). A combination of canal paresis with directional preponderance towards the opposite side is commonly found.

2. Cold tap-water test

Should the minimal temperatures above fail to produce nystagmus in either ear, cold tap-water at a temperature of approximately 10°C may be used under the same conditions as those described. Failure to elicit nystagmus from one ear indicates severe depression of its function.

3. Cold air test

If there are contraindications to irrigating the ear with water (e.g. active middle ear infection or a mastoidectomy cavity) a simple qualitative test using cold air will demonstrate whether the vestibular labyrinth is functioning.

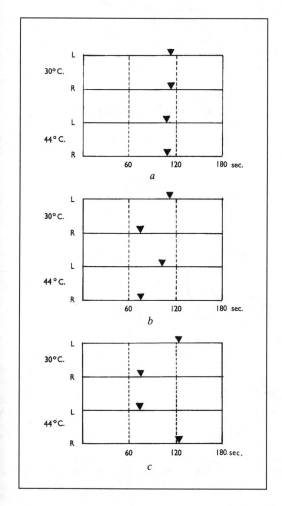

Figure 3.3 Calorograms. a, Normal; b, right canal paresis; c, right directional preponderance

Oxygen or compressed air from a cylinder is allowed to flow through a coil of copper tubing (Dundas Grant's tube) which is cooled by an ethyl chloride spray. The emerging jet of cold air is held just inside the auditory meatus, and will elicit nystagmus within 30–60 s if the labyrinth is active.

Rotation test

The patient is seated in a Bárány chair with the head erect. With eyes closed, the chair is turned round ten complete circles in 20 s, then suddenly stopped. Nystagmus results if the labyrinths are active and is always opposite in direction to that of rotation, e.g. rotation to right produces nystagmus to left. Whereas it is possible to stimulate each labyrinth separately in caloric tests, the rotation test has the disadvantage of always stimulating both together. The test is also open to criticism on the grounds that the stimulus is excessively violent, and is even capable of causing damage to the labyrinth. Used with care, however, it can be very valuable in determining the presence or absence of labyrinthine function in patients with bilateral total or subtotal sensorineural deafness, particularly in young children on whom caloric tests may be difficult to do satisfactorily.

Cupulometry

This is a more delicate form of rotation test in which subjective vertigo and objective nystagmus resulting from very gentle rotational stimuli are recorded electrically. The test is performed in the dark.

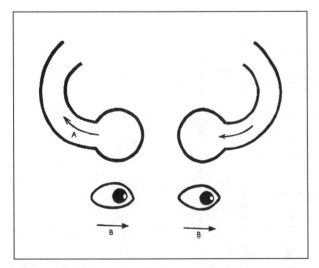

Figure 3.4 Physiology of rotational stimulation. A, After-effect of rotation to the right. Endolymph moves away from right ampulla, and towards left ampulla; B, nystagmus is to the left

Physiology of rotational stimulation (Figure 3.4)

The patient is turned to the right (clockwise). Law of inertia dictates endolymph does not accelerate nor decelerate as fast as the walls of the semicircular duct. When rotation is stopped endolymph continues to move (away from the right ampulla) and displaces the crista. This produces nystagmus to the left (since flow towards the ampulla always produces nystagmus to the same side; away from the ampulla, to the opposite side).

Fistula test

A fistula in the bony wall of the horizontal semicircular canal may result from erosion by cholesteatoma or from the fenestration operation. In either case, compression of air in the external auditory canal will produce movement of endolymph in the duct, hence vertigo and nystagmus, as long as the vestibular labyrinth is still functioning. If the labyrinth has been destroyed, the test may be negative even though a fistula is present. Air in the canal can be compressed mechanically either by pushing in the tragus with a finger or by compression of the bulb of Siegle's speculum.

Test for positional nystagmus

This is described under Positional vertigo.

Gait

Gait is noticeably unsure and 'wide-based' in severe bilateral vestibular disorders. After compensation from unilateral lesions it may be normal.

Romberg's test

With incompletely compensated unilateral lesions, or with bilateral vestibular damage, eye closure results in a dramatic loss of balance, even if proprioceptive sensory (posterior column) function is intact (cf. tabes dorsalis).

Unterberger's test

Detects compensated unilateral lesions. Rotation to the left or right while marching on the spot, eyes closed, indicates the weakest labyrinth, on the side to which the patient turns. More than 30° in 30 s is pathological.

Walking to a target eyes closed

Sensitive test of vestibular symmetrical function and of gait.

Electronystagmography and optokinetic nystagmography

These can give additional information on the functional status of the vestibular system.

Other tests

The patient's centre of gravity can be continually recorded and displayed on a television screen by placing the patient on a platform sensitive to pressure. If the platform is moved then the patient's posturing to maintain his balance can be recorded. The degree of movement at the hips compared to the ankles can indicate certain abnormalities.

Chapter 4

Diseases of the external ear

CONGENITAL MALFORMATIONS

Congenital defects of the external ear may be associated with others in middle and inner ear. Development of the face and lower jaw may also be defective.

Types

1. *Complete or partial absence of auricle.* Due to failure of development of the six auricular tubercles.
2. *Pre-auricular sinus and/or cyst.* Found in the region of the crus helicis. Due to incomplete fusion of the tubercles. A cyst may develop in the track and may become infected.
3. *Accessory auricles.* Due to tubercles sited on other parts of the first or other cleft depressions.
4. *Atresia of external auditory meatus.* Due to a defect in the inward growth and canalization of the epithelial anlage. Often associated with microtia.
5. *Fistula or sinus of visceral cleft origin.* May grow into, or towards, the pharynx or middle ear cleft (rare).
6. *Abnormalities in size or shape of auricle.* Including the protruding ear ('bat ear' and 'lop ear').
7. *High jugular bulb.* May be accidentally opened during tympanoplasty.

Treatment

1. *Minor auricular defects.* Plastic operations may improve appearance.
2. *Major auricular defects.* Prosthesis is more effective. This may be glasses mounted, attached by adhesive or by transcutaneous osseous-integrated bolts.
3. *Pre-auricular sinus and/or cyst.* May become infected, when it must be excised completely.
4. *Protruding ear.* Can be corrected through a vertical incision on the cranial surface of the auricle. The cartilage is so incised (and reduced if necessary) as to weaken its outwardly projecting 'springiness' and to create a new strong antihelix. A cartilage scoring technique has been described by Stenström and Mustardé recommends a method with simple permanent sutures.

5. Deafness. Surgical attempts to relieve the deafness of congenital malformations are justifiable, if cochlear function is present, especially when they are due to atresia, with or without middle ear deformities. Surgical correction is however fraught with problems especially stenosis of the surgically created external auditory canal and infection. If a conventional hearing aid cannot be used then an implantable hearing aid may be suitable.

INJURIES

Lacerations

All degrees are encountered including complete avulsion of auricle.

Treatment

In repairing lacerations sutures should not pass through cartilage. Complete avulsion usually requires a prosthesis but immediate suture has been successful.

Blows

Haematoma auris

Due to rupture of vessels in the perichondrium, especially on the external aspect of the auricle. This leads to effusion of blood. Haematoma or serous effusion may sometimes arise spontaneously in the elderly. Failure to treat results in fibrosis of the clot, with permanent thickening of the auricle ('cauliflower ear').

Treatment

Consists of:

1. Aspiration (when small) or incision (when larger).
2. Shirt buttons or a moulded splint secured by a through monofilament suture in pairs astride the haematoma.

Frostbite

Clinical features

Red or blue areas first appear on the helix. These later become white. The whole ear except the lobule swells and becomes painful, red, vesicated, and finally gangrenous.

Treatment

In the early stages. Gentle rewarming.
In the later stages. As for gangrene.

Foreign body

Clinical features

Hard or soft objects, some hygroscopic, get into the external auditory canal. Live insects may enter, to cause intense irritation and noise. When the canal is blocked, deafness (conductive) and tinnitus follow sometimes with pain. There may be a reflex cough.

Treatment

Smooth round foreign body. Remove by a hook if it cannot be removed by syringing. Forceps must not be used as they only push the foreign body further in. A general anaesthetic is essential in children and sensitive adults. Operating microscope always a help.

Other foreign bodies can usually be removed by:

1. Hartmann's 'crocodile' forceps if there is an edge or,
2. Syringing (insects may be killed before syringing, by instilling spirit drops into the meatus), or
3. Suction.
4. A strong magnet for ferrous items.

Swelling of canal walls may result from irritation by the foreign body or unskilled use of forceps. A postaural incision must be made, to allow extraction of the foreign body via the posterior wall of the canal.

OTITIS EXTERNA

Definition

An acute or chronic reaction of the whole or a part of the skin of the external ear arising from local or general causes, or from a combination of both.

General considerations

Many diseases of the skin found elsewhere may produce lesions in the external ear. These may be:

1. *Dermatoses,* such as psoriasis,
2. *Infections,* such as impetigo, carried by direct spread or contamination.
   Some special forms of systemic infection cause characteristic skin lesions

in the ear, e.g. syphilis. It is not customary to include all these as separate clinical types of otitis externa, but rather to select certain of them which chiefly involve the external canal and are of special concern to the otologist.

Aetiology

The causative factors may be:

1. *Local.* Due to bacterial or fungal infection.
2. *General.* Allergic or seborrhoeic states, and systemic infection by bacteria or viruses.

These are frequently combined, hence:

1. Infection may produce an allergic (eczematous) response.
2. Eczema may become secondarily infected.
3. Infection and allergy may complicate the seborrhoeic state.

Clinical types

The following clinical types are described:

1. *Furuncle of external canal.*
2. *Diffuse infective otitis externa.*
3. *Otomycosis.*
4. *Eczematous otitis externa.*
5. *Seborrhoeic otitis externa.*
6. *Granular myringitis.*
7. *Myringitis bullosa haemorrhagica.*
8. *Herpetic lesions of external ear.*
9. *Otitis externa malignans.*

1. Furuncle of external meatus

Pathology

A staphylococcal infection of a hair follicle in the cartilaginous portion of the external canal. Usually single, may be multiple. Recurrence common. Spontaneous evacuation usually occurs in a few days. Abrasion and maceration facilitate infection but often no predisposing factor is evident. Diabetics are especially susceptible to uncontrolled spread of the infection.

Clinical features

Irritation is the first symptom which may lead to scratching.
Pain follows. It is often intense and is aggravated by movement of the auricle or attempts to pass a speculum.
Trismus may occur when the boil is anterior.
Deafness. Conductive in type, follows if the canal is occluded by swelling.
Regional lymphadenitis is often present.
Spread of infection. Occasionally pus may track from a furuncle:

1. *Backwards.* Superficial to the periosteum over the mastoid, with obliteration of the postauricular sulcus.
2. *Forwards.* Into the parotid region.
3. *Inwards.* Through the notch of Rivinus, to infect the tympanic cavity (rare).

Differential diagnosis

At times the diagnosis between furunculosis and mastoiditis may be difficult; the two conditions occasionally coexist.

Herpetic lesions may cause difficulty, especially after rupture of the vesicles.

Mastoiditis	*Furuncle*
Preceding history of otitis media	Usually no preceding history of otitis media
Deafness present	No deafness unless canal occluded
Tympanic membrane shows signs of middle ear cleft infection	Tympanic membrane normal (if visible)
Pain on pressure over mastoid, not on moving auricle	Pain on moving auricle, not on pressure over mastoid
Postauricular groove tends to remain	Postauricular groove tends to be obliterated
Fistula into canal forms in bony portion (posterior wall)	Fistula into canal forms in cartilaginous portion (any part of circumference)
Radiographic changes in mastoid.	No radiographic changes in mastoid.

An *exostosis* should not be mistaken for a furuncle, as it is a painless swelling, hard to the probe, in the deep bony portion of the canal.

Treatment

Antibiotics

Usually flucloxacillin. The most valuable therapy and often all that is required.

10% ichthammol in glycerin. Applied locally as a gauze wick, is soothing before rupture.

Heat and sedation

May relieve the pain. Analgesics must also be used.

Incision

Seldom required, though it may be necessary when infection has extended beyond the canal.

Aural toilet

After spontaneous discharge. Suction cleansing under the microscope is especially useful.

2. Diffuse infective otitis externa

Definition

An infective dermatitis, usually starting in or near the external auditory canal and sometimes spreading to involve the whole auricle. Two clinical forms may be distinguished but their separation is arbitrary and they tend to merge.

1. *Infiltrative.*
2. *Desquamative.*

Aetiology

Predisposing causes are maceration, scratching and clumsy instrumentation. It occurs less often with the discharge of an otitis media than might be expected.

Pathology

In the acute stage there is a spreading infection of the epithelial and subepithelial layers of the canal. Usually due to a streptococcal infection, but staphylococci, *Pseudomonas aeruginosa, Bacillus proteus* and *Escherichia coli* are not infrequently found. Occasionally it may spread as a cellulitis of the face and neck and may involve the deeper structures.

Clinical features

Itching. The first symptom.
Pain. Follows.
Redness, swelling and serous oozing are found in the lining of the canal.
Infiltration, crusting, desquamation and discharge. Present in varying degrees.
Toxaemic symptoms. Present in severe acute cases with pyrexia and lymphadenitis.
Scaling, fissuring and stenosis. Seen in all gradations in the chronic form.

Treatment

General

Systemic antibiotics. Required in severe cases.

Local

Ribbon gauze wicks. Soaked with a mild astringent (aluminium acetate 8%) may be introduced to separate the walls. 10% ichthammol in glycerin is helpful in reducing the oedema.

Aural toilet. Suction removal of pus and debris under the operating micro-scope with special attention to the anterior recess of the deep meatus.

Antibiotics. When applied locally, may cause a local reaction. If used, they should be in combination with hydrocortisone. Neomycin, gentamicin and chloramphenicol are the commonest sources of an iatrogenic allergic reaction. Topical antiseptics such as chlorhexidine or the use of clioquinol reduce the risks of developing such a complication.

Calamine lotion usually allays residual itching. 1% phenol may be added to increase the antipruritic effect.

Special forms

1. Infiltrative otitis externa

Probably follows contamination with a dirty finger-nail in most cases. In the acute phase, the canal is occluded by a generalized, tender, brawny swelling. Discharge is scanty and may lead to crust formation. In severe cases, it may spread to cause thickening of the auricle. Scaling occurs as the condition subsides. Treatment follows the lines indicated above.

2. Desquamative otitis externa

In hot, humid climates, otitis externa commonly assumes a highly desquama-tive form. Bathing in these climates may lead to maceration of canal skin and so predispose to infection. *Ps aeruginosa* and *B. proteus* are the organisms most commonly found, so that gentamicin drops would appear to be indi-cated. However, astringent drops or wet wicks of 3% silver nitrate or 8% aluminium acetate help to form a protective coagulum and are very effective and free from allergic reactions.

3. Otomycosis

Otitis externa due to fungal infection may resemble the desquamative form of diffuse infective otitis externa but is much less common in this country and is associated with the presence of fungi. However, it is becoming more common with the widespread use of topical antibiotic preparations. The mycotic infection may be primary or secondary to a bacterial one (*Ps. aerug-inosa).* Many varieties of fungi are found, but aspergilli (especially *Aspergillus niger)* and *Candida albicans* are the commonest in temperate climates.

Clinical features

Otomycosis usually presents as a discharging ear in which the canal is lined by a mass like wet newspaper and has a peculiar musty odour. In a propor-tion of cases granules containing the mycelium, hyphae and spores can be shown microscopically. Occasionally, an inactive dry form occurs in which the canal is lined by a mould giving a fluffy appearance. It is then either symptomless or produces only irritation. Pain is unusual in the absence of associated pyogenic infection.

Diagnosis

Diagnosis is made by the identification from swabs and cultures of conidiophores (like pin heads).

Treatment

1. Removal of mass

By forceps or suction.

2. Fungicides

- Nystatin cream is effective for candida infection.
- *Clotrimazole* as 1% cream.
- *Amphotericin cream.*
- Econazole 1% drops or cream. Econazole also has an antibacterial action against Gram positive organisms.
- *Gentian Violet.* Effective for all types but has the disadvantage of staining the skin and bed-linen.

4. Eczematous otitis externa

Definition

An allergic dermatitis of the external ear.

Aetiology

The exciting factor is either:

Extrinsic

1. *General.* As in food or inhalation allergy.
2. *Local.* Known as 'contact dermatitis'. Examples are:

- Eczema of the postauricular sulcus due to nickel in spectacle frames.
- Eczema due to local application of antibiotics.
- Eczema due to presence of bacterial and/or fungal infections in the external ear.

Intrinsic

In the 'psychosomatic' type.

Clinical features

Irritation, redness and oedema are severe. They affect the skin of the canal, sometimes of the entire auricle.

Vesication, weeping and crust formation follow, sometimes spreading to the face and neck.

Secondary infection is usual and may mask the true nature of the condition. The condition is recurrent. Between attacks the skin becomes stiff and shiny, especially in the concha.

Scaling and fissuring occur at the canal entrance in the chronic state.

Stenosis results from thickening and fibrosis, and may be permanent.

Treatment

It is essential to recognize, and if possible to remove, the allergic cause of the condition and to appreciate the emotional element in the psychosomatic variety.

Acute stage

Hydrocortisone acetate ointment may lead to dramatic improvement and may prove to be the treatment of choice in both acute and chronic cases. More potent steroids such as beclomethasone or fluocinolone may be required to reduce the inflammation in stubborn cases.

Antihistamine drugs should be given systemically, to allay the irritation.

Drops or wicks. Astringent or coagulative lotions, such as aluminium acetate 8%, are of particular use in healing weeping skin that is not oedematous.

Chronic stage

Silver nitrate. 10% solution is applied to fissures.

Coal-tar ointment. Used for scaling.

Dilatation. By indwelling polythene tubes of increasing sizes, when the canal is stenosed. Restenosis is common and secondary infection is a frequent complication due to the presence of a foreign body.

Plastic operation. Sometimes necessary when stenosis is severe. Over correction with stenting is required as restenosis is common.

5. Seborrhoeic otitis externa

Definition

A greasy, scaling and crusting condition of the skin of the external ear.

Aetiology

Not fully understood. Probably due to abnormal quality and/or quantity of the sebum and wax. *Staphylococcus aureus, Microbacillus cutis communis* and *Pityrosporum* (Mallasey) are thought to be causative agents but have not been proved. The aural condition is best regarded as part of that affecting the scalp.

Clinical features

Greasy yellow scales line the canal. The postauricular sulcus and lobule are commonly affected, the scalp always.

Itching is usually present. Secondary infection results from scratching.

Treatment

Shampoo. The scalp must be treated. Selenium sulphide and ketoconazole containing shampoos are effective.

Ointment. Salicylic acid and sulphur 2% in aqueous cream BP is very effective.

Aural toilet.

6. Granular myringitis

Granulations are seen on the superficial aspect of the tympanic membrane:

1. As a localized form of otitis externa.
2. As a result of contact with a plug of hard wax, a grommet, or other foreign body.
3. In association with influenza.

Aluminium acetate 8% due to its astringent action often brings the condition under control. Florid granulations may hide a perforation and coincidental otitis media. If granulations are slow to heal after removal of the cause, they may be cauterized with silver nitrate on a very fine probe. Many cases, however, prove intractable.

7. Myringitis bullosa haemorrhagica

Aetiology

Unknown. The condition is usually seen as a complication of influenza.

Clinical features

Haemorrhagic blebs form on the tympanic membrane and adjoining deep canal. They rupture quickly.

Pain is a prominent symptom.

Deafness is conductive in type. It may be caused by:

1. Obstruction by bulla formation.
2. Accompanying otitis media.

Symptoms due to a non-suppurative encephalitis may occur.

Treatment

1. Relieve pain.
2. Prevent secondary infection.
3. Treat otitis media, if present.

8. Herpetic lesions of external ear

Aetiology

Probably caused by neurotropic viruses. Sometimes associated with changes in the nervous system, such as cranial nerve paralysis and encephalitis.

Varieties

There are two varieties:

Herpes simplex

May occur about the external ear as elsewhere. Severe cases may require treatment with acyclovir.

Herpes zoster oticus

Pain is usually severe and may be persistent (postherpetic neuralgia). It may be present for several days before the rash.

Vesication occurs but disappears early and may therefore not be seen. Later the epithelium of the collapsed vesicles may present as white plaques on the surface of the tympanic membrane. The vesicles appear on the tympanic membrane, or on the skin of the meatus and auricle, particularly in the conchal region.

Cranial nerve lesions sometimes accompany the other symptoms:

1. Deafness, sensorineural in type.
2. Vertigo.
3. Facial nerve (and occasionally other) palsies.

The Ramsay Hunt syndrome can include all the above features.

Treatment

Oral and topical acyclovir, with analgesics in the early stages. Cranial nerve palsies due to herpes zoster have such a poor prognosis that if one is seen in the first 3 days hospital admission for intravenous acyclovir is recommended.

9. Otitis externa malignans

Definition

A pseudomonas infection, not infrequently fatal, occurring in elderly diabetic patients and in the immunosuppressed.

Pathology

The original infection in the meatus may spread, usually at the junction of its bony and cartilaginous portions, to adjacent bone, causing osteitis and/or osteomyelitis.

Involvement of the stylomastoid foramen may affect the VIIth cranial nerve, and spread to the region of the jugular foramen may involve any or all of the last four cranial nerves. Extension to the petrous apex may affect the Vth and VIth cranial nerves.

A fatal outcome may result from spread of infection to the sigmoid venous sinus and meninges.

Clinical features

1. *Pain in the ear.* May be severe and resistant to analgesics.
2. *Discharge.* May be seropurulent.
3. *Granulations.* May be seen in the meatus, especially on its floor.
4. *Cranial nerve paralyses.* May affect the VIIth, IXth, Xth, XIth and XIIth cranial nerves.

Rarely a Gradenigo's syndrome may result, from involvement of the Vth and VIth cranial nerves.

Treatment

Must be combined, both medical and surgical.

1. Medical

- *Control the diabetes.*
- *Cefotaxime 2g 6-hourly.*
- *Gentamicin or netilmicin*, according to sensitivities of organism. Pre- and post-dose serum levels are measured to prevent ototoxicity with aminoglycosides, in consultation with a bacteriologist. (Renal function is impaired in diabetics.)
- *Topical application of gentamicin.* To meatus or mastoid cavity.

2. Surgical

May range from:

- Removal of granulations, to
- *Radical mastoidectomy.*

Treatment may have to be continued for weeks or months.

Prognosis

This condition may be fatal. Early treatment is essential to survival. Outlook is much worse when cranial nerves are involved.

Perichondritis of the pinna

An infection of the auricular cartilage, which may lead to necrosis. Shrinkage and deformity result. It may follow:

1. Haematoma auris, frostbite.
2. Operations involving the auricular cartilage, especially operations for chronic otitis media (*Ps. aeruginosa*).
3. Furuncle of external auditory canal and other forms of otitis externa.

Treatment

Consists of:

1. Systemic antibiotics.
2. Incisions for drainage.
3. Removal of necrotic cartilage.
4. Subsequent plastic surgery may be needed.

NEOPLASMS OF THE EXTERNAL EAR

Benign

Pathology

Papillomas, angiomas, fibromas, adenomas (including ceruminomas) and keloids all occur but are rare. The commonest benign tumours are the exostoses of the bony canal.

Ceruminoma

Clinical features

Firm masses. Appear under the skin of the outer meatus. They may become malignant.

Treatment

Wide excision. Essential.

Exostosis

Definition

A new bone formation projecting into the lumen of the bony canal.

Clinical types

Sessile. Type most frequently seen. Usually bilateral and formed of ivory bone. Can be single or double, but is usually in a trefoil arrangement. It is debatable whether this is a true osteoma or a hyperostosis.

Single pedunculated. Rare and usually unilateral. Formed of cancellous bone. Regarded as a true osteoma.

Diffuse. There is a generalized circumferential thickening of the tympanic plate. Probably a hyperostosis.

Aetiology

The role of wetting and temperature changes is uncertain, but the condition appears to be more common in swimmers.

Clinical features

The sessile variety may appear around puberty and grow slowly to form a trefoil arrangement. In the course of years, they may fuse to hide the tympanic membrane. Collection of debris may cause:

1. *Irritation.*
2. *Deafness,* when it collects between the exostoses and the tympanic membrane.

Treatment

Aural toilet. The canal must be kept free of collected debris as often as necessary.

   Removal. Only when the degree of stenosis is so great that deafness can no longer be relieved by toilet. Removal is best effected by an electric burr. It is always difficult and the tympanic membrane is easily damaged. If approached from the mastoid and removed with a chisel, the facial nerve is easily damaged. The pedunculated form is readily severed at its attachment.

   Mastoidectomy. Necessary when chronic suppuration of the middle ear cleft is complicated by obstructing exostoses.

Malignant

Pathology

Adenocarcinoma, rodent ulcer, squamous-cell carcinoma.

Adenocarcinoma

Pathology

May be primary, or due to malignant change in adenomas (including ceruminomas).

Treatment

By *radical surgery* followed by postoperative *irradiation.*

Rodent ulcer (basal-cell carcinoma)

Clinical features

Occurs more commonly on the auricle than in the external canal. Found particularly in countries where there is strong sunlight. Tends to become a squamous-cell carcinoma.

Treatment

1. *Local excision.*
2. *Irradiation.*

Squamous-cell carcinoma

Clinical features

Usually presents as:

1. *Bleeding polypus.*
2. Ulcerated area, in the meatus or on the auricle.
3. *Serosanguineous discharge,* in which malignant cells may sometimes be detected, is usually present.
4. Some cases are associated with xeroderma pigmentosa.

The middle ear may be secondarily invaded, or it may be the primary site. All aural polypi must be examined histologically.

Treatment

1. *Irradiation.* Failure requires excision.
2. *Wide excision* of the auricle, canal and bone, sometimes the whole petrous bone, sacrificing the facial nerve. Grafting the cavity allows subsequent inspection. Large defects are obliterated with a scalp pedicle flap or free flap.

Prognosis

Poor due to spread to inaccessible lymph nodes or cranium.

MISCELLANEOUS CONDITIONS OF THE EXTERNAL EAR

Wax

Wax (cerumen) is a mixture of the secretions of the ceruminous glands, pilosebaceous glands and sheets of desquamated keratin. These are situated in the cartilaginous portion of the canal. The consistency of wax is determined by the proportions in the mixture. Normally it is expelled from the canal in flakes, aided by movements of the jaw. Plug formation is encouraged by excessive formation of wax and its retention by stiff hairs, desquamation, exostoses and other stenosing conditions.

Clinical features

Deafness is caused only when occlusion of the canal is complete.
   Tinnitus, 'reflex cough', earache and vertigo may all occur. Symptoms are sudden and severe when a plug is impacted against the tympanic membrane, as in washing, swimming or attempts at removal.

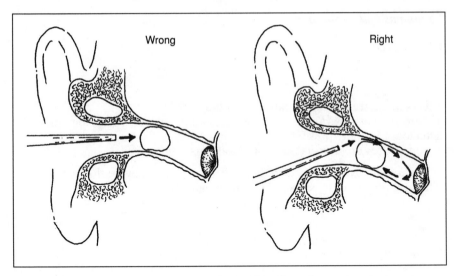

Figure 4.1 Technique for syringing. The nozzle should be directed upwards or backwards

Treatment

Syringing with water at body temperature will usually remove wax easily. (Figure 4.1).

Removal with ring probe, hook and forceps is often better with old, dry, hard plugs.

Softening of such plugs can be effected by repeated instillation of a saturated solution of sodium bicarbonate or dilute hydrogen peroxide.

Suction through the operating microscope if necessary under general anaesthesia, is the safest way to remove wax when a perforation is present or suspected, or if syringing causes pain.

Keratosis obturans

Clinical features

A plug of desquamated epithelium fills the deep canal. This becomes expanded though the tympanic membrane remains intact. It resembles a cholesteatoma of the middle ear. It may be bilateral. Sometimes it is associated with chronic sinusitis and bronchiectasis. It may follow radiotherapy to the ear.

Deafness. Usual.

Pain. Common.

Treatment

Removal and *regular* inspection are required as recurrence is to be expected. This may sometimes be prevented by the regular use of *keratolytic substances,* such as sodium bicarbonate ear drops or salicylic acid 2% in alcohol.

General anaesthesia may be required.

Tophi

Due to subperichondral deposits of sodium biurate crystals in gout. Controlled by treating the underlying condition.

Chondrodermatitis nodularis chronicis helicis

These are small painfull nodules on the superior free margin of the pinna thought to be due to local vasoconstriction as a result of cold.

Sebaceous cysts

These usually occur on the back of the auricle and in the lobule. They should be dissected out completely if causing symptoms.

Acquired atresia and stenosis of external auditory meatus

Aetiology

Acquired atresia and stenosis may result from:

1. *Chronic otitis externa.* Usually of the eczematous type, in which an excess of fibrous tissue causes thickening of the auricle and stenosis of the canal.
2. *Operation.* Especially where suppuration continues after a radical mastoidectomy.
3. *Perichondritis.*
4. *Exostoses.*
5. *Injury.* Especially after corrosive burns, or fractures of the tympanic plate.
6. *Idiopathic.* A dense fibrosis can form in the deep meatus with only minimal stenosis. A false tympanic membrane can form or the true membrane can be markedly thickened (up to 1 cm or more). There may be coincidental fibrosis of the tympanum. There is rarely any significant discharge. The condition is usually refractory to treatment.

Treatment

Indwelling polythene tubes will sometimes overcome minor degrees of stenosis due to fibrosis. They are introduced in increasing sizes, and retained as long as possible.

Surgical treatment is only indicated if the condition results in deafness, especially when it is bilateral or when toilet and inspection of a radical mastoidectomy cavity are rendered impossible.

Meatoplasty is usually performed through a postaural incision. Webs, scar tissue and thickened meatal skin are excised, and the bony meatus enlarged if necessary. The enlarged meatus is then packed and allowed to epithelize spontaneously, or with the help of grafts pedicled from the meatus, or by split-skin grafts.

Chapter 5

Diseases of the middle ear cleft

CONGENITAL MALFORMATIONS

Various degrees of developmental failure of the tympanic cavity and ossicles can occur, causing deafness. They may be unilateral or bilateral.

Severe abnormality of gill-cleft structures is usually associated with deformities of the external ear but the relationship is haphazard.

The inner ear, being of different origin, may not always be involved. (*See also* pp. 136 and 137.)

The great variations in degree of mastoid pneumatization are not classed as malformations.

Aetiology

These deformities may be either genetic or teratogenic but the origin cannot be identified in every case. Teratogenic factors include viruses or toxic chemicals operating in the early months of pregnancy; the best known is thalidomide. When exposure to the teratogenic factor occurs after the third month the pinna and middle ear may reach normality and there may be only a fibrous atresia of the external auditory meatus.

Pathology

1. Abnormal osicles

The ossicles are deformed, most commonly the incus and malleus, the long process of the former and handle of the latter not being present. The ossicles may be fused together, and sometimes to the bony wall of the tympanic cavity. The handle of malleus, long process of incus and head of stapes may be united by a long bar, or the stapes head may be fixed to the promontory by a strut.

The stapes may be absent or deformed and the undeveloped ossicle may abut against an unopened oval window, or the footplate may fuse into the window.

2. Crouzon's syndrome (craniofacial dysostosis)

Conductive deafness is due to external canal atresia and middle-ear abnormalities.

3. Wildervanck syndrome

In which a conductive deafness due to fusion or other malformation of the ossicular chain is associated with pre-auricular sinuses (marginal pits), pre-auricular appendages and malformations of the auricle.

4. Treacher Collins syndrome

An hereditary malformation of the lower face in which the malar bones, maxillae and mandible are hypoplastic, together with varying degrees of developmental failure of the external and middle ears. It may be unilateral or bilateral.

5. Klippel–Feil syndrome

In which malformation of the cervical vertebrae, resulting in a short webbed neck, is associated with congenital anomalies of the ear. The hearing loss is sensorineural or mixed.

6. Marfan's syndrome

The soft auricles collapse and obstruct the auditory canals.

7. Other anatomical abnormalities

Not causing deafness, may be encountered during operations on the middle ear, and include:
● *Dehiscence in floor of tympanic cavity.* Exposing jugular bulb.
● *Dehiscence of the facial nerve canal (6%).* Facial nerve crowding the oval window or situated on the promontory, or bifid with a division passing on to the promontory. The second bend of the facial nerve may be acutely angled posteriorly. Bifurcation of the vertical part of the facial nerve is rare.
● *Persistent stapedial artery.* Sometimes sizeable, passing between the crura.

Clinical features

Conductive deafness, unless inner ear is also involved. The deafness dates from memory of early childhood and may be unilateral or bilateral.

External ear deformities may or may not be present.

Sometimes other non-otological congenital defects are present and a family history of such may be obtained.

Diagnosis

Easy when an external ear abnormality accompanies the deafness.

A conductive deafness, unilateral or bilateral since early childhood, even in the absence of abnormalities on clinical otoscopy, should lead to suspicion of a congenital malformation and calls for exploratory tympanotomy. X-ray examination, tomography or high-definition CT scan will show an ossicular mass and the outline of the labyrinth, but rarely shows the exact pathological state.

Treatment

The surgical objectives are to provide:

1. A functioning ossicular mechanism.
2. A tympanic membrane.
3. A wide meatus.

The new tympanic membrane and meatal lining are made from a bag-shaped split-skin graft which makes contact with a mobile ossicular mechanism.

When ossicular deformity is present tympanoplastic procedures with or without prosthetic devices are adapted as necessary.

Stapedectomy or labyrinthine fenestration is usually reserved as a separate operation as also is plastic reconstruction of the pinna.

In bilateral cases surgery is desirable as early as 2 years of age so that speech can be learnt. The alternative is the use of bone-conduction hearing aids, bone anchored aids stay in place better than traditional 'Alice band'. Air conduction aid is satisfactory if a meatus can be constructed but discharge is a problem.

In unilateral cases operation is rarely indicated. If hearing impairment exists in the so-called 'good' ear a hearing aid should be fitted to it at once.

INJURIES

Foreign bodies

Foreign bodies may cause:

1. Rupture of tympanic membrane.
2. Indentation of tympanic membrane with injury to underlying ossicular chain.

Matchsticks, hairpins and syringe nozzles are frequently concerned as are attempts to remove such smooth, round objects as a bead or ball bearing.

Traumatic rupture of tympanic membrane

Aetiology

1. Perforation

By foreign body or unskilled instrumentation or syringing.

2. Sudden air compression

As in boxing, hand-slap, blast or rapid descent in non-pressurized aircraft.

3. Sudden fluid compression

By a blow, on the ear when the canal is filled with water, as in water polo or underwater swimming.

4. Inflation of eustachian tube

If this is overforceful or if the membrane is frail.

5. Fractured base of skull

When the fracture line involves the attachment of the membrane.

6. Lightening strike

The electric shock causes rapid heating of intracorporal gas. The air in the middle ear can expand and rupture the tympanic membrane.

Clinical features

Pain. May be severe at the time of rupture, but is often slight.
Deafness. Usually minimal with a small, simple perforation but more marked with a larger one.
Tinnitus and vertigo. Usually transient.
Perforation. Has a red margin, usually irregular.
Blood. Usually present in the meatus.

Treatment

Foreign material should be removed. Welding slag can often be removed with an electromagnet.

Prevent infection with antibiotics. Leave blood clot in situ for 10 days or more.

Never syringe.

Myringoplasty. Must be considered if the perforation has failed to heal after 3 months. Fascia or vein grafts may be used. Immediate repair is sometimes justifiable if the pars tensa is seen to be 'rolled up on itself'. Unrolling and supporting it in a position of function may close a large perforation in days instead of months.

Fracture of temporal bone

Types

1. Longitudinal fracture (common type – 80%)

Fracture line is in long axis of petrous bone and involves the tympanic cavity, tympanic membrane and bony external auditory canal.

Clinical features
Deafness is conductive in type and usually recovers.

Bleeding from a lacerated meatal skin or through a ruptured tympanic membrane. If the fracture does not reach and tear the tympanic membrane the blood is retained in the tympanic cavity (haemotympanum) and shows as a black or blue drumhead.

Traumatic bony deformity of the deep meatus may be apparent on otoscopy.

Facial paralysis may occur. Usually the nerve is damaged in the region of the geniculate ganglion.

Cerebrospinal otorrhoea. Rare and usually of short duration.

2. Transverse fracture (Less common type)

Fracture line runs at right angles to the long axis of the petrous bone involving the labyrinth or internal auditory meatus.
Clinical features
Deafness. Sensorineural in type and usually permanent.

Vertigo and nystagmus usually present for a variable period until the loss of homolateral vestibular function is compensated.

Haemotympanum may be seen when the fracture line involves the inner tympanic wall.

Facial paralysis not uncommon. Usually recovers spontaneously, when the paralysis is incomplete and delayed in onset, due to mild compression. Severe and immediate paralysis indicates gross neural damage with poor prospects of spontaneous recovery. The labyrinthine portion is the commonest site of injury (80%).

3. Fracture of bony meatus

Results from indirect injury as from a blow on the chin. The anterior meatal wall is often displaced posterosuperiorly and the tympanic membrane torn. Closing the mouth may produce pain in the ear.

Diagnosis

Bleeding from the ear following a head injury indicates the presence of a fracture until proven otherwise. Plain radiography is often insufficient to demonstrate the fractures adequately even with a range of views. Polytomography in two planes will often show fractures that are not easily visible on plain films.

The minimal nerve excitability test and electromyography can be useful in confirming the continuity of the facial nerve in cases of facial paralysis.

Treatment

In the first instance the treatment is that of the head injury. The treatment of a ruptured tympanic membrane (*see* pp. 44, 101) is at first strict non-interference. Fracture of the bony meatus may need reduction or excision of the displaced fragment at a later date.

Failure of a conductive deafness to recover after temporal bone fracture should suggest possible disconnection. In cases of immediate and total facial paralysis surgical exploration of the nerve must be considered. Prophylactic antibiotics are obligatory. When the fracture involves an ear which is the site of active chronic suppurative otitis media systemic antibiotics must be given and a mastoidectomy may be advisable to prevent infection passing through the fracture line.

Rarely as a delayed complication a cholesteatoma can develop due to inclusion of epithelium into a fracture.

Traumatic disconnection of the ossicular chain

Aetiology

Disconnection may be caused by head injury, direct or indirect, with or without fracture of the temporal bone; surgical procedures in the tympanic cavity or mastoid antrum; foreign bodies indenting or perforating the tympanic membrane; or lightning.

Pathology

Separation of the incudostapedial joint is the commonest lesion, and derangement of the malleo-incudal joint is seen rarely. The displaced ossicles may become fixed to the bony walls of the tympanic cavity. Fracture of both stapedial crura may occur in head injuries.

In old-standing cases the lenticular process of the incus is often atrophied. Dislocation of the footplate from the oval window leads to progressive sensorineural hearing loss unless treated immediately.

Diagnosis

Ossicular disconnection is suspected when a *conductive deafness* persists in the presence of a normal or healed drumhead after a head injury or the other causes mentioned.

Typically the *audiograph* indicates normal bone conduction but an air/bone gap of up to 60 dB. Tympanometry shows a high compliance and absent stapedial reflex.

Tomography may demonstrate the lesion, but confirmation is by exploratory *tympanotomy*.

Treatment

1. Repositioning of the long process of the incus to the stapedial head.
2. Interpositioning of a homograft ossicle between the long process of incus and the stapedial head or footplate.
3. The usual stapedial operations are necessary should the footplate be fixed but incus mobile.

Barotraumatic otitis media

Synonyms

Aero-otitis, otitic barotrauma.

Definition

A non-infective inflammatory reaction produced in the lining of the middle ear cleft when the air pressure within it is considerably below that of the surrounding atmosphere, i.e. a relatively negative intratympanic pressure. The condition is caused by rapid rise in extracorporal pressure such that the body is unable to adapt.

Aetiology

The eustachian tube is normally opened by muscular action. This allows the air pressure within the middle ear cleft to be raised to that of the surrounding atmosphere. When the tube cannot be so opened, it is said to be 'locked'. 'Locking' occurs when there is a difference of 80 mmHg (critical pressure difference) which cannot be overcome by muscular action. If the tubal lining is oedematous or contains excessive lymphoid tissue, 'locking' occurs at a smaller difference of pressure.

The physical conditions required to produce 'locking' occur during rapid descent in non-pressurized aircraft, in a diver's rapid descent, or in pressurization in a chamber. A perforation of, or grommet in, the tympanic membrane prevents 'locking'.

Pathology

The tympanic membrane retracts inwards with the relative decrease of pressure in the cleft.

Vascular engorgement occurs throughout the cleft lining.

Oedema, ecchymosis and transudation of serum, which may be sanguineous in severe cases, follow. With sudden and intense pressure changes, the tympanic membrane may split.

Secondary infection is uncommon.

Clinical features

Increasing discomfort and pain usually disappear in a few hours.

Deafness. May remain for several days or even longer. There may be autophony and a sense of fluid in the ear. In rare cases a permanent sensorineural deafness (barotraumatic otitis interna) is associated.

Tinnitus. Commonly.

Vertigo. Sometimes.

Otoscopy. Five grades of severity are described:

1. Reddening over the malleus handle.
2. Redness of the whole tympanic membrane.
3. Bubbles and yellowish middle ear fluid seen through the membrane.

4. Haemotympanum with dark tympanic membrane.
5. Perforation.

Treatment

'Unlocking'. When possible, a return to the height (i.e. pressure) at which the tube 'locked' will often allow it to be opened. If available a decompression chamber would be ideal.

Subsequent descent should be slow and auto-inflation should be performed frequently. If the tube has been 'locked' for more than an hour, this treatment is unlikely to be effective.

Eustachian catheterization will usually cure if fluid is absent.

Myringotomy is justified if fluid is present. It can be evacuated by suction with Siegle's speculum. This is followed by gentle and repeated inflation of the tube.

Systemic antibiotic is necessary if secondary infection threatens.

Prevention

Avoidance of flying with an upper respiratory infection. Particularly in non-pressurized aircraft.

Avoidance of sleep during descent. The Eustachian tubes are not opened by swallowing during sleep.

Application of a vasoconstrictor before descent. By nasal spray or inhaler. This facilitates opening of the tube in minor cases of congestion.

Auto-inflation. By the method of Valsalva. This should be performed regularly as the atmospheric pressure rises. Previous instruction may be necessary and divers must be especially trained. In older people dental malocclusion may exist, when auto-inflation may be helped by holding a dental prop between the molar teeth.

Insertion of grommets. May be called for in recurrent cases.

Relative positive intratympanic pressure

Results from interference with the usual passive adjustment of raised intratympanic pressure and lower pressure in nasopharynx by air flow down the Eustachian tube. Occurs when under-water swimmers surface, and, under general anaesthesia, from build-up of nitrous oxide in the middle-ear cleft.

The symptoms are:

Vertigo. Usually short-lived but may be severe and may cause drowning.
Deafness. Sensorineural. May only affect high frequencies but may be total and permanent.
(*See also* Trauma due to decompression, p. 147.)

Delayed barotraumatic otitis media

After using oxygen on long flights, the gaseous contents of the cleft have a high percentage of oxygen. After landing, this oxygen is absorbed. Sleep soon after landing prevents active opening of the tube, so that symptoms (usually mild) are noticed on waking.

OTITIS MEDIA

Acute suppurative otitis media

An acute infection can spread very rapidly over the whole lining of the middle ear cleft, but the symptoms form an ordered progression suggesting successive infection of separate sites. It is best, however, to assume that some degree of infection is present throughout the whole cleft.

The type of inflammatory reaction and its progress (i.e. whether suppurative or non-suppurative) depends not only on the virulence of the infecting organisms and the resistance and age of the patient, but also on drainage and therapy, particularly with antibiotics. In addition, the clinical course is influenced by previous infections and the degree of pneumatization of the mastoid.

Effect of pneumatization

A high degree of pneumatization provides both a large surface area for the production of inflammatory exudates and a large capacity for their retention. Consequently a high degree of pneumatization often results in a severe clinical picture. Conversely, in the acellular type, the symptoms tend to be mild.

Aetiology

The cleft usually becomes infected by:

1. Extension of a nasopharyngitis via submucosal lymphatics.
2. Direct spread via an infected surface exudate, later.

The common precursors, mostly virus infections, are:

1. Rhinitis. Usually the common cold, less often the allergic type, with secondary infection later.
2. Sinusitis.
3. Nasopharyngitis.
4. Pharyngitis and tonsillitis.
5. Influenza and the acute infectious diseases.
6. Nasopharyngeal tumours and ulcerations. Less commonly.
7. Other causes. Infection may enter the tympanum as a result of rupture of the tympanic membrane, or through a wetted grommet or a perforation. Swimming and diving can force water up the Eustachian tube, and nasopharyngitis due to irritation by chlorinated water also occurs.

Operations on the nose and throat may give rise to infection, especially when a postnasal pack has been retained for more than 24 hours. Excessive nose blowing acts similarly.

Bacteriology

A wide range of organisms is found, the commonest being:

1. Haemolytic streptococcus.
2. *Strep. pneumoniae.*
3. *Staphylococcus aureus.*
4. *Haemophilus influenzae.*

Pathology

Tubal occlusion occurs quickly.

Engorgement and *oedema* of the cleft lining.

Exudation follows. As the exudation increases, a collection of fluid forms in the tympanum and may be found in the mastoid cells at an early stage.

It is:

1. *Serous* at first.
2. *Mucopurulent* later.

Bulging of tympanic membrane proceeds to the point of rupture.

Rupture by pressure necrosis. This usually takes place in the lower half, and the fluid contents escape as an otorrhoea.

Hyperaemic decalcification. At around 10 days or later, the infected fluid in the mastoid cells causes the thin bony intercellular septa to disintegrate, with coalescence of the infected cells.

Osteitis later causes erosion of the mastoid cortex.

Subperiosteal abscess follows. While infection is limited to the lining of the cleft it remains an otitis media, but strict adherence to this pathological definition is not customary when describing the clinical condition. For this reason, mastoiditis is here included in the clinical phases of acute otitis media.

Clinical features

Phase I. Acute tubal obstruction (acute Eustachian salpingitis)

Fullness in the ear is felt.

Deafness. Conductive in type and accompanied by autophony.

Retraction of tympanic membrane may be seen in the very early stages, but is transitory.

Phase II: Acute infection of tympanic cavity (acute tympanitis; commonly described as 'acute otitis media')

1. Before perforation
- *Deafness* increases.
- *Bubbling sounds* are heard in the ear.
- *Discomfort* progresses.
- *Earache* of a stabbing or boring character follows.
- *Constitutional disturbances* are present. They include malaise and pyrexia which are more marked in children who often complain of abdominal pain.

- *Tympanic membrane.* Dilatation of blood vessels around the handle of malleus and periphery of the membrane is seen on otoscopy. This increases until the whole membrane is red and lustreless, with gradual loss of landmarks as it thickens and bulges.

2. *After perforation*

- *Otorrhoea.* Follows rupture. It may be serous, bloodstained, mucopurulent, or purulent.
- *Relief of pain.* Immediate. Mastoid tenderness, if present. usually disappears. Only a few hours may pass between invasion of the cleft and rupture of the tympanic membrane. Little pain occurs when a thin scar closing a previous perforation allows early rupture.

Phase III. Retention of pus in mastoid (acute mastoiditis – rarely seen today)

- *Pain* develops in the mastoid region.
- *Tenderness* can be elicited over the mastoid antrum and/or tip. A thick cortex lessens the tenderness.
- *Oedema.* The posterosuperior wall of the deep meatus (which is in close relationship to the antrum) sags from oedema. Later oedema appears over the mastoid in thin and well-pneumatized bones from a periostitis. This is not usually seen before a week or more following onset of infection. These signs indicate that infection has passed beyond the lining of the cleft.
- *Constitutional disturbances.* Increase.

Differential diagnosis

Furuncle or diffuse otitis externa. Radiograph will usually show clouding and loss of the mastoid pattern on the affected side in mastoiditis.

Referred otalgia. The tympanic membrane and hearing are normal.

Herpetic lesions of ear may also cause difficulty especially after rupture of the vesicles.

Postauricular adenitis from an abrasion or infected scalp particularly with head lice, will produce a swelling over the mastoid. but it is not accompanied by deafness or otoscopic changes.

Treatment

Symptomatic treatment includes:

1. *Rest*
2. *Analgesics.*
3. *Sedation.*
4. *Local heat* (hot-water bottle).

Antibiotic therapy is the most important form of treatment and must be used in all stages of the infection. A culture must be made of pus in ear, nose or throat and a wide-spectrum antibiotic should be used until sensitivity tests show that it is necessary to substitute another. Inadequate dosage, insufficient period of administration, and inappropriate antibiotic may explain an incomplete resolution (masking effect). If a child vomits on oral antibiotics the first dose should be by intramuscular injection. When doubt exists, operation is the safest procedure.

Local treatment

1. Before rupture
- *Myringotomy*: required when pain is intense.
- *Ear drops are not usually recommended:* given before rupture, they are of no use for disinfection and may obscure the otoscopic picture. However, drops containing glycerin and benzocaine may have a soothing effect.

2. After rupture
- The discharge rapidly abates in most cases. Antibiotic drops and systemic antibiotics need be used only if spontaneous healing is delayed and purulent discharge persists.
- *Aural toilet:* this can be followed by antibiotic drops, or by the insertion of a wick moistened with an antibiotic solution.
- *Vasoconstrictor nasal drops or spray:* should be applied every 4 hours. They help by reducing congestion around the pharyngeal orifice of the eustachian tube.
- *Audiometry* after 2 or 3 weeks will indicate if the hearing has returned to normal.
- *Operative treatment: conservative: (cortical) mastoidectomy.* If the general condition is good a trial of conservative treatment is justified in uncomplicated mastoiditis.
- *Mastoidectomy* should be performed, however, unless rapid recovery occurs, and promptly if subperiosteal abscess or other complications appear.

Sequelae

The infection may be halted at any stage.

Healing

May be complete, with return of hearing to normal. The perforation may be closed by a scar that is virtually invisible. Sometimes it is closed by a thin veil-like membrane. Dense fibrotic and adhesive changes are not often seen after a single attack of acute suppurative otitis media.

Open perforation

A perforation may remain open, though sometimes adherent to the inner tympanic wall for a portion of its circumference. Open perforations may be *dry* or *moist.* Their position is non-marginal.

Residual deafness

The degree of deafness in the presence of a perforation is variable but anterior small ones are less deafening than larger central ones.

Tympanosclerotic plaques are usually though not always indicative of past suppurative infection. They are compatible with normal hearing.

Special forms of acute infection of middle ear cleft

1. Infection of the pneumatized petrous apex (petrositis)

When present, the cells in the petrous bone can take part in a cleft infection. They usually recover with the treatment applied to the concomitant mastoiditis.

Rarely, the infection in them is not so controlled and they coalesce to form an abscess in the petrous apex. This abscess may connect with the cleft at one of a number of possible sites in the base of the petrous pyramid. This usually shows as a fistulous tract.

Suppuration in the petrous is usually accompanied by a serous meningitis generally in the middle, rarely in the posterior, cranial fossa. Later the intrapetrous abscess perforates the cortex either anteriorly or posteriorly to form an extradural abscess. Septic meningitis follows. Rarely, infection may track along the internal carotid artery to form a parapharyngeal abscess.

Clinical features

Petrositis is always associated with an established mastoiditis, which may or may not have been operated upon.

- *Deep temporal and retro-orbital pain* is always suspicious and is due to irritation of the Vth cranial nerve.
- *Otorrhoea* persists and is accompanied by worsening of the general condition.
- *Paralysis of lateral rectus muscle* is usual but not inevitable. It is due to compression of the VIth cranial nerve between the petroclinoid ligament and the swollen dura over the petrous apex.

The deep pain, paralysis of the VIth cranial nerve and mastoid infection together constitute *Gradenigo's Syndrome*.

Diagnosis

The presence of Gradenigo's triad with radiographic demonstration of a petrous abscess is conclusive.

Treatment

Mastoidectomy may be followed by spontaneous recovery of petrositis, but this cannot be relied upon.

Systemic antibiotics: In high dosage.

Drainage may be established by following any obvious track from the base of the pyramid to the abscess. When no track exists, one should be excavated or drilled, by forward extension through the canal for the tensor tympani muscle.

Other classical approaches, now rarely used, are:

- Through the anterior wall of the carotid canal after retraction of the artery (Ramadier).
- Under the arch of the superior semicircular canal (Frenckner).
- Through the anterior surface of the petrous, via an extradural approach to the middle cranial fossa (Eagleton).

2. Zygomatic mastoiditis

Produces swelling above or in front of the ear. It may simulate mumps.

Treatment
By antibiotics and/or mastoidectomy.

3. Infection in infants

Otitis media is a common cause of pyrexia and meningeal irritation in infants. There may be no obvious symptoms directed to the ear. Possibly the wide, short Eustachian tube predisposes to infection. It is possible that contaminated milk may enter the Eustachian tubes as a result of bottle-feeding in the supine position. Teething, with its associated rhinitis, is also a cause.

Association with gastroenteritis. In weak babies otitis media may be associated with gastroenteritis, diarrhoea being the presenting symptom.

The tympanic membrane may be grey and not obviously bulging yet have pus behind it. When in doubt myringotomy is indicated. If pus is found or if the child is not improving with conservative measures the mastoid antrum must be opened. Infection, may pass through the unclosed petrosquamous suture.

4. Infection in children

Usually follows the adult course, but there may be a *very high temperature* in the earlier stages causing febrile convulsions. Hypertrophy and infection of the adenoids and cleft palate are potent factors in starting or maintaining the infection. Virus infections produce conditions favourable to the growth of pathogenic bacteria. Poor housing and overcrowding are contributory factors and should be rectified.

Treatment
- Antibiotics chosen by reference to local laboratory reports.
- Treatment of recurrent attacks. Removal of adenoids is often indicated and the tonsils must be removed also if they are infected. Treatment of sinusitis is essential. Antibiotics must be relied upon if the attacks continue after removal of all sources of infection in the nose and throat. Fortunately attacks become less frequent as age increases.

5. Infection complicating acute infectious diseases

Measles, scarlet fever and, rarely, diphtheria and typhoid. The haemolytic streptococcus is the organism responsible for the tympanic infection in all of these, but it is accompanied by the specific organism of the disease in some and by a virus in others. A synergic effect may be responsible for the extensive destruction of the tympanic membrane.

Clinical features
The infection in some cases is exceptionally severe and causes massive necrosis of the tympanic membrane. Its almost complete destruction results in a large kidney-shaped perforation (*otitis media necrotica*).

6. Infection complicating influenza

This usually pursues the normal course, but a *haemorrhagic bullous eruption* is seen in some cases on the outer surface of the tympanic membrane and the walls of the adjacent deep external auditory meatus. Haemorrhagic exudate and ecchymosis of the cleft lining are described.

7. Infection by pneumococcus type III

Characterized by its *insidious progress* leading to a quiet necrosis. A sudden and unexpected complication may arise in exactly the same way as from a mastoiditis masked by antibiotics.

Chronic otitis media

Chronic otitis media embraces several clinical entities which differ in aetiology, pathology, and in the part of the middle ear cleft principally involved.

Chronic otitis media may be suppurative or non-suppurative, Specific infections are occasionally responsible, cessation of active disease may be followed by healing which may be accompanied by permanent residual changes conveniently termed extinct otitis media.

Chronic suppurative otitis media (CSOM)

Clinical types

1. Tubotympanic disease

Regarded as safe.
Aetiology
This is the residue of an acute suppurative infection usually acquired in infancy or early childhood and often associated with the acute infectious diseases. Lack of attention and re-infection either from the nasopharynx (in adenoids or cleft palate) or through the perforation allow active infection to persist or to recur.
Pathology
The *perforation* of the tympanic membrane can be of any size or shape – sometimes large and kidney-shaped (subtotal) but situated in the pars tensa sparing the fibrous annulus (Figure 5.1) frequently antero-inferiorly. The *ossicular*

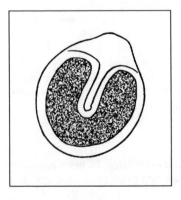

Figure 5.1

chain often remains intact. *The mucosa of the tympanic cavity* is velvety and pink and may be oedematous. Occasionally a polypus, pedunculated and sometimes of considerable size (when it is then partially covered with squamous epithelium), arises from the inner tympanic wall.

Areas of ulceration and cholesterol granulation tissue may occur, although rarely. Areas of the normal pavement cell epithelium may be replaced by columnar secreting (goblet) cells either by metaplasia or by extension of the mucosa from the eustachian tube.

The mastoid is usually cellular but may be acellular. The mucosa of the mastoid cells may show changes similar to those of the tympanic cavity, and the cells may act as a reservoir for secretions.

Clinical features

- *Discharge:* mucoid, often scanty and usually intermittent but becoming purulent and foul smelling during exacerbations and in the presence of secondary invaders, particularly *B. proteus* and *Ps. aeruginosa.* It is more profuse during upper respiratory infections.
- *Deafness:* Conductive in type. The degree varies with the size and position of the perforation, usually relatively slight when it is small and anterior. Sometimes hearing is better when the ear is moist than when dry owing to a favourable shielding of the labyrinthine windows by mucus.

Treatment

- *Topical antibiotics* are given when the discharge is active. Intravenous antipseudomonal antibiotics are occasionally required.
- *Aural toilet* should be performed meticulously under direct vision and daily if necessary. Preferably it should be performed by controlled suction under the operating microscope. *Removal of polypi and excessive granulation tissue* should precede other forms of local treatment, if necessary under general anaesthetic. A firm antiseptic ribbon gauze pack (BIPP) is helpful in some cases.
- *Elimination of adjacent foci of infections* if present in tonsils, adenoids and sinuses.
- *Mastoid operation* is seldom required as the condition is 'safe', and is generally amenable to conservative treatment though this may need to be prolonged. In unilateral cases failure to improve and the presence of a profuse discharge with clouding of mastoid cells on radiography may require cortical mastoidectomy to eradicate a reservoir of infection in the cells.
- *Myringoplasty* may be performed for a persistent dry perforation. Systemic antibiotics may dry up a wet perforation long enough for a graft to heal.
- *Ossiculoplasty* may be performed at the same time, or as a secondary procedure, if conductive hearing loss remains.

2. Attico-antral disease

Associated with cholesteatoma and regarded as dangerous. Granulation tissue may or may not be present. At first the keratin is relatively free of infection, but later intense infection may take place and render the danger of serious complications much greater.

Synonyms. Cholesteatosis; Epidermosis; Keratosis of the middle ear; Non-malignant destructive ear disease.

Relevant definitions
- *Cholesteatoma:* the traditional name given to the epidermoid cyst containing layers of keratin.
- *Cholesterol granuloma:* a non-specific granulation tissue. Cholesterol crystals, foreign-body giant-cells, and blood pigments (haemosiderin) are present in the fibrous matrix.

Theories of the pathogenesis of cholesteatoma
- *Congenital (primary).* Arising from embryonic epithelial tissue. This might explain the excessively rare cholesteatoma found in the petrous bone and that isolated in the mastoid. These 'congenital cholesteatomata' may involve the otic capsule. They cause facial paralysis, severe unilateral sensorineural deafness, and some vestibular dysfunction.

The 'pearly tumour' causes characteristic rounded or lobulated areas of rarefaction with sclerosed edges when seen radiographically. A white 'pearl' or sausage may be seen with the otoscope beyond an intact tympanic membrane.

Diagnosis is confirmed by operation.

- *Acquired (Secondary)*

(a) Blocked Eustachian tube. Usually in infancy or very early childhood, due to adenoids or upper respiratory infection, with subsequent retraction pockets in the attic or posterosuperior marginal area.

(b) Collection of keratin. In pocket, due to disturbance of migration.

(c) Perforation. Of weakened area.

(d) Invasion of attic with keratin. To form a cholesteatomatous 'pearl'.

(e) Gradual expansion of sac. Which may surround the ossicles and invade the aditus, antrum and mastoid process.

Pathology
The encysted and concentrically laminated keratin which forms the cholesteatoma is at first limited to the attic. The capsule or matrix of the cyst is covered by tympanic mucosa at any surface projecting freely within the lumen of the cleft. Exploratory tympanotomy has occasionally shown an attachment from a small cyst to the deep surface of Shrapnell's membrane by a narrow stalk and this point is marked externally by a dimple.

Increase in the amount of accumulated keratin may lead to the following pathological processes:

- *Extrusion of a small attic or antral cholesteatoma* into the external auditory canal. If the evacuation is total then healing of the site of evacuation and natural cure can result.
- *Protrusion of finger-like processes of the cyst* into the tympanic cavity between the ossicles and also between these and the bony tympanic wall.
- *Filling of the tympanic cavity by the sac* with disruption of ossicular chain and dissolution of the individual ossicles, the long process of the incus being the most susceptible.
- *Encroachment into mastoid structure (usually diploic or acellular) as the sac progresses from the antral region:* there is absorption of bone as the sac expands – perhaps from an enzymatic action. A 'natural' radical mastoidectomy cavity may be so excavated.
- *Interference with ventilation:* obstruction by the cholesteatoma together with some pre-existing tubal obstruction encourages a secretory otitis. This

takes the form of a glairy fluid stained with blood pigments, sometimes termed 'black cholesteatosis'.

- *Active infection of the keratotic mass:* formation of granulations and polypi and increased exudation follow active infection of the cholesteatoma.
- *Provision of pathways facilitating the spread of infection and/or transference of pressure:* the absorption of surrounding bone provides direct pathways for infection to the labyrinth and to the meninges and for the transference of pressure from the expanding sac to the facial nerve and perilymphatic system. Active infection becomes increasingly dangerous because of infective necrosis (caries) of thinned bony barriers. The tegmen antri and tympani and sinus plate are the commonest sites from which infection reaches the meninges in this way. Fistularization of the labyrinth via the lateral semicircular canal and exposure of the facial canal in the region of the second genu are the commonest areas for symptoms of compression by cholesteatoma.

Clinical features

Deafness. Conductive in type, may be the only symptom when the cholesteatoma is small. Sometimes the deafness may be very slight, even unnoticed – the 'silent cholesteatoma'. A portion of cholesteatoma may bridge a gap in the ossicular chain allowing conduction to be maintained.

Malodorous otorrhoea. Noticed in varying amounts after secondary infection. Sometimes bloodstained when granulations present. Even bleeding may occur.

Perforation. Situated either in Shrapnell's membrane (Figure 5.2a) or marginally in the posterosuperior quadrant of the pars tensa with destruction of the fibrous annulus (Figure 5.2b). Adherent flakes or crusts on the tympanic membrane and meatal wall may hide small perforations. Later cases show a perforation expanded so as to occupy the greater part of Shrapnell's membrane and posterior half of pars tensa.

Cholesteatoma may be visible through the perforation as a greyish paper-like substance or as the typical pearly sheets of keratin which are easily recognized. Cholesteatomas in the attic are sometimes seen to invaginate downwards behind an intact tympanic membrane.

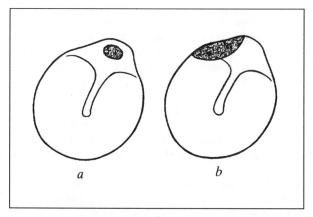

a   b

Figure 5.2

Headache, earache, vertigo and facial paralysis all indicate complications. Advice may not be sought by patients until one of these symptoms is present. Facial paralysis is often mislabelled Bell's palsy and wrongly treated with steroids.

Diagnosis

The onset is insidious. Usually there is no history of acute infection but if obtained it is likely to be associated with the exanthemata in childhood.

The marginal position of the perforation and the presence of offensive discharge and granulations are all suggestive; visible pieces of cholesteatoma are diagnostic.

Suction-clearance under the operating microscope is desirable for proper viewing in doubtful cases. *Radiography* usually but not necessarily shows an acellular mastoid. Bone destruction is only seen with certainty in the more advanced cases. Tomography and CT are informative but not necessary. A negative finding does not exclude cholesteatoma. Granulations should be submitted to histological examination to exclude carcinoma.

Treatment

1. Conservative. Where no complication is suspected and if the cholesteatoma is *small* and *accessible,* a trial of conservative treatment is permissible. This includes:

● Removal of cholesteatoma employing fine crocodile forceps, and suction clearance under magnification.
● Removal of polypi and/or granulation tissue with cup forceps.
● Lifelong periodical inspection is essential.

2. Surgical. Operation is indicated when conservative treatment fails or when complications are present or threatening. Primarily the objective is to remove the disease; secondly to improve or to retain hearing, tubal patency being an essential condition for any reconstructive surgery.

Principles of surgery. Surgery must be excisive. Surgical exposure and clearance of the middle ear cleft should begin where the disease starts, namely, in the attic. The extent of the subsequent surgery is determined by the extent of the disease.

Types of operation

● Atticotomy. When disease is limited to the attic, a limited atticotomy may suffice.
● Antrotomy. If the cholesteatoma is seen to extend backwards into the aditus, the mastoid antrum should be exposed with cutting burrs.
● Intact canal wall mastoidectomy. It may be possible to remove the whole sac without disturbing the bony meatal walls. Recurrence of disease is common, however. A second look in one year is needed before the patient can be discharged.
● Posterior tympanotomy. If doubt exists as to the presence of residual disease, the middle ear may be exposed from the mastoid through a posterior tympanotomy – a triangular opening between the facial nerve posteriorly, the chorda tympani anteriorly, and the short process of the incus (or fossa incudis) superiorly.

Any remains of malleus or incus surrounded or eroded by cholesteatoma must be removed. The stapes should be disturbed as little as possible. Granulations around it settle down when the cholesteatoma is gone.

- Modified radical mastoidectomy. If doubt still remains about the completeness of removal of the sac, the 'facial bridge' should be reduced completely, thus producing a modified radical mastoidectomy.
- Radical mastoidectomy. Involves the removal of any remnant of the tympanic membrane, malleus and incus.
- Tympanoplasty. Plastic reconstruction of the tympanic apparatus consists of reconstruction of the deficient tympanic membrane (*myringoplasty*) plus reconstruction of a sound-conducting ossicular chain (*ossiculoplasty*).

The perforation may be closed by connective tissue (e.g. temporalis fascia) placed either deep to the tympanic membrane (underlay) or between its middle fibrous and outer epithelial layers (overlay). The ossicular reconstruction may be made with the patient's own, cadaver (homograft) or synthetic ossicles.

Preserved homograft tympanic membrane plus ossicle(s) may also be used in these reconstructive procedures especially when the patient's malleus is missing.

Such operations may be staged. Functional results are better when the bony canal wall can be kept intact, but safety must never be sacrificed to technical virtuosity.

Complications of suppurative otitis media

Spread of infection beyond the bony walls of the cleft may occur during acute or chronic otitis media.

Serious intracranial complications are most frequently seen during acute exacerbations of chronic suppurative infections associated with cholesteatoma.

The antibiotics have lessened the incidence and improved the prognosis of these complications.

Mode of spread of infection

1. *Direct spread through bone* may be caused by:
- *Osteitis* which has caused a large area of destruction, sometimes sequestrated. Rarely osteomyelitis.
- *Caries.* A limited osteitis, forming a track in the bone.
- *Erosion,* by cholesteatoma.

2. *Venous spread.* Venous channels convey the septic process by retrograde thrombophlebitis, sometimes to a distance from the focus, e.g. across the subarachnoid space, by small veins which leave the brain substance and connect with the Haversian canals in the bone by way of veins in the dura mater.

3. *Spread via labyrinth.* The labyrinth itself becomes infected first through a fistula or through its windows. The latter provide a pre-formed pathway. Infection extends from the labyrinth through:
- *Internal auditory canal*
- *Aqueduct of vestibule or of cochlea.* Less frequently.

4. *Other routes* include:
- *Fracture lines.* Basal fractures, including old ones with fibrous union, facilitate passage of infection from the cleft.

- *Un-united cranial sutures.* Most often petrosquamous, less often squamo-mastoid or occipitomastoid.
- *Vascular foramina.* Of the mastoid emissary vein or of vessels opening on to the suprameatal triangle.
- *Congenital dehiscences.* May occur in the floor of the tympanic cavity or into the canal of the facial nerve.

Types of complication

Extracranial
1. Subperiosteal abscess
- *Postauricular abscess:* lies over the external surface of mastoid and is the commonest type, especially in children. The auricle is displaced outwards, forwards, and downwards. The postauricular sulcus tends to be retained. Pus has often tracked outwards through minute vascular channels in the suprameatal (Macewen's) triangle.
- *Zygomatic abscess:* pus escaping from zygomatic cells near the squama forms an abscess deep to the temporal muscle and makes a swelling above and in front of the ear. This may be confused with a parotid swelling. Pus escaping from more distal cells in the process forms an abscess superficial to the temporal muscle. Pus tracking outwards under the periosteum of the roof of the bony canal can reach the subtemporal position (Luc's abscess).
- *von Bezold's abscess:* perforation of the tip or inner surface of the mastoid may give rise to an abscess in the sternomastoid muscle (von Bezold's) or in the digastric triangle (Citelli's).
- *Pharyngeal abscess:* pus tracking from peritubal cells may form a parapharyngeal or retropharyngeal abscess.

Note: sites of perforation of the cortex of the temporal bone on its intracranial aspects lead to intracranial complications (*see* p. 119). They are:
- Middle fossa, through the tegmen antri and tympani and through the anterior surface of the petrous.
- Posterior fossa, through the lateral sinus plate and posterior surface of the petrous (Trautmann's triangle).

2. Osteomyelitis of temporal bone
Rare. Infection spreads to the marrow-spaces of a poorly pneumatized mastoid and is then propagated to any part of the temporal or other cranial bones by thrombosis of the medullary venous channels. It may be acute or chronic, leading to necrosis and sequestration. Treatment is by systemic antibiotics and removal of sequestra. Meningitis is the usual termination in unsuccessful cases.

3. Bloodstream infection
Some degree of bloodstream infection probably occurs in all cases of acute suppurative otitis media, but is controlled by natural process or treatment. Clinical septicaemia is therefore uncommon.

In cases of extreme virulence, organisms may enter the venous sinuses by passing through their walls or via small tributaries, without thrombosis occurring. Otogenic infection may cause thrombosis of the larger venous sinuses, from periphlebitis or retrograde spread.

If the clot becomes infected, organisms or infected emboli may enter the bloodstream. *Septicaemia* or *pyaemia* results.

Metastatic abscesses develop in the lungs, joints, bones and elsewhere in pyaemic cases.

Treatment
- Antibiotics.
- Drainage of the infecting focus, if necessary.
- Blood transfusion may be required when toxaemia is severe.

4. Paralysis of facial nerve
Described under Facial paralysis (p. 277).

5. Labyrinthitis
Described under Infections of inner ear (*see* p. 148).

Intracranial
These are all described under Neurological diseases (*see* p. 545). They include:
- *Pachymeningitis.* Inflammation of the dura, with or without extradural or subdural abscess.
- *Leptomeningitis.* Inflammation of the pia-arachnoid, serous or purulent, localized or diffuse.
- *Thrombophlebitis of sigmoid sinus.*
- *Otitic hydrocephalus.*
- *Brain lesions.*
(a) Non-suppurative encephalitis.
(b) Brain abscess, cerebral or cerebellar.

Non-suppurative otitis media

The term 'non-suppurative otitis media' is applied to the clinical conditions characterized by the presence of a non-purulent fluid in the middle ear cleft. Conductive deafness is the principal feature. Acute and chronic forms can sometimes be distinguished according to the mode of onset or by their duration, but the distinction may not be clear and the condition is often recurrent. One in four children in the UK entering school has 'a glue ear'.

Synonyms

There are many but the following have been used most often: 'glue ear'; otitis media with effusion; 'catarrhal' otitis media; serous otitis media; mucinous otitis media; secretory otitis media.

Aetiology

Not completely elucidated. Several factors may be concerned. (Effusion into the middle ear following barotrauma is considered separately under Barotraumatic otitis media, p. 104.) The following are relevant factors:

1. Occlusion of the Eustachian tube

May result from:
- Adenoids and other accumulations of hypertrophied lymphoid tissue in and around the pharyngeal mouth of the tube.

- Tubal infection. This is an extension of bacterial infection from the respiratory tract and represents the pre-suppurative stage of an acute otitis media but not progressing to suppuration, as the result of immunity or treatment.
- Thick mucoid fluid plugging the tubal isthmus.
- Other causes of tubal occlusion:
(a) Stricture or adhesion after adenoidectomy.
(b) Ulceration or neoplasm of the postnasal space involving the orifice of the tube.
(c) Paralysis of palatal muscles from myopathic or neuropathic causes, e.g. myasthenia gravis.
(d) Nasopharyngeal atresia, congenital or acquired.
(e) Postnasal packs.

2. Unresolved acute otitis media

Infection inactivated but not entirely resolved, either from failure of natural immunity or from inadequate antibiotic therapy.

3. Viral infections of the middle ear cleft lining

The adenoviruses and rhinoviruses causing nasopharyngitis and rhinitis are considered likely to be responsible for many cases of non-suppurative otitis media.

Viral haemorrhagic myringitis is often accompanied by a middle ear effusion.

4. Allergy

Allergic changes, including effusion, occur in the middle ear cleft due to seasonal or perennial forms of hypersensitization, e.g. hay fever may be associated with a middle ear effusion.

5. Cleft palate and its repair

If the pterygoid hamulae are fractured, cause poor Eustachian tube function.

Clinical features

Deafness

Conductive in type, is the principal and often the only symptom. One or frequently both ears affected in children. Onset may be sudden or gradual and may be unrecognized for a long period in young children. Adults often refer the onset to a recent head cold or even to one acquired months previously. Changes of position of the head often cause changes in degree of deafness when the fluid is thin. Hearing is usually better in bed when supine but it clouds over when getting up (erect position). There are three types of audiometric curve:

1. Retraction of tympanic membrane causes increased stiffness which leads to a loss in the low frequencies (curve slopes to left).

2. Subsequent effusion adds mass to the tympanic membrane to cause a loss in the high frequencies (curve is now flattened).
3. Equalization of the negative intratympanic pressure occurs as the effusion increases so that there is increased mass but without increased stiffness. There is a high tone loss only (curve slopes to right).

Acoustic impedance measurements show a reduction in compliance and negative middle ear pressure.

Tinnitus

Buzzing and whistling, variable. Usually crackling and bubbling noises and sensation of fluid in the ear, especially on blowing nose and swallowing.

Vertigo and pain

Are typically absent.

Otoscopic appearances

The tympanic membrane is usually dull and retracted, the malleus short process prominent, the handle foreshortened, and more horizontal. When the tympanic cavity is completely filled with fluid the tympanic membrane may not be distorted. Partial filling produces a meniscus which shows as a horizontally disposed crescentic hairline. Bubbles, even to the extent of foam formation, may be seen in the fluid.

The colour of the tympanic membrane depends on that of the effusion behind it and is usually pale yellow, sometimes slate grey or even blue, but may be near normal. On release of suction applied by use of Siegle's speculum there is a characteristic snap back of the tympanic membrane owing to the surface tension of the fluid.

The fluid varies in quantity and viscosity. It may be only a small foamy collection in the tympanic cavity or enough fluid to fill the tympanic cavity and mastoid cells.

It may be clear or opaque, colourless, yellow or dark brown. It varies from a serous to a glue-like consistency. The fluid is generally bacteriologically sterile but may become secondarily infected. Eosinophils swarm in the effusion of allergic cases.

Thin serous fluid usually results from passive transudation due to tubal obstruction, as in barotraumatic otitis media or carcinoma of the nasopharynx; thick 'glue' usually results from active exudation due to infection, as in incompletely resolved acute suppurative otitis media. The fluid in non-suppurative otitis media may be serous, seromucinous, seropurulent, mucoid, mucopurulent or frankly purulent, the character of the fluid being determined by the relative degrees of transudation and exudation.

Diagnosis

The condition is suspected in all children suffering from varieties of the 'tonsils and adenoids syndrome' and in adults when conductive deafness follows influenza or a head cold. Audiometric screening of school children detects many cases.

A meniscus, bubbles, or fluid found on myringotomy confirm it.

Treatment

Eliminate aetiological and predisposing factors as far as possible. *Surgical measures* may be necessary if the effusion persists.

1. Myringotomy and evacuation of fluid, under general anaesthesia. The operating microscope and suction should always be used. Noise trauma is minimized by use of an 18 SWG (0.8 mm i.d.) suction tip. Evacuation can also be effected into the external auditory meatus by suction exerted by Siegle's speculum.

2. Indwelling Teflon tubes or grommets are commonly inserted through the membrane. They are left in position until rejected spontaneously, usually after nine months.

3. Intratympanic injection of urea solution may help to facilitate the evacuation of excessively thick 'glue'.

4. Cortical mastoidectomy may be indicated very rarely. Recurrences occur in about 20% of cases.

Extinct or healed otitis media

The term denotes the various permanent structural changes found in the middle ear cleft after the inactivation and subsequent healing of either suppurative or non-suppurative forms of otitis media. The resultant deformities, which may occur singly or in combination, include:

1. Perforations of the tympanic membrane

Vary in size, shape and position. Perforations of the pars tensa eroding the fibrous tympanic annulus are *termed marginal* and those sparing the annulus are *termed central.* Perforations of the pars flaccida are marginal as the annulus is deficient superiorly.

The edges may be free or may be attached to the inner wall of the tympanic cavity over varying amounts of the circumference of the perforation. Open perforations can become *closed* by a thin membrane. Such a closed perforation has no middle layer of fibrous tissue and is often seen as a saucerized depression. This can sometimes be distended on inflation. The degree of deafness depends upon the size and position of the perforation, posterior ones causing more deafness than anterior ones. Closed perforations often have little deafness associated with them. Surgical closure of an open perforation by myringoplasty is usually possible.

2. Thinning of areas of the tympanic membrane

Especially in the posterosuperior quadrant, appears to occur without prior perforation, probably from degeneration of the fibrous layer. The weakened area tends to become invaginated. When the invagination is sharp the appearance resembles a perforation. The true state is shown by the eversion of the sac on inflation or by suction with Siegle's speculum if the sac is not adherent to the inner tympanic wall. Hearing may be temporarily improved when the sac is everted. Excision and grafting a retraction pocket fails if the Eustachian tube is blocked.

3. Tympanosclerosis

A white snow-like layered thickening produced by calcification of the fibrous tissue of the lining of the middle ear cleft which has undergone hyaline degeneration, initiated by infection. The familiar calcareous plaque of chalk patch in the tympanic membrane is the result of this process. Surgical removal of tympanosclerosis from the region of the oval window is not infrequently followed by a sensorineural hearing loss.

4. Chronic adhesive otitis media

Synonyms include: chronic adhesive process (CAP); intratympanic adhesions; fibrotic otitis media.

The formation of adhesions in the middle ear is often bilateral and may follow either suppurative otitis media or non-suppurative otitis media, especially if the latter is of long standing. However, fluid is known to have existed in the tympanic cavity for years without the formation of adhesions.

The tympanic membrane which may show areas of both atrophy and of thickening, often with chalk patches, is frequently adherent to the inner wall of tympanum.

Treatment

Inflation is unavailing, and attempts to sever adhesions are usually unsuccessful. However, the recurrence of adhesions after division may sometimes be prevented by the use of Silastic or other plastic sheeting. A hearing aid is the most certain way of improving the patient's hearing.

5. Loss of portions of the ossicular chain

The long process of the incus is the part most susceptible to atrophy but the stapedial crura and handle of malleus may also be absorbed. The incus has not uncommonly been completely extruded. The bodies of the malleus and incus are sometimes stuck to the roof of the middle ear (attic fixation).

Treatment

Treatment by surgery employs a variety of ossiculoplastic techniques, e.g. the interposition of an incus between the malleus and stapedial head or foot plate.

Tuberculous otitis media

Aetiology

This increasingly rare disease is secondary to severe pulmonary tuberculosis, usually in children and young adults. It is generally carried up the Eustachian tube from the nasopharynx but rarely may be blood-borne. A bovine type in the very young has been almost eliminated by milk sterilization and testing cows.

Pathology

Tubercle formation and caseation occur in the submucosa of the middle ear cleft.

Multiple perforations develop quietly and usually without pain. These tend to coalesce later.

Quiet caries of the mastoid and ossicles. Not infrequently, this leads to an unexpected *facial nerve paralysis* and to a *cold subperiosteal abscess.* A mild chronic type of *labyrinthitis* may be a further complication. *Secondary pyogenic infection* usually supervenes.

Symptoms

Conductive deafness and otorrhoea are characteristically so insidious that serious complications may first call attention to the condition.

Diagnosis

A painless conductive deafness and otorrhoea in a tuberculous patient should arouse suspicion. The tympanic membrane may appear thick and sodden at first, but later shows multiple perforations and possibly flabby granulations. Detection of tubercle bacilli in the discharge is conclusive. Sensorineural deafness and vestibular symptoms which may result from the toxic effects of aminoglycoside antibiotics must be distinguished from symptoms arising from a middle ear infection in the patient with pulmonary tuberculosis.

Treatment

Treatment is that of the pulmonary condition by systemic antituberculous chemotherapy supported by:

Aural toilet when otorrhoea is present.

Mastoidectomy is necessary when sequestration or other complications are present.

Syphilitic otitis media

Pathology

The usual aural manifestation of syphilis is a meningoneurolabyrinthitis, but occasionally the middle ear cleft is involved by a *gummatous osteoperiostitis.* The combination of middle and inner ear infection is known as an *otolabyrinthitis.* It is a rare condition today. Otolabyrinthitis is usually bilateral and can occur in both early and late forms of *congenital syphilis,* more commonly the latter. In these cases the osteoperiostitis may precede changes in the vestibule but these organs are always 'dead' before an otorrhoea is evident. Otolabyrinthitis is also found in the *tertiary stage* of acquired syphilis. The gummatous change leads to a foul discharge and extensive destruction of the mastoid. A part of the labyrinth is sometimes sequestrated. Secondary pyogenic infection supervenes.

Diagnosis

Foul, painless otorrhoea, in the presence of sensorineural deafness, is suspicious.

Congenital stigmata or positive serological tests are confirmatory.

Treatment

1. *Antisyphilitic treatment* is required.
2. *Operation* may occasionally be needed for the removal of sequestra, whose presence may be demonstrated by radiography.

NEOPLASMS OF THE MIDDLE EAR CLEFT

General considerations

All are relatively uncommon. Squamous-cell carcinoma is the most frequent primary neoplasm and glomus tumour (chemodectoma) the next. The following are extremely rare:

Malignant: adenocarcinoma; sarcoma; melanoma.
Benign: osteoma; neurinoma of VIIIth and VIIth cranial nerves; intratympanic meningioma.

Secondary neoplasms occur by invasion from neighbouring sites and by metastatic deposits from distant primaries. Included in the latter group is multiple myelomatosis.

Middle ear neoplasms may be simulated by histiocytosis-X, malignant granuloma and intratemporal epidermoids.

Glomus tumour *(chemodectoma)*

Definition

A very slowly growing tumour arising from non-chromaffin paraganglionic (chemoreceptor) tissue situated in, or in close relationship to, the middle ear. Metastases are rare (4%).

Pathology

The tumour may originate in:

1. The tympanic cavity, from the paraganglion tympanicum on the tympanic branch of the IXth cranial nerve on the promontory.

2. The glomus bodies in the adventitia of the dome of the jugular bulb.
3. The paraganglion juxtavagale related to the ganglion nodosum of the Xth cranial nerve.

It resembles the carotid body tumour. The glomus cells are large polyhedral cells which appear in cords, columns, or clusters and are surrounded by a reticulovascular network in which are non-myelinated nerves. The vessels vary in size from capillaries to cavernous spaces. Rarely vasoactive substances may be produced.

Fibrosis occurs in varying degrees. The jugular bulb tumours invade the middle ear through its floor. Slow spread from the initial site takes place into the mastoid and petrous bones.

The tumours are usually seen after the age of 40 and more commonly in females. Sometimes there is coincidental occurrence of carotid body tumours on one or even both sides.

Clinical features

Tympanic tumours give aural symptoms at first. Jugular bulb tumours may present the syndrome of IXth, Xth, XIth, and/or perhaps XIIth cranial nerve paralysis before tympanic symptoms.

Deafness is the earliest symptom in tympanic tumours. It is conductive at first from invasion of tympanum, later sensorineural from involvement of the labyrinth.

Tinnitus also early in tympanic tumours, 'swishing' in type and synchronous with the pulse.

Vertigo. Dizziness is not uncommon but is not severe.

Pain sometimes present but not severe.

The above symptoms may be present for some time before there is anything definite to be seen on otoscopy in the jugular bulb tumour.

Red flush with or without bulging of the tympanic membrane is the first sign of the tympanic tumour. Compression with Siegle's speculum causes the intratympanic tumour to blanch.

Polypus. A red fleshy polypus is seen in the external auditory canal after the tumour has perforated the membrane. It bleeds readily and profusely on touch.

Cranial nerve palsies may be multiple. May range from VIth to XIIth (VIIth and VIIIth relatively early in tympanic tumours while the lower bulbar ones are earlier in the jugular bulb cases) and are expected in all cases in which deafness has exceeded 10 years.

Audible bruit can sometimes be heard over entire skull with a stethoscope in advanced cases.

Pulsating tumour over mastoid or in nasopharynx in very advanced cases.

Diagnosis

Radiography (tomography and high definition CT scanning) may show erosion of temporal bone. Arteriography shows the tumour as a 'blush' while retrograde venography may show a filling defect in the jugular bulb. The radiological features are virtually diagnostic. Biopsy conclusive and distinguishes it from simple inflammatory or malignant polypus, haemangioma or meningioma. Tympanotomy is required in cases where tympanic membrane is intact. Biopsy may produce severe haemorrhage.

Treatment

1. Surgery. Most of these tumours can be completely excised with low risk of mortality. Glomus tympanicum tumours can usually be removed by a tympanotomy whereas glomus jugulare tumours require an infratemporal fossa approach as described by Fisch. Tumours involving the carotid syphon or with an intradural extension are best dealt with by the few surgeons that have been trained to handle them. Preoperative arterial embolization of the tumour which is usually fed by the ascending pharyngeal artery can reduce intraoperative haemorrhage.

2. Radiotherapy. Cases with neurological signs are best treated by telecobalt or megavoltage X-rays. Regression may be due to radiosensitivity of some tumours or to reduced vascularity from fibrosis in others.

Prognosis

The patient may survive for years untreated but death can occur from haemorrhage or from invasion of the cranial cavity. Radiotherapy may cure some glomus tumours but probably slows the progress of all.

Carcinoma

Pathology

Usually a squamous-cell carcinoma, very rarely an adenocarcinoma. Long-standing middle ear suppuration thought by some to predispose; it sometimes develops in a radical mastoidectomy cavity. Local spread is early and can go in any direction, usually accompanied by sepsis:

- *Outwards* into meatus and thence into parotid or into postauricular region.
- *Upwards* into middle cranial fossa.
- *Backwards* into mastoid.
- *Downwards* into jugular fossa.
- *Inwards* into inner ear and petrosphenoid angle. It may invade the facial nerve in its tympanic course.
- *Forwards* in tissue planes around the Eustachian tube to the postnasal space. Lymphatic metastases are late and usually in retropharyngeal glands – Rouvière's node over the transverse process of the atlas.

Incidence

Though rare it is the commonest malignant primary tumour of the middle ear. Most commonly in sixth decade. Males and females equally affected.

Clinical features

Cases may be grouped as petromastoid or tubotympanic when the site of origin can be identified. When the meatus and middle ear are involved simultaneously the disease should be assumed to have started in the latter.

Bloodstained otorrhoea is present. More than half of the patients will have had long-standing middle-ear infection.

Granulations and polypi bleed readily on touch. This should always arouse suspicion of malignancy.

Pain may be absent at first but intense later, from meningeal involvement.

Deafness is conductive in type, until the labyrinth is involved in later stages.

Facial palsy of lower motor neurone type. Not uncommon and usually late but can be early.

Other cranial nerve palsies are late signs and preclude any chance of cure.

Diagnosis

Biopsy will always distinguish it from inflammatory conditions or from glomus tumour. Biopsy may entail tympanotomy. Routine cytology of discharge will often detect presence of malignant cells. Radiographic examination may show extension of bony destruction. Polytomography and CT scan are especially useful.

Treatment

Radiotherapy is used:

1. Curatively in early cases without evidence of bone or cartilage invasion. Supervoltage techniques have largely eliminated the need for surgery (*see below*).
2. Postoperatively in more extensive cases in which hope of cure is still entertained.
3. Purely as palliation provided a trial does not increase the pain.

Surgery. The standard treatment of carcinoma of the middle ear is radical mastoidectomy, followed by radiotherapy, but this view is not advocated by all. The advantages claimed for surgery before irradiation are the better appreciation of the extent of the tumour; drainage and elimination of pain and sepsis; and improved access for subsequent observation. Surgery for recurrence after irradiation has been extended so as to include total petrosectomy and block dissection of the neck, the defect being covered by a scalp rotation flap.

Chemotherapy is only palliative but may relieve pain.

Selective nerve-blocking injections may help in pain relief.

Prognosis

Bad. About 25% or less can expect 5 years' survival after treatment at specialized centres. No cure can be looked for when cranial nerve palsies are present or X-ray examination shows the disease beyond the confines of the temporal bone. Death results from involvement of brain and meninges by direct spread, or from inanition due to intractable pain.

Chapter 6

Diseases of the otic capsule

OTOSCLEROSIS

Definition

A localized disease of the otic capsule in which new spongy bone causes ankylosis of the footplate of stapes or invades the cochlea. The French synonym *otospongiose* is highly descriptive.

Aetiology

Many theories have been advanced.

Heredity

There is a family history in about 50% of cases. Affected members belong to the same blood group. If both parents have otosclerosis, the chances of the children having it are high. If only one parent is affected, the odds are unpredictable.

Incidence

Otosclerosis accounts for about one-half of the cases of bilateral conductive deafness in adults. Incidence about the same in females as in males. White races are more commonly affected than coloured. Fair complexioned persons are said to be more prone than dark.

Age of onset

Clinical manifestations usually begin between 20 and 30 years of age. It rarely starts before 10 years or after 40. Post-mortem examinations have shown that many people have 'histological otosclerosis' which has never progressed to 'clinical otosclerosis'.

Effect of pregnancy

Pregnancy may accelerate the condition but never causes it. The contraceptive pill and hormone replacement therapy may have similar effects.

Effects of focal infection and trauma

Neither has any direct effect on its initiation but they may accelerate the condition. This may be of medicolegal importance.

Associated conditions

1. Familial association of osteogenesis imperfecta, blue sclerotics, and otosclerotic deafness (van der Hoeve's syndrome). Inherited as a Mendelian dominant characteristic.
2. Osteitis deformans (Paget's disease) shows some similarities.

Pathology

Normal bone is absorbed and replaced by spongy osteoid bone at one or more scattered but constant sites. This occurs in the middle (endochondral) layer of the bony otic capsule. The commonest site is on the tympanic promontory, immediately anterior to the oval window *(fissula ante fenestram)*. Vestigial cartilaginous 'rests' have been demonstrated there. Its proximity to the foot-plate of the stapes explains the ankylosis which develops later. 'Silent' areas may be present which do not involve the oval window region, and therefore do not cause the clinical manifestation of deafness. Spread of osteoid bone is usually limited, but the cochlea may become involved.

Spongy otosclerotic bone is formed in stages. Histologically, immature bone contains much cementum and few fibrils. It stains markedly blue with haematoxylin and eosin, giving the 'blue mantles of Manasse' which are seen to advance in active areas. With increased maturity, the bone stains more red and finally becomes sclerotic.

Clinical features

Deafness is the predominant symptom and is usually bilateral (80% of cases). It may be limited to one ear at first. It starts insidiously and the rate of progress is usually slow but may be rapid.

It is conductive in type. High tones are affected later if the cochlea becomes involved. Rarely, a sensorineural deafness may be the first manifestation when osteoid bone invades the cochlea rather than the footplate. Even when this occurs, there is usually remarkably good bone conduction for lower tones. The voice is soft at first but becomes loud if and when a sensorineural loss ensues.

The deafness becomes an appreciable handicap when loss of hearing by air conduction exceeds 30 dB in the better hearing ear.

Paracusis is often experienced. Patient hears better in a noise.

Tinnitus is nearly always present, sometimes to a troublesome degree. It may indicate rapid progress of disease.

Vertigo is uncommon and minimal in degree. More likely to be provoked by sudden changes of posture.

Tympanic membrane is normal in most cases. A *'flamingo pink'* tinge (Schwartze's sign) may be seen through the membrane, due to hyperaemia of the promontory. This usually indicates rapid progress. Signs of previous otitis media or distension from excessive auto-inflation may coexist.

Eustachian tube is patent.

Pure-tone audiometry shows flat loss in most cases. In the early stage, there is an upward slope to the right: but with cochlear involvement, there is a downward slope to the right. The bone conduction curve shows a dip at 2 kHz ('Carhart's notch').

Stapedius reflex as shown by impedance measurement, is ineffective.

Acoustic impedance is increased (reduced compliance), and middle-ear pressure normal.

Radiography. Tomograms or CT may show thickening of the stapes foot-plate and/or evidence of bony cochlear involvement.

Differential diagnosis

1. *Chronic non-suppurative otitis media.*
2. *Healed suppurative otitis media.*
3. *Ossicular disconnection or fixation.* Congenital, traumatic or inflammatory.
4. *Sensorineural deafness in young adults.* This may be difficult to distinguish from otosclerosis involving the cochlea, especially if minor degrees of trauma have occurred.

Treatment

1. *Regular observation* is indicated in early stages. Guidance is given to overcome social and vocational handicaps. No drugs or physiotherapy will improve the prognosis, or relieve the deafness. Eustachian inflation is useless.
2. *Hearing aid and lip-reading tuition* may be combined with rehabilitation at work. They are indicated when operation is contraindicated or opposed by the patient. Patients hear well with aids unless a sensorineural element exists. An air conduction receiver should be tried before a bone conduction one.
3. *Stapedectomy* with total or partial removal of the footplate.

Assessment of patients for operations

(a) 'Favourable' cases. Those in which the air–bone gap is large and:

- Loss of hearing by air conduction is not more than 70 dB in the speech frequencies of the worst ear.
- Loss of hearing by bone conduction is not more than 30 dB. A greater loss suggests cochlear involvement, though in some such cases an improvement in bone conduction has followed stapedectomy. (Filling of Carhart's notch.)
- Progress of the disorder has not started very early nor been very rapid.
- Psychological adjustment to failure has been assured. 'Dead' ear occurs in about 5% of stapedectomies.

(b) Less 'favourable' prognosis likely if:

- Above criteria are not complied with exactly but no definite contraindication is present.

- Marked occlusion of the footplate is found at operation, and a 'drill-out' has to be employed. Many patients do profit by operation even though not gaining perfect results.

(c) Contraindications are usually:

- Small air–bone gap.
- Presence of marked cochlear involvement.
- Only one ear with operative possibilities.
- Previous stapedectomy in the other ear.

Operative technique

The smallest part of the footplate consistent with the insertion of a prosthesis should be removed. If the whole stapes becomes mobile it is best left in this condition rather than completely removed (stapes mobilization). After total stapedectomy, if unavoidable, the oval window should be covered, preferably with fascia or other connective tissue and a prosthesis placed between the incus and the sealed oval window. After partial removal of the footplate, a stainless-steel or Teflon or Teflon/wire piston may be used and surrounded by fat. Gelatin sponge is better avoided as an oval window seal.

The fenestra can usually be made with needles and picks, but it may be necessary to thin it with a very fine (1 mm) burr in obliterative cases.

In the stapedotomy technique, a 0.5 mm hole is drilled in the footplate using either a hand drill or laser. This is preferably done with the stapes superstructure still in place. The prosthesis is positioned then the superstructure removed. This technique gives added stability when inserting the prosthesis and is claimed to reduce the risk of a 'dead ear'.

The operation is usually performed under general anaesthesia in the UK, but elsewhere it is commonly done under local analgesia. Systemic antibiotic 'cover' should be given.

Sequelae and complications of operations

i. Sensorineural hearing loss. The most serious complication of stapedectomy.
ii. Vertigo. Usually minimal and lasts only for a few days.
iii. Otitis media, infected granulations may form around the footplate. Rarely.
iv Damage to facial nerve. Very rarely. Can be transient from effects of local anaesthetic.
v. Perilymph fistula. With fluctuating hearing loss and sometimes vertigo, usually slight.
vi. Infective labyrinthitis. Extremely rare.
vii. Inexplicable failure to gain improvement in hearing in spite of apparently successful operation. A persistent or delayed conductive loss is usually due to displacement of the prosthesis.
viii. Actual operative hazards, such as dislocation of the incus, bleeding, or loss of part or whole of footplate into the vestibule. Avoided with skill gained by dissecting in a temporal bone laboratory. Uncontrollable profuse perilymph flow may require abandonment of operation.
ix. Meningitis has been reported.

Operation results

'Favourable' cases can be offered 90% chance of closure of the 'bone–air' gap.

Treatment of complications

Persistent hearing loss, whether conductive or sensorineural, will usually call for further surgical exploration of the middle ear. Risk of 'dead ear' doubles with the second procedure.

Infections may be treated with appropriate antibiotics, but facial paralysis will often require immediate surgical exploration, unless it is known with certainty that the facial nerve is physically intact.

Because of the risk of sensorineural deafness, sometimes years after a successful operation, it is doubtful whether stapedectomy should be performed in both ears.

Fluoride therapy may be tried in cochlear or combined otosclerosis, provided that the patient can tolerate it. There is no firm evidence of the effectiveness of fluoride in retarding the progress of otosclerosis.

MISCELLANEOUS CONDITIONS OF THE OTIC CAPSULE

Osteogenesis imperfecta

Definition

Autosomal dominant disease where collagen fails to mature into strong bone.

Clinical features

1. *Fragile bones.* Pathological fractures are common.
2. *Blue sclerotics.*
3. *Deafness* may occur. It presents as an otosclerotic deafness with stapes fixation. Combination of above symptoms is known as the van der Hoeve-de Kleyn syndrome, sometimes incomplete by virtue of the absence of bone fragility.

Paget's disease

Aural manifestations

Deafness is a frequent symptom but is due to the disease itself and not to otosclerosis. Otosclerotic foci have been demonstrated in cases of Paget's disease but they are probably unrelated. Osteitis begins in the periosteal layer of the otic capsule when the ears are affected. The deafness may be:

1. *Conductive,* possibly due to calcium deposition in the vestibulostapedial joint; increased bulk of the ossicles.
2. *Sensorineural,* probably due to mechanical interference with the nerve fibres by new bone or to serous labyrinthitis.

Tinnitus and vertigo may be associated with the deafness. Treatment with calcitonin may sometimes arrest the progress of the deafness.

Histiocytosis-X

This name is given to a group of diseases of the reticulo-endothelial system, in which there are focal accumulations of larger macrophages in various organs.

Types

1. Letterer–Siwe disease

A rare acute illness of infancy and early childhood. Destructive accumulations of reticuloendothelial cells are formed in many organs. Pyrexia, splenomegaly, hepatomegaly, lymphadenopathy and skeletal lesions are often accompanied by a purpuric rash and a secondary hypochromic anaemia. The condition is fatal.

2. Hand–Schüller–Christian disease

A less severe and more chronic form in children and young adults. In addition to similar but less severe lesions of the more acute types, exophthalmos and diabetes insipidus from involvement of the sphenoid bone are characteristic. Mortality is about 30%.

When the temporal bone is affected (besides the labyrinth or middle ear) the facial nerve or jugular foramen may be involved.

Histology
The characteristic finding is the presence of lipoid-filled histiocytes (foam cells).

Treatment
Irradiation and chemotherapy.

3. Eosinophil granuloma

A less acute condition in children and young adults. Characterized by localized skeletal lesions in the early stages, sometimes of one bone, often of the *temporal* or *frontal* bones and seen radiographically as an area of destruction.

Otological manifestations
Swelling over mastoid process, otorrhoea, granulations in the external canal, deafness and facial palsy. They may mimic a tuberculous mastoiditis.

Histology
The yellowish-grey granulation tissue contains:

- Large, pale mononuclear histiocytes with mitotic figures.
- Eosinophils.

Treatment
- Surgical excision by curettage of individual lesions.
- Radiotherapy of recurrences and inaccessible lesions. Useful for relieving pain.
- Steroids, ACTH and cytotoxic drugs may be given a trial.

Prognosis
- Guarded, but most patients recover.

Wegener's granulomatosis

Wegener's granuloma affects the otic capsule as well as the middle ear. It is a collagen disease, with associated periarteritis nodosa and can affect any part of the respiratory tract. It can present with a conductive hearing loss due to mucosal disease with or without an effusion. Often there is a sensorineural hearing impairment when there is an arteritis affecting VIIIth nerve or the cochlea. Radiologically it is indistinguishable from malignant neoplasms. The disease is described in more detail on page 227.

Other rare disorders of the temporal bone

1. Fibrous dysplasia

Present with progressive hearing impairment, localized swelling, and progressive bony occlusion of the external auditory canal. The monostotic form is the commonest. Treatment is conservative.

2. Osteopetrosis

Two forms of this inherited disorder. A benign dominant and an aggressive recessive form. The skull may become very thick with stenosis of the foramina. The otic capsule is unaffected. The recessive form causes sensorineural deafness before death intervenes. The dominant form usually has a conductive hearing loss due to ossicular mass. Facial nerve paralysis can occur; this may require a decompression of the internal auditory canal.

3. Neurofibromatosis

The skull may become deformed.

4. Osteomalacia.

Chapter 7

Diseases of the inner ear

CONGENITAL DEAFNESS

The bony and membranous part of the cochlea may be absent or show only rudimentary development, with or without partial deficiency of the spiral ganglion. These defects may rarely be associated with congenital abnormalities of the external canal and middle ear cleft.

Anatomical types

1. Scheibe dysplasia

Involves only the phylogenetically newer parts of the inner ear (i.e. saccule and cochlea). The stria vascularis shows areas of aplasia alternating with hyperplasia. Reissner's membrane is usually collapsed and lying on the stria and a rudimentary organ of Corti. The supporting elements of the organ are distorted and collapsed, and hair cells are sparse or missing. The cochlear neurones are spared and accessible to electrical stimulation by a cochlear implant if there is no aidable hearing. This type accounts for 70% of cases of hereditary deafness.

2. Mondini dysplasia

Dysplasia of bony and membranous structures. This occurs in the heredodegenerative type of deafness. The cochlear duct may be reduced to one and a half turns; the organ of Corti may be absent or reduced to a flat mound of undifferentiated cells. This type is clearly detectable by CT scanning.

3. Bing–Siebenmann dysplasia

There is a normal bony labyrinth but an underdeveloped membranous labyrinth, both cochlear and vestibular. It is often associated with retinitis pigmentosa (Usher's syndrome).

4. Michel dysplasia

Total absence of both labyrinths. Extremely rare.

Syndromes of hereditary deafness

Sensorineural

1. Waardenburg

Additional features are white forelock, broad nasal bridge, lateral displacement of medial canthus and heterochromia iridium (different coloured irises). Due to a dominant hereditary factor.

2. Alport

Associated with hereditary, familial, congenital haemorrhagic nephritis.

3. Pendred

Associated with sporadic goitre.

4. Usher

Associated with retinitis pigmentosa.

5. Jervell and Lange-Nielson

Associated with electrocardiographical abnormalities and syncope.

6. Ballantyne

Familial heredodegenerative with progressive high-tone loss and ash-blonde hair and blue eyes. Begins in youth.

7. Cockayne

Associated with dwarfism and retinal atrophy.

Conductive (See also pp. 81, 98, 99)

1. Crouzon

Hearing loss associated with exophthalmos, divergent squint, underdeveloped maxillae, hypertelorism and 'parrot-beak nose'.

2. Klippel–Feil

Associated with a short neck (due to fusion of two or more cervical vertebrae) and a low hair line.

3. Marfan

Associated with hypotonic muscles, laxity of joints and anomalies of heart and lungs.

4. Treacher Collins–Franceschetti

Mandibulofacial dysostosis, due to congenital deformity of structures arising from the first branchial arch (Meckel's cartilage).

5. Pierre–Robin

Conductive hearing loss associated with cleft palate, micrognathia and glossoptosis. At birth the face has a small receding mandible, and the airway is readily obstructed by the tongue.

Aetiology

1. Hereditary

The incidence of deafness is determined by Mendelian law. Probably recessive in severe deafness, dominant in milder degrees. Small proportion sex-linked. Occurs in about 4 in 10 000 live births.

2. Prenatal

Due to maternal illness in the first 3 or 4 months of pregnancy, after which the cochlea is fully developed.

- Rubella is the commonest of these causes. Opinions differ on percentage of infants involved; probably about 30%. Deafness varies in degree from moderate to subtotal with chief loss usually in the middle frequencies.
- Toxic influences of influenza, nephritis or drugs (e.g. aminoglycosides, thalidomide) upon the pregnant woman and fetus.
- Congenital syphilis is a less common cause than was previously thought.
- Congenital cytomegalovirus. 12% of a UK series of deaf children.

3. Natal

Prematurity and birth injury are both suspected causes.

4. Neonatal

- *Kernicterus* from Rhesus incompatibility between infant (if Rh-positive) and mother (if Rh-negative) may lead to deafness, characteristically for high tones; 20% have severe deafness. Histologically the dorsal and ventral cochlear nuclei are damaged: also the superior and inferior colliculi and medial geniculate ganglia. There is usually a history of severe jaundice at or soon after birth (erythroblastosis fetalis) and athetosis is commonly associated.
- *Anoxia.* May also produce high-frequency hearing loss and athetosis.

Clinical features

Deafness occurs in various degrees:
1. *Severe or total* leads to deaf-mutism unless residual hearing is used to the uttermost with bilateral high powered aids and special training is given. Even

then academic attainments are usually limited and many embrace sign language. If only one ear is affected the condition may not be noticed until later in life, usually between the fifth and tenth years, education is not impaired.

2. *Lesser degrees* lead to late development or defects of speech and delayed progress at school, even though intelligence is normal.

Vestibular symptoms are not usually evident.

Diagnosis

May be very difficult, but in severe cases should be possible before the age of 1 year, certainly before 2. Less severe forms of bilateral deafness may not be evident until school age. Accurate diagnosis may need several unhurried consultations, to obtain details of:

1. *Family and personal history* includes hearing for certain sounds, use of voice, behaviour, and 'milestones' (such as talking and walking). Mother's opinion never to be ignored.

2. *Otoscopic appearances* to ascertain defects of external ear and signs of previous otitis media.

3. *Degree of hearing loss*

- Total.
- Subtotal, with response only to very loud sounds.
- Partial.

4. *Objective audiometry* (ERA): electrocochleography by transtympanic approach (TTECoG) is the most sensitive objective test. Gets within 25 dB of threshold at 3 kHz. General anaesthetic required but this allows rapid treatment of glue ear if present and impressions for hearing aid moulds without child struggling. Brainstem evoked response audiometry (BSER, BERA) less sensitive but does not require anaesthetic. Struggling a problem in the babies and young children for whom objective audiology can be crucial.

5. *Vestibular tests* to determine the presence or absence of vestibular activity.

- Rotation.
- Caloric. In older children.

6. *Radiographic appearances* to determine the number of turns of the cochlea and if the cochlear duct is patent, ossicles, or bony external auditory canals, when operation is contemplated.

7. *Psychological assessment* to exclude mental retardation as a cause of speech delay or defect.(Often impracticable until hearing loss if any has been rectified.)

Differential diagnosis

1. *Acquired deafness* (as in meningitis) before speech has developed.
2. *Mental defectiveness,* Down's syndrome and cretinism.
3. *Aphasia* of central origin. (Congenital auditory imperception, i.e. 'word deafness'.)

4. *Dyslexia ('word blindness')*. Child has difficulty in reading (words, not numbers), and partial deafness must be excluded.
5. *Autism.*

Treatment

Prophylactic

1. *Avoidance of predisposing factors.* These include consanguinity, intermarriage of the born deaf, and exposure to ototoxic drugs or rubella during early pregnancy. Rubella vaccination is combined with measles and mumps and is available widely in the UK as MMR. The risk of a pregnancy ending with a deaf child in a hearing family is considered by many medical authorities to be an indication for termination.
2. *Estimation of parents' Rhesus groups* should always be done. Desensitization of susceptible mothers and immediate postnatal replacement transfusion have reduced the incidence of deafness from this cause.
3. *Screening tests* should be performed on all children between 7 and 9 months of age, and again soon after school entry, between 5 and 6 years of age.

Therapeutic

Normal hearing cannot be restored by any form of treatment.

Cochlear implants delivering coded pulses of electrical energy to the inner ear can transmit recognizable samples of speech sounds across a range of frequencies but are as yet largely untried in congenital deafness. Parents must be warned against unwarranted claims of cures. Guidance must be given on obtaining early educational help.

Educational

The importance of the *early* training of a child born deaf is becoming increasingly recognized. The principles of special training include:

1. *Auditory training.* Hearing aids chosen to make the best use of residual hearing are required. So-called 'phonic ear' permits short-wave radio reception with amplification from speaker to child.
2. *Lip-reading* provides visual clues to the meaning of speech and language and forms a useful supplement to auditory training in children with partial deafness.
3. *Sign language* allows early and easy reply to the questions a child needs to ask, and provides a language for intellectual development when this cannot be obtained by auditory input. It does not preclude parallel development of speech.
4. *Speech training* is required to correct defects of speech resulting from congenital or early acquired deafness.
5. *Family guidance* is essential for the families of all children born deaf or partially hearing.

Conclusions

An increasing number of children born deaf or partially hearing are now receiving education in normal schools, thanks to earlier assessment of the handicap and earlier training.

This special training should be given by a trained Teacher of the Deaf and special schools are available for Deaf and Partially Hearing children. The ultimate aim of all such training, however, should be to keep the deaf or partially deaf child in a normal hearing environment or to return him to that environment as often as possible and as soon as possible.

TRAUMA

Direct trauma

Rarely, missiles or sharp implements may pass through the external canal and middle ear to injure the labyrinth. *Deafness* and *vertigo* occur at once. Acute suppuration often supervenes.

Treatment

As for injuries of the middle ear cleft, together with rest in bed, systemic antibiotics, and sedatives for the vertigo.

Fractured base of skull

Fractures involving the petrous bone result from direct or indirect trauma. They are of two main types:

1. *Longitudinal.* Parallel to the long axis of the petrous bone. More common type. Involve the middle ear cleft but not the labyrinth.
2. *Transverse.* At right angles to the long axis of the petrous bone. Less common type. Fracture line crosses the floor of the middle and posterior cranial fossae anteroposteriorly, involving either the internal meatus or the inner ear and medial wall of tympanum.

Pathology

1. *Haemorrhages* of varying degrees occur in the cochlea, vestibule, or internal meatus.
2. *Rupture of organ of Corti* or fractures of the osseous spiral lamina.
3. *Microscopical fractures* of the otic capsule have been demonstrated post mortem. These may account for the permanent type of deafness following tangential blows on the skull with high-velocity bullets.

Clinical features

Deafness. Sensorineural in type, usually severe and permanent, though lesser degrees are known to occur.
  Tinnitus. Often permanent.
  Vertigo. Present at first, but usually disappears.

Tympanic membrane intact (in uncomplicated cases). If fracture involves deep bony canal a step-like displacement may be apparent at the site of fracture.

Radiographs. Ideally tomograms in two planes, may demonstrate the presence and position of fracture. Negative findings do not exclude a fracture.

Complications

1. *Involvement of middle ear.* With haemotympanum or rupture of tympanic membrane.
2. *Tearing of dura mater.*
3. *Damage to facial nerve.* Causing a lower motor neurone type of paralysis.
4. *Cholesteatoma.* May develop as a late complication.

In the first two complications, blood and cerebrospinal fluid may flow from the external canal or into the nasopharynx.

Differential diagnosis

1. *Concussion deafness.*
2. *Conductive deafness* due to middle ear injury or suppuration.

Treatment

This is determined at first by the general condition of the patient and the extent of the injuries.

Never syringe lest infection be introduced. The ear must be examined as soon as possible to determine the state of the tympanic membrane. There must be no instrumentation, or any interference which could predispose to secondary infection. Above all caloric tests must not be done before any perforation has healed soundly.

Antibiotics, systemically, are given prophylactically to prevent intracranial infection through the fracture lines from the ear.

Prognosis

Risk to life depends on the extent of intracranial damage.

Purulent leptomeningitis may follow immediately after injury, or at a later date if an acute otitis media occurs.

Gradual increase in deafness may develop if not complete at once.

Vertigo disappears gradually as 'compensation' at brainstem level occurs.

Facial paralysis usually recovers spontaneously, though a few cases require surgical exploration of the nerve (*see* p. 278).

Concussion of labyrinth

Definition

A temporary loss of cochlear and/or vestibular function without fracture. Due to trauma but distinct from the effects of blast and noise.

Pathology

Exact pathology is unknown. The diagnosis is a clinical one.

Clinical features

Deafness. Sensorineural in type but recoverable. Degree may bear no relationship to severity of the blow (e.g. severe deafness from a 'box on the ear'). The audiogram may show a dip most marked at 4 kHz.

Tinnitus and vertigo also occur, the latter especially if cerebral concussion has been marked. Brainstem haemorrhages have recently been shown to be a cause of persistent vertigo. Difficulty may be caused by a superadded functional element ('psychogenic overlay').

Prognosis

Deafness and vertigo usually disappear. Tinnitus may persist. If the hearing has not returned in 6 months, haemorrhages into the organ of Corti are the probable pathology.

Differential diagnosis

1. *Traumatic deafness* of a permanent nature due to unrecognized and minute fracture of the otic capsule.
2. *Pure psychogenic deafness.*

Treatment

Rest in bed, if complicated by cerebral concussion. Mild sedation.

Deafness and noise

1. Acoustic trauma

Definition

Sensorineural hearing-loss due to very brief exposure to very loud noise.

Aetiology

Small arms gunfire and magazine explosions, all associated with explosive pressure waves, or single, very loud sounds unassociated with explosion, may cause aural damage.

Acoustic trauma may arise from short-term intense exposure, or sometimes from one single exposure. The greater an explosive force, the greater the degree of damage. Explosions in closed spaces have more effect than those in open spaces. Underwater explosions lead to 'immersion blast'. The intensity of the sound pressure wave is four times greater than it would be in air at the same distance.

Clinical features

Deafness. A sensorineural deafness occurs. More often it is mixed. It is permanent and shows a severe and often abrupt loss for higher frequencies, such as 5500 Hz.

Tinnitus. Variable in intensity and duration.

Differential diagnosis

1. Blast deafness of conductive type (traumatic rupture of tympanic membrane and disconnection of ossicles).
2. Psychogenic deafness.

Treatment

Preventive. Use of protective earplugs or ear muffs. Silencers on weapons.
Therapeutic

1. *Rest and sedation, with avoidance of further trauma.*
2. *Hearing aid and auditory training will be necessary in severe cases.*

Prognosis

Must be guarded, as a slow increase of deafness may be initiated.

2. Noise-induced hearing loss

Definition

Injury to the inner ear caused by prolonged exposure to loud noise in certain industrial occupations. The cochlea is affected: vestibular function remains normal in almost all cases. Tinnitus is usually a feature.

Aetiology

Continued exposure to sounds above a sound pressure level of 85 dB is unsafe (sounds of lesser intensity may cause deafness with prolonged exposure in a few susceptible workers). Degree of deafness is proportionate to duration of exposure, though there is marked variation in individual susceptibility. Small arms gunfire comes in this category. Examples are to be found in many occupations (e.g. mining, drop forging, pile driving, chipping, hammering, riveting or drilling).

Clinical features

 Initially after exposure to loud noise there is an elevation of the threshold of hearing in the higher frequency range. After a period away from noise the hearing usually returns to normal. This is called the *noise induced temporary threshold shift.* After some time a permanent threshold shift can be observed.

Characteristically, the hearing loss is greatest at 4 kHz. A recurve can be present on the audiogram anywhere between 2 kHz and 6 kHz.

Pathological changes

The initial changes are in the basal turn of the cochlea, responsible for perceiving frequencies about 4 kHz. This area of the basilar membrane is more rigid and subject to more tension: the bony capsule is weaker here. Degeneration occurs first in the outer hair cells, and a split occurs in the supporting structure between Deiters's and Hensen's cells. In the cochlear nucleus the cochlear nerve endings can degenerate within days of exposure.

Experimental work

This indicates that oxygen tension is reduced and the glucose content of the perilymph increased. The microphonic response is impaired.

Unless prevented by short recovery periods, exhaustion of metabolites occurs with decrease of nucleic acid and protein in cell cytoplasm, and loss of intracellular potassium and glycolytic activity.

There is reduced stiffness of the stereocilia after acoustic trauma and fractured, fused and giant stereocilia have been described.

Mechanical factors may be present, with whirlpool eddies in the perilymph causing minor displacements of the basilar membrane.

Susceptibility

An idiosyncrasy or increased sensitivity in the individual may be an hereditary trait. Previous exposure to acoustic trauma may increase liability. The effect of previous middle ear disease and stapedectomy operations may depend on a critical sound pressure level below which conditions protect the cochlea, but above which the harmful effect of noise is accentuated. Older workmen appear more susceptible than younger.

Differential diagnosis

Mainly from psychogenic deafness. Changes due to presbycusis should be considered only if they contribute to the sufferer's handicap.

Treatment

1. *Preventive.* Most important.

- 'Screening' of personnel in noisy occupations, for increased liability to auditory damage.
- Use of efficient earplugs or muffs.
- Sound insulation in factories and workrooms. 'Silencers' on noisy machines.
- Resting and rehabilitation of personnel complaining of early symptoms.

2. *Therapeutic.* Rest and avoidance of causal factors may arrest progression to a permanent or more severe deafness.

3. Otitic blast injury

Definition

Trauma to external, middle and inner ear from the sudden explosive force of blast, e.g. from bursting shells, detonating minefields, exploding bombs and mortars, or roaring guns.

Mechanism of trauma

The blast wave is an intensely powerful arrhythmic wave occurring in two phases; first, a sharply-rising wave of positive pressure; followed by a secondary wave of slowly declining negative pressure. The positive wave damages the middle ear, the negative wave the inner ear.

Pathology

Reissner's membrane. May be ruptured.
Outer hair cells. May be damaged, especially in the mid-position of the basal turn of the cochlea.

Clinical features

Tympanic membrane. May or may not be ruptured. The cochlea may still be damaged even though the drumhead be deficient.

Differential diagnosis

Mainly from functional deafness.

Prognosis

Many cases have at least partial, some complete recovery.

Noise and the law

The law related to compensation for noise-induced hearing loss varies a great deal from country to country. The plaintiff may have a source of redress through compensation from the employer and/or through social security provisions provided by the state.

In the UK, industrial noise-induced hearing loss has been added to the list of prescribed industrial diseases under the 1975 Social Security Act. To qualify for benefit a claimant must show that he has worked in any occupation involving:

1. The use of pneumatic percussive tools or high-speed grinding tools in the cleaning, dressing or finishing of ingots or blooms; or
2. The use of pneumatic percussive tools on metal in the shipbuilding and ship-repairing industries; or
3. Work wholly or mainly in the immediate vicinity of drop-forging press plant engaged in the shaping of hot metals.

For the purposes of a claim occupational deafness is defined as 'substantial permanent sensorineural hearing loss due to occupational noise amounting to at least 50 dB in the better ear, being the average after exclusion of hearing losses not due to occupational noise, of pure tone losses measured by audiometry over the 1, 2 and 3 kHz frequencies.'

However, the American Academy of Otolaryngology–Head and Neck Surgery recommend that hearing handicap should begin at 25 dB average of 0.5, 1, 2, and 3 kHz. Australia has adopted a complex system of assessment. There are great variations from one legal system to the next as to what frequencies should be used and at what threshold compensation should begin. Furthermore there is a great variation between how X% auditory handicap should be converted to Y% total body handicap.

Individuals may also claim compensation by commencing an action for negligence (under the law of torts in the UK) as well as under social security law. In addition there are compensation agreements for out of court settlements; these are usually between a trade union and an employer's insurers.

Labyrinthine window rupture

Definition

Fluctuating deafness following a blow on the head or ear or after flying or diving, or unaccustomed exertion.

Clinical features

The hearing fluctuates and there is a sense of vague disequilibrium.

Pathology

The round or oval window membranes are ruptured with leakage of perilymph.

Treatment

If several days' bed rest with sedation in 30° head-up posture fails to improve the results of daily audiometry or if Fraser's test (*see* p. 65) is positive, the ear should be explored for fistulae, and the windows plugged with body fat.

Prognosis

A third of cases recover hearing after surgery.

Trauma due to compression

Caisson disease ('bends')

Follows too rapid decompression in diving and submarine work. Bubbles of nitrogen are released suddenly as emboli, leading to disruption with haemorrhages and subsequent necrosis in organ of Corti.

Sudden severe deafness, tinnitus and vertigo are complained of, and are accompanied by vomiting. The middle ear is involved as well (haemotympanum). Recovery is possible, but percentage of cures is uncertain.

Barotraumatic otitis interna

Though the effect of barometric trauma is predominantly on the middle ear, some cases of inner ear deafness have occurred after subjection to raised atmospheric pressure.

Surgical trauma

Damage may be inflicted on the labyrinth accidentally during operations on the ear. It is a recognized hazard of stapedectomy, with a suddenly and completely 'dead ear', or a slowly progressive but partial sensorineural loss. Deafness may appear suddenly weeks, months or years after operation. Fluctuating hearing loss after stapedectomy should suggest a perilymph fistula, and tympanotomy may be indicated. Tinnitus and vertigo also result. Deafness is permanent, but tinnitus and vertigo usually disappear.

Electrocution

Most cases occur through lightning strike, or while holding a conversation on the telephone in a thunderstorm. The most frequent damage is due to sonic rupture of the ear drum but a temporary sensorineural hearing loss can occur. There is usually burning of the skin at the entry and exit sites.

Radiation injury

Radiotherapy involving the Eustachian tube or middle ear cleft can cause an effusion with a conductive hearing loss. Late onset osteoradionecrosis of the temporal bone can occur. There is some evidence that a sensorineural deafness can occur after radiation exposure.

INFLAMMATORY CONDITIONS

Otitic labyrinthitis

Definition

The inner ear is infected by extension of acute or more commonly chronic suppurative otitis media (CSOM).

Aetiology

In *acute ear disease,* labyrinthitis either complicates acute suppurative otitis media or accompanies a myringitis bullosa haemorrhagica of virus origin.

In *chronic ear disease,* this condition, in its milder forms, remains one of the commonest complications of CSOM, in spite of antibiotics (in about 1–2% of cases of CSOM). Severe labyrinthitis is uncommon. Infection may result from:

1. *Bony erosion.* Commonly of lateral semicircular canal, rarely of the tympanic promontory, in chronic disease with cholesteatoma.
2. *Petrositis.*
3. *Trauma.* Less commonly. It may be:

● *Accidental* as in fractured base of skull in the presence of middle ear suppuration.
● *Surgical* as in mastoid and stapedectomy operations or removal of polypi.

4. *Direct spread.* Very occasionally, through the fenestra ovale or rotunda. This occurs in acute infections.

Pathology

Changes occur in varying degrees.

1. Circumscribed labyrinthitis

A localized perilabyrinthine inflammatory process, i.e. lying outside the endosteal lining. Results from erosion of the bony wall of the horizontal semicircular canal.

2. Diffuse serous labyrinthitis

With only a few round cells in the perilymphatic spaces. In the above two types there are no organisms in the perilymph.

3. Manifest diffuse purulent labyrinthitis

With massive purulent infection of the peri- and endolymphatic spaces, in which organisms are present.

4. 'Dead' labyrinth (so-called latent diffuse labyrinthitis)

This is a later stage of the above, with obliteration by granulation or fibrous tissue later replaced by bone.

Clinical features

Vary according to the degree of pathological changes. They are due to:

Vestibular irritation

This may occur in:

1. *Circumscribed labyrinthitis.* Symptoms are slight and intermittent, often precipitated by such minor events as manipulation of the pinna or sudden movement of the head.

Vertigo is the predominant complaint. It may be accompanied by nausea and vomiting ('labyrinthine storms'), which may be confused with gastric disturbances, especially in children.

Nystagmus also occurs. It is horizontal with the fast component to the affected side, or rotatory. Caloric tests should never be performed in the acute phase.

Hearing loss is no greater than that due to the causative otitis media.

'Fistula' test is positive in the chronic form with fistulous erosion of the bony canal.

2. *Diffuse serous inflammation.* There is a sudden dramatic onset of:

Vertigo, nausea and vomiting: The patient lies curled up in bed on the affected side, with eyes closed. All movement is avoided. If standing, he falls towards the opposite side.

Nystagmus is fast, horizontal or rotatory. It is spontaneous, and increased by looking to the affected side.

Deafness increases in this stage but may still recover.

Loss of cochlear and vestibular functions

Irritation gives way to paralysis as the inflammation becomes purulent.

1. *Manifest diffuse purulent labyrinthitis. Vertigo, nausea and vomiting* are marked. Toxaemia is present.

Nystagmus is towards the affected side at first, but changes to the opposite side when vestibular paralysis is complete.

Deafness becomes absolute.

Deep-seated temporal headache is common.

2. *'Dead' labyrinth.* Approximately two weeks after onset the labyrinth 'dies'. This leaves a total sensorineural deafness, with an inactive vestibular apparatus whose lost function is gradually compensated by the brainstem.

It may be discovered later, either at routine examination of an old chronic suppurative otitis media, or less commonly with the onset of meningitis ('latent labyrinthitis').

Differential diagnosis

From cerebellar abscess. Both conditions may be present. The cerebellar lesion causes coarse persistent nystagmus, more marked to the affected side; vertigo becomes more persistent and independent of the degree of nystagmus; tendency to fall towards side of lesion; past pointing only in hand on side of lesion; dysdiadokokinesis marked; joint sense impaired.

Treatment

In acute infection, antibiotic therapy and sedation. *In chronic infection,* mastoid surgery also is necessary, for removal of cholesteatoma and exposure of fistula. Exploration of the petrous bone may be indicated. Only rarely need the vestibule be drained.

Other forms of infective labyrinthitis

Aetiology

Infection may enter the labyrinth by routes other than the middle ear cleft. These are:

1. *Meningeal,* via internal auditory canal, aqueduct of vestibule, or ductus cochleae.
2. *Haematogenous.*

Bacteriology

Many different infections may affect the labyrinth and sometimes the VIIIth cranial nerve also. They are:

1. *Pyogenic meningitis*
2. *Meningococcal infection,* especially in infancy, as epidemic cerebrospinal meningitis.
3. *Tuberculosis* as a complication of tuberculous meningitis, as distinct from a tuberculous otitis media.
4. *Syphilis.* Both congenital and acquired.
5. *Scarlet fever.*
6. *Typhoid fever.*
7. *Typhus.*
8. *Virus infections* such as influenza, measles, mumps, herpes and others not readily definable.

Pathology

Though the whole labyrinth is usually involved, the cochlea alone may be affected. Small epidemics of unexplained vertigo suggest that the vestibular apparatus may also be involved separately.

A *'neurolabyrinthitis'* is set up, with either serous or purulent exudate in the chambers of the cochlea and vestibular labyrinth.

Degeneration of the ganglion cells occurs in severe cases, with marked destruction of nerve tissue. Replacement by granulation tissue follows if the patient survives.

Clinical features

The local disturbance is similar to that of severe diffuse otitic labyrinthitis but may be masked in the acute phase by the general and mental conditions of the patient in septic cases.

Treatment

Aimed at the primary infection. Lumbar puncture may be indicated for diagnostic or therapeutic reasons. Vestibular sedation (e.g., cinnarizine) may help the vertigo.

Prognosis

Vestibular irritation usually subsides. Partial recovery of hearing appears to occur more often than previously thought. In typhus, complete recovery can occur during the convalescent stage. Only one ear is usually affected in mumps and herpes.

Syphilitic labyrinthitis

Incidence

Syphilitic deafness is rare except in the congenital and neurosyphilitic types of the disease. Approximately 1 in 3 patients with congenital syphilis develops otological manifestations, but cochlear or vestibular disturbances due to late acquired syphilis are less common. About three cases of congenital syphilitic deafness are encountered for each case due to acquired syphilis.

Pathology

Syphilis of the labyrinth may be congenital or acquired. In either type, all parts of the auditory system are involved – brainstem, VIIIth cranial nerve, spiral ganglion, organ of Corti and its vessels, and all three layers of the otic capsule.

1. Macroscopic changes

Meningoneurolabyrinthitis occurs. Sometimes associated with a gummatous periostitis. When the middle ear is involved it is termed an otolabyrinthitis.

2. Microscopic changes

Include:
- Periostitis.
- Hydrops of cochlear duct, saccule and utricle.
- Atrophy of neuro-epithelial elements.
- Obliterative endarteritis.
- Gummatous formation.

Clinical features

Deafness. There is a sudden onset of sensorineural deafness which increases rapidly to a severe degree.

Congenital form

Deafness begins in one ear but ultimately involves both. There are two types.
- *Early:* deafness occurs in first two years of life.
- *Late:* deafness usually begins in the third, fourth or fifth decades and may progress by sudden and irregular steps, but more commonly the natural history is of slow relentless progression to profound bilateral deafness.

Acquired form

Deafness is usually bilateral but may be unilateral. It can occur at any time from early secondary to late tertiary stage, rarely before the age of 35 years. The contention that bone conduction is disproportionately reduced is not generally accepted. There is no constant type of hearing loss but it is usually a progressive one for higher frequencies. Less frequently a flat audiograph or a low-tone loss is found.

Vertigo and tinnitus. Common. They tend to disappear as deafness increases.

Vestibular reactions. Vary enormously. Often they are lost completely, but there may be a loss to caloric but not to rotational stimulation ('vestibular paradox').

Hennebert's sign. Present in many cases of the late congenital form. There is a 'fistula sign without a fistula', due to an abnormally mobile footplate of stapes. It is invariably transient and occurs when the hearing-loss is minimal.

Diagnosis

Reliance must be placed chiefly on the clinical picture and history. The condition is easily mistaken for Meniere's disease. The most reliable serological test is the fluorescent treponemal antibody absorbed test (FTA–ABS), which is positive in 98% of congenital cases and 100% of acquired cases. It should be requested in all suspected cases.

Treatment

Intensive antisyphilitic treatment. The patient should be admitted to hospital for 17 days of intramuscular benzylpenicillin 500 000 units 6-hourly, together with probenecid 05–1 g 6-hourly to block the excretion of penicillin and raise the blood levels. Concurrently, prednisolone 10 mg t.d.s. is administered in the first week, followed by 25 mg daily for 3 weeks.

By thus reducing the immune responses of the body both systemically and in the local lesion, the treponemes are more effectively destroyed. A possible Herxheimer reaction is also minimized or obviated.

Residual hearing is assisted by hearing-aids, lip-reading and auditory training, which should be started as soon as possible.

MISCELLANEOUS CONDITIONS OF THE INNER EAR

Menière's disease

Definition

A common disorder of the endolymphatic labyrinth characterized by attacks of vertigo with deafness and tinnitus. It accounts for approximately 5% of referrals to an average vertigo clinic.

Aetiology

Unknown.

There may be a genetic predisposition. On HLA typing of 41 patients, 75% where found to have the HLA-Cw7 antigen.

Pathology (Figure 7.1)

Menière first confirmed in 1861 that an affection of the labyrinth could cause vertigo, but it was not until 1938 that Hallpike and Cairns demonstrated *distension of the membranous labyrinth,* most marked in the scala media of the cochlea and the saccule. Fibrosis but not dilatation of the saccus endolymphaticus has been found. Distension of the scala media causes bulging of Reissner's membrane into the scala vestibuli, and frequently herniation through the helicotrema. The distended saccule may spread over the stapedial footplate: the utricle may herniate into the perilymphatic space of the semicircular canals. Rupture of the distended portions may occur, with fistula formation.

Degenerative changes have been recorded in the sensory elements, though Schuknecht *et al.* (1962) found normal hair cell and neurone populations, when histological fixatives were applied within 3 hours of death, and Wüllstein and Rauch (1961) found normal biochemical analysis of the labyrinthine fluids.

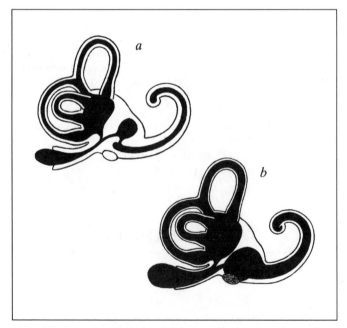

Figure 7.1 Hydrops of labyrinth – diagrammatic representation of the labyrinth. a, Normal; b, in Menière's disease. Note distension of the endolymphatic system with herniations at ampulla, and helicotrema. The saccule is in contact with footplate

Mechanical factors due to distension of endolymph system may explain:

1. Early and reversible low-frequency deafness from distortion of broad part of basilar membrane.
2. Vertigo from herniation and rupture of Reissner's membrane.

Biochemical factors are present due to mixing of the endolymph and perilymph following rupture of part of endolymphatic tube, and possible formation of minute fistulae. The cochlear microphonics and action potentials of the cochlear nerve are upset.

Clinical features

The disorder is usually unilateral at first, but the opposite labyrinth is eventually affected in possibly more than 50% of cases. It is slightly more common in males, with the onset of symptoms usually between the ages of 30 and 55. Paroxysms of attacks may be described as the *acute phase,* with vertigo as the predominant feature. Remissions with variable intervals constitute the *chronic phase,* where increasing deafness may become more noticeable. Patients become extremely apprehensive of attacks.

Vertigo

Occurs in attacks. The onset is sudden and may be severe enough to render the patient helpless. Unconsciousness and diplopia do not occur.

There may be no warning, but other symptoms may give an 'aura', with increase or change in quality of the tinnitus and deafness, and a fullness in or behind one ear.

The vertiginous feeling is usually one of rotation, either of the patient himself or of objects about him. The direction of these movements is indeterminate, and no guide to the ear affected. Some patients experience up-and-down and to-and-fro sensations, and others very severe 'storm-like' episodes.

The duration of the vertigo is variable, from 20 minutes to 24 hours or so; the collapse which follows may make the patient describe the attack as lasting much longer. Between attacks of formal vertigo there may be a trivial amount of unsteadiness. Horizontal or horizonto-rotatory nystagmus is always present during the attack.

Partial recovery of vestibular function occurs after each attack, but gradually to a lesser degree until eventually there may be complete loss of function and attacks cease.

Deafness

Is sensorineural in type, but at first it tends to affect the lower frequencies. This early loss is reversible. With each attack deafness tends to progress, and the higher frequencies are increasingly involved. The loss becomes permanent. Recruitment (and sometimes 'over-recruitment') is present. Marked distortion is particularly troublesome. Hearing aids may not be tolerated.

Tinnitus

May be very troublesome, and is usually described as a constant high-pitched 'hissing noise', except in early cases when it is usually low-pitched. It may be exaggerated during an attack. In many patients it is present, with deafness, months or even years before any vertiginous episodes occur.

Additional features

1. *Vagal disturbances* leading to:

● Nausea and sometimes vomiting and even diarrhoea.
● Pallor, cold sweats and lowered blood pressure.

2. *Headaches* may be considerable. Migraine may be associated with the condition in 7–20% of cases.
3. *Anxiety* may be marked, due to fear of recurring vertigo and/or possibility of 'brain cancer'.
4. *Phobic and other neurotic illness* is common.

Diagnosis

May be confirmed by tests of cochlear and vestibular functions.
   1. *Vestibular tests* cannot be carried out during an attack. *Caloric tests* between attacks usually show a 'canal paresis' on the affected side. Directional preponderance may be demonstrated.
   2. *Audiometry.* Pure-tone audiometry demonstrates the sensorineural nature with low-tone loss in the early stage and high-tone loss later. *Recruitment* may be recorded. Békésy audiometry usually shows a Type II response (Jerger). *Speech reception threshold* very closely matches the threshold on pure-tone audiometry. Transient improvement occurs during the glycerol dehydration test. Electrocochleography shows increased summating potential.

Differential diagnosis

Many disorders irritate the labyrinth to give similar symptoms. They were formerly included under the term 'Menière's syndrome'. Brainstem lesions including basilar artery migraine must be excluded.
   The conditions most likely to be confused are:

1. Labyrinthitis from cholesteatoma, neoplasm, virus infection, syphilis, drugs and trauma.
2. Cogan's disease, probably a rare collagen disorder affecting the eyes as well as the labyrinth.
3. Vestibular neuronitis.
4. Benign paroxysmal positional vertigo.
5. Acoustic neuroma.
6. Disseminated (multiple) sclerosis.
7. Epilepsy, with vertiginous aura.
8. Otosclerosis with co-existing endolymphatic hydrops.

Treatment

Conservative

1. *Reassurance.* Concerning the nature of the disorder.
2. *Sedation.* Relaxation and freedom from stress are essential. Benzodiazepines should be avoided because of the risk of dependence. In an acute attack promethazine theoclate, cinnarizine, dimenhydrinate, perphenazine, prochlorperazine, or promethazine hydrochloride may be given. Suppositories and sublingual preparations are useful if vomiting in attacks precludes oral medication.
3. *Vasodilator drugs* have been found helpful in some cases. Betahistine hydrochloride, nicotinic acid derivatives, naftidrofuryl and cyclandalate are used.
4. *Improve the general physical and mental health.* Any infections should be dealt with. Excessive smoking is curtailed. Any psychological illness is investigated and treated.
5. *Diuretics* can be helpful if attacks are related to the menstrual cycle. Restricted salt and fluid intake benefits some patients.
6. *Ototoxic therapy.* Streptomycin can be given either locally or systemically. There is a risk of cochlear damage.

Surgical

Indicated if the vertiginous attacks are crippling and unrelieved by the above measures.
1. *Grommet* — harmless, though of debatable efficacy. Any benefit is probably due to placebo effect.
2. *Decompression or drainage* of saccus endolymphaticus (Portmann), by (i) simple exposure or (ii)incision. A Teflon drainage tube may be inserted (House). This conservative surgery is planned to conserve hearing, but very commonly fails to relieve the vertigo. An improvement can be expected in about 75% of patients. However, in 1981, Thomsen has shown no difference in efficacy between sac surgery and a simple mastoidectomy.
3. *Cervical sympathectomy.* Rarely done. Resection must be from C3 to T3. Probably best suited to those patients with Menière's disease in an only remaining ear.
4. *Endolymph-perilymph shunting operations.* The saccule decompressing operations described by Fick in 1964 and Cody in 1968 have not been widely accepted because of the high risk to hearing.
5. *Selective labyrinthine destruction.* Ultrasonic energy or extreme cold can be applied to the labyrinth, usually via the lateral semicircular canal, with a special probe. Excellent results have been reported, however, it has not been widely accepted due to difficulties in obtaining and maintaining equipment.
Destruction of labyrinth
- *Ablation:* by removal of membranous canal (Cawthorne). Performed through lateral semicircular canal or stapedial footplate. Alternatively, the membranous canals, utricle and saccule can be avulsed by a more extensive transmastoid osseous labyrinthectomy, behind, above and medial to the facial nerve. Ablation is reserved for unilateral cases, as it involves loss of the residual hearing in the ear operated upon, but it is very effective in curing the vertigo.

6. *Division of vestibular nerve.* First done by Parry (1904) and extensively by Dandy (1941). Selective division may be made by way of a middle fossa approach, by a retrolabyrinthine approach, or by a posterior fossa approach. Some authorities hold that Scarpa's ganglion must be included in the neurectomy.

Prognosis

Spontaneous remissions occur and add to the difficulty of evaluating any particular form of treatment. Non-surgical measures control about 75% of cases in whom only slight attacks are experienced. Destruction of the labyrinth gives complete relief from vertigo in the majority of uncontrolled unilateral cases. Labyrinthectomy will deny a patient with increasing bilateral deafness the chance of a cochlear implant in that ear. With bilateral condition, selective surgery directed to preservation of cochlear function is indicated: early intervention might avert the irreversible changes that occur in the disorder. Deafness tends to be progressive even if vertigo is controlled. Tinnitus persists.

Presbycusis

Many persons over 55 complain of some degree of 'senile' deafness. Many more have a considerable degree without being aware of any deterioration. Deafness is characteristically bilateral and symmetrical. Sex ratio is about equal.

Aetiology

Individual susceptibility and inherited predisposition. Causal factor, besides age, may be exposure to noise ('sociocusis').

Pathology

Degenerative changes occur as a result of vascular insufficiency from sclerosis or thrombosis. Opinions differ on association with atherosclerosis.

1. Atrophy of *epithelial* tissue in basal turn of cochlea. The number of hair cells is reduced. Affects both afferent and efferent nerve fibres. Leads to high-tone loss, and recruitment.
2. Atrophy of *neural* tissue in spiral ganglion cells. Loss of 'neurone population' occurs. Leads to gradual high-tone loss and loss of speech discrimination.
3. Atrophy of stria vascularis. Gives a flat audiogram. Known as 'metabolic presbycusis'
4. Loss of elasticity of basilar membrane. Degeneration of the spiral ligament.This alters the microphonics of the cochlea. The cells of the basal coil are subjected to more 'wear and tear' than the others.

Clinical features

Deafness. Is sensorineural in type, with increasing loss for tones above 1 kHz. Bone conduction is reduced correspondingly. The patient hears low and medium tones well, but not higher ones (e.g. bells, birds and watch). Speech is difficult to understand, especially if fast, too loud, or in a noisy background, because recruitment and auditory fatigue are present and central reaction time is slowed. Deafness is progressive and the resulting handicap may be severe both socially and vocationally. Additional conductive loss due to wax, eustachian obstruction, etc., causes disproportionate increase of subjective handicap.

Treatment

Modern hearing aids offer great help to the majority unless marked recruitment is present. Environmental aids can be very useful. Non-electrical aids may help a limited number. Speech to a person with sensorineural deafness must be clear, relatively slow, and not too loud. Lip-reading and auditory training can be helpful.

Ototoxicity

Definition

Damage to the cochlear and/or vestibular part of the inner ear by drugs.

Ototoxic drugs include:

1. *Aminoglycoside antibiotics.* Including streptomycin and gentamicin (mainly vestibulotoxic); neomycin, kanamycin, vancomycin, framycetin and tobramycin (mainly cochleotoxic). More recent drugs (e.g. netilmycin) are claimed to be less ototoxic, though not free from risk.
2. *Diuretics.* Including:
● Ethacrynic acid.
● Frusemide (Lasix).
3. *Antiprotozoal agents.* Including:
● Quinine.
● Chloroquine.
4. *Salicylates.* Rarely.
5. *Cisplatin.*
6. *Phenytoin.* In overdosage may cause disequilibrium.

Routes of access to inner ear

Ototoxic effects are produced by:
1. *Parenteral administration.* Usually.
2. *Oral administration.* Much less commonly.
3. *Topical application.* To ears, joint cavities, wounds and burns, rarely. When applied topically to the ears themselves, the ototoxic antibiotics probably reach the inner ear by permeating the round window membrane, into the perilymph and thence through Reissner's membrane to the endolymph; when administered systemically or applied topically to areas other than the ears, they reach the labyrinthine fluids via the bloodstream. It must be borne

in mind that pus is ototoxic and a short course of aminoglycoside ear drops is probably less toxic than months of chronic sepsis.

Pathology

The main changes are:

1. *Degeneration of stria vascularis.* With all ototoxic drugs.
2. *Degeneration of sensory epithelia.* In the organ of Corti and vestibular labyrinth, with aminoglycoside antibiotics. Outer hair cells are affected more than inner hair cells, and the degenerative changes diminish from base to apex of cochlea.
3. *Degeneration of ganglion cells.* Secondary to degeneration of the sensory epithelia.

Clinical features

1. *Tinnitus.* Often the first symptom, and should be a warning of probable deafness in any patient receiving ototoxic drugs.
2. *Deafness.* Sensorineural in type and affecting high tones more than low tones.
3. *Vertigo.* Occurs with vestibulotoxic drugs.

The symptoms of ototoxicity may develop and/or progress after cessation of administration. They are more severe in the very young and very old, and in patients with renal or hepatic failure.

Ototoxic drugs given to a pregnant woman may pass the placental barrier to affect the fetus.

Treatment

1. Preventive

- *Avoid or discontinue ototoxic drugs.* Whenever there is a satisfactory alternative.
- *Monitor treatment.* With regular estimation of serum levels of drug and/or creatinine, and/or with nomograms.
- *Monitor hearing.* With regular audiometric checks in patients receiving ototoxic drugs.
- *Pretreatment audiometry and calorics should be considered.*

2. Therapeutic

No medical or surgical treatment is effective. A *hearing aid* may be helpful.

Endogenous causes of sensorineural deafness

Aetiology

A number of constitutional diseases may cause deafness:

1. *Hypothyroidism.* Deafness may be marked in endemic cretinism, less so in adults.

2. *Avitaminosis.* In humans subject to lack of vitamin-B 'complex' (not common in classic beri-beri or pellagra but in 'mixed' cases as in prisoners of war). Often associated with retrobulbar neuritis and ataxia. Deafness never complete; usually associated with tinnitus, never with vertigo. Onset sudden after long latent period.

3. Diabetes mellitus, leukaemia, pernicious anaemia, Niemann–Pick disease, Hand–Schüller–Christian disease, nephritis, sarcoidosis, osteitis deformans (Paget's disease) may cause partial deafness.

Cogan's syndrome

Definition

A condition in which auditory and vestibular symptoms coexist with a non-syphilitic interstitial keratitis.

Aetiology

Not definitely known, but it may be a local manifestation of polyarteritis nodosa.

Pathology

Endolymphatic hydrops, with degeneration of the organ of Corti and cochlear neurones, has been reported. Necrotizing vasculitis affecting the heart, kidneys, aorta and gastrointestinal tract is associated.

Clinical features

1. *Deafness.* Sensorineural, and usually bilateral. It is commonly sudden in onset and tends to progress in successive 'attacks' at regular intervals. It may ultimately be total.

2. *Vestibular symptoms.* Include *vertigo, nausea* and *vomiting,* usually of sudden onset.

3. *Ocular symptoms.* Consist of *lacrimation,* a *sensation of foreign body, blurring of vision* and *blepharospasm.* Impairment of vision is usually not severe.

Diagnosis

Serological tests for syphilis are negative.

Treatment

Urgent, and large doses of *steroids* should be given at the onset. Azothiaprine, or cyclophosphamide are effective in severe cases.

Deafness due to vascular insufficiency (ischaemia)

Aetiology

1. Vasculitis. In polyarteritis nodosa and Wegener's granulomatosis. Infective vasculitis.
2. *Embolization.* Microemboli arising from heart and vascular surgery have been implicated. Emboli from other sources.
3. *Thrombosis.* Hypercoagulation states e.g. macroglobulinaemia, cryoglobulinaemia, multiple myelomatosis.
4. *Hypoxia.* Reduced tissue oxygen tensions can arise in polycythemia rubra vera due to sluggish blood flow. Tissue hypoxia also occurs in sickle cell disease, iron deficient and megaloblastic anaemia.

There is no definite evidence that atherosclerosis, hypertension or hyperlipidaemia is associated with the development of sensorineural deafness.

Pathology

Ischaemia causes degeneration in ganglion cells, stria vascularis and spiral ligament. Hair cells not involved extensively; basal turn not specially affected.

Some effects are due to anoxia, causing changes in cochlear microphonics, and cumulative depression of electrical potentials.

Symptoms

Deafness may be sudden in onset or chronic and insidious. Usually permanent, but may be temporary and recurring due to spasm. Condition is one of the commonest causes of sudden sensorineural deafness. Recruitment usually absent. Deafness may be unilateral or bilateral.

Tinnitus and *vertigo* may be present, though not usually severe.

Differential diagnosis

From all causes of sudden deafness, Menière's disease and psychogenic conditions.

Treatment

Often the patient presents with a sudden decrease in hearing and the diagnosis is inferred from the history and lack of positive findings for other diagnoses. Treatment has been aimed at relieving any associated vascular spasm and reducing inflammation. Thrombolytic agents could be tried but as yet there is little published data on their efficacy.

1. Drugs. Vasodilators in large doses. Histamine i.v. drips may be helpful.
2. Low molecular weight (Dextran 40) infusions.
3. Steroids.

Psychogenic deafness

Definition

Deafness without organic cause.

Types

There are three types:

1. *Functional (hysterical).* The deafness is subconscious and therefore outside voluntary control. Onset is usually due to some acute stress.
Clinical features
- Deafness is usually bilateral and complete.
- Other evidence of psychological disturbance is often present, in the form of mutism or tremors.
- Anaesthesia of the external ear may be present.
- Cochleopalpebral reflex (blinking) is absent in total functional deafness though present in malingering (unless suppressed by practice).
- Deafness persists during sleep but not during hypnosis.
- Lip-reading is learnt quickly.
- Voice remains unaltered.
- Vestibular reactions are normal.
- Responses to audiometric tests are sluggish and results vary from day to day.
- ERA shows normal responses.
- Improved hearing will result from hypnosis and posthypnotic suggestion.

2. *Malingering (feigned type).* Patient is aware of the deception. The malingerer listens intently but endeavours not to respond. This 'acting the part' of a deaf person leads to considerable mental strain. After an unhurried examination is thought to be finished he may relax and then be caught out. Complete unilateral deafness is common as is partial bilateral deafness especially in efforts to avoid call-up for military service and compensation claims.
Diagnostic tests. No single test is diagnostic, but it may be possible to uncover the condition by means of one special test. The examiner must not appear suspicious. In most of the tests described below, it is assumed that only one ear is 'deaf'.
- *General examination:* Behaviour is watched, especially when the patient is off guard. Inspection is made for artefact burns or wounds. Examination is made with the patient alone. Ears are tested separately and several times. Inconsistent results are suspicious.
- *Stenger test:* See page 52.
- *Lombard's test:* a Bárány noise box is placed over the normal ear and the patient is asked to count or read in his normal voice. With true deafness, the voice is markedly raised. In malingering, and sometimes in functional deafness, the voice remains the same or only slightly raised.
- *Double speaking tubes:* two persons speak, one into each tube, on different subjects and at different rates. Prerecorded tapes and earphones may be used instead of live voices. If the patient hears with both ears, he will be confused and unable to repeat either of the sentences spoken.

- *Doerfler-Stewart test:* this also depends on the fact that persons with normal hearing raise the voice in the presence of background noise. The subject reads a passage while 'white' masking noise is introduced to the reputedly deaf ear. If deafness is feigned the voice will be raised when masking note exceeds 35 dB.
- *Pure-tone audiometry*

(a) Markedly inconsistent readings are suggestive of malingering.
(b) Denial of hearing intensity of over 60 dB (with good ear unmasked) shows disregard of air-conducted sound crossing the midline of skull.
(c) Békésy audiometry. Jerger and Herer maintain that there is suspicion of a psychogenic cause if the continuous trace is better than the interrupted one.

- *Delayed speech 'feedback':* the patient is asked to read a simple text and as he reads this, aloud, his speech is 'fed back' through a microphone, into a special apparatus which plays it back to the patient after a delay of about 0.1 sec. If he hears what is played back after this very short delay his speech becomes confused and blurred.
- *Stapedius reflex* is a reliable objective proof of hearing in the stimulated ear when it is detected as a change in the impedance of the ear as a response to acoustical stimulation.
- *ERA* may also provide objective evidence of hearing and show the true thresholds.
- *Hypnosis:* This and pentothal abreaction produce complete relaxation and will usually reveal a functional deafness. Several sessions may be necessary.

3. *'Psychogenic overlay'*. A functional element may complicate some cases of temporary or permanent organic deafness.

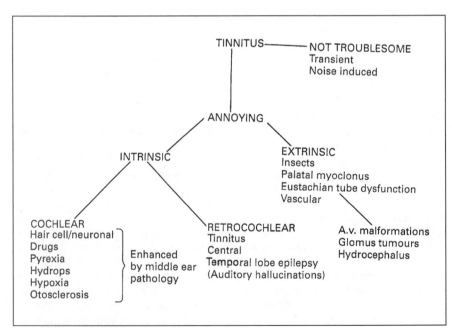

Figure 7.2 A classification of tinnitus

Treatment

The patient with functional deafness must be treated by psychotherapy. Malingerers are 'cured' once tests have exposed the fraud.

Tinnitus

Definition

A sensation of noises in the ear or head. The term does not include hallucinations of voices, which are of psychogenic origin. Tuneful or rhythmical sounds may indicate a temporal lobe epilepsy or other focal lesion. Tinnitus is usually subjective, but occasionally objective clicks or buzzings may be heard by the observer. Vascular bruits must be excluded.

Nature of tinnitus

Tinnitus may occur in two clinical forms:

1. With deafness

Some measurable hearing loss is present in the great majority of cases, even when the sufferer is not conscious of subjective difficulty in hearing. Examination must be made for an aural lesion and this must be treated if possible. Tinnitus pitch often corresponds with the frequency of maximal hearing loss.

Tinnitus may accompany any hearing loss but it tends to be particularly troublesome in presbycusis and Menière's disease and is often the first warning symptom of ototoxicity, acoustic trauma or industrial noise-induced hearing loss.

Unilateral tinnitus is not infrequently the first symptom of an *acoustic neuroma*. Unilateral *pulsatile* tinnitus suggests the possibility of glomus tumour.

2. Without deafness

Sometimes no cause may be found but certain extra-aural lesions must be considered, such as focal sepsis, carious or impacted wisdom teeth, migraine, anaemia, atheromatous plaques in the carotid artery, cerebral vascular disease and intracranial vascular tumours. Auscultation of the skull may detect an audible bruit in cases due to vascular conditions. Hyper- or hypotension may be associated with tinnitus. Rarely, clonic contractions of the intratympanic or palatal muscles may cause objective tinnitus.

Research has shown that coincidental affective disorders may be present in as many as 40% of patients referred for a specialist opinion. Usually the patient is complaining of the annoyance of the symptom or asking for reassurance that there is no serious cause. Where no definite organic disease can be found, or when patients first attend many months or years after the onset then there is a higher likelihood that the condition is complicated by an affective disorder, usually depression.

Treatment

Tinnitus may disappear when a causative aural condition responds to appropriate medical or surgical treatment, but when this is impossible or ineffectual the noises usually persist. Explanation about the cause of the symptom and reassurance about its harmless nature will usually enable the patient to accept it, and he should be encouraged to avoid undue stresses.

Minor tranquillizers help in the short term but are detrimental in the long term, so should be avoided. Active treatment of any affective disorder often dramatically reduces the annoyance of the symptom and improves the patient's general sense of well being. However, many of these patients with a psychological illness have refused to accept this as a possible diagnosis and that is why they are attending with a physical complaint. Coincidental social problems such as a recent bereavement, business problems, marital or sexual problems and loneliness should be explored. Help from a trained councillor, psychiatrist or psychologist can be invaluable. Hawthorne and his co-workers have shown that many hours of counselling may be required.

Tinnitus maskers

A tinnitus masker is a small electronic generator that provides noise that is used to mask out a patient's tinnitus. Most maskers are similar in design to a 'behind the ear' hearing aid and deliver their sound into an ear mould. The power source is a hearing aid battery. The criteria for optimum performance are not yet defined and each patient has to be fitted individually. Generally a pure tone or narrow band of noise is selected in consultation with the patient which is just loud enough to make the tinnitus inaudible. A few fortunate patients find that tinnitus suppression occurs and that this continues even after the device is removed; sometimes relief obtained lasts all day. Some find the masking noise worse than the tinnitus. Computer-assisted characterization and masking of tinnitus allows a wide range of sounds to be scanned in search of the most effective. A pillow radio may help the patient to get to sleep.

Intravenous lignocaine, or naftidrofuryl oxylate (Praxilene – a vasodilator) will produce temporary relief, in some cases. Long-term medication with Tocainide helps a few, however it is doubtful if the effect is better than placebo.

Section of the cochlear division of the VIIIth cranial nerve may alter the character of a tinnitus but only rarely abolishes it. Deterioration of the hearing increases the patients perception of the tinnitus in most cases.

PART II
The nose and paranasal sinuses

Chapter 8

Surgical anatomy

DEVELOPMENT OF THE NOSE

Frontonasal process

This is a mesenchymal structure covered with ectoderm which grows between the floor of the primitive forebrain and the roof of the stomodeum.

Olfactory placodes

These appear as thickened patches of ectoderm on the ventral surfaces of the processes during the fifth week of fetal life. They soon become depressed to form the *olfactory pits* (Figure 8.1). The frontonasal process can now be divided into:

1. *A median nasal process.* Between the pits.
2. *Two lateral nasal processes.* Lateral to each pit.

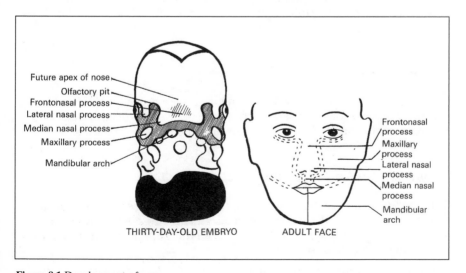

Figure 8.1 Development of nose

Maxillary processes

These are also mesenchymal structures covered with ectoderm, which grow ventrally from the dorsal end of the *mandibular (first visceral) arch* to fuse with the lateral nasal process.

Nasolacrimal duct

Formed by the canalization of a solid rod of ectodermal cells which develops in the line of fusion of maxillary and lateral nasal processes, and sinks beneath the surface. Should these processes fail to fuse, the nasolacrimal duct forms an open furrow along the side of the nose; or it may empty on the face as a fistula in this line.

Primitive nasal cavity

The apices of the maxillary processes fuse with the median nasal process, so converting the olfactory pits into short tubes. These are the primitive nasal cavities. *Primitive anterior nares* open on to the face. *Primitive posterior nares* (choanae) open into the stomodeum. The primitive posterior nares are closed for a time by a plug of epithelial cells. This is the *bucconasal membrane,* which normally ruptures about the 27th day.

Primitive nasal septum

Develops as a partition between the primitive nasal cavities. This partition is usually regarded as a single midline structure, but the rare incidence of a bifid nose with a split septum suggests the possibility of a bilateral origin. Furthermore, a median groove has been demonstrated between the developing olfactory pits in young embryos.

Primitive palate

Formed by the backward growth of the lower deep aspect of the frontonasal process, which becomes separated from its more superficial aspect by the extension of the maxillary processes towards the midline (Figure 8.2).

Formation of definitive palate

During the sixth week of fetal life, the inner surfaces of the maxillary processes give rise to the palatine processes. These fuse with each other and with the free caudal border of the primitive nasal septum. Later, ossification extends into the palate to form:

1. *Premaxilla.* In the primitive palate.

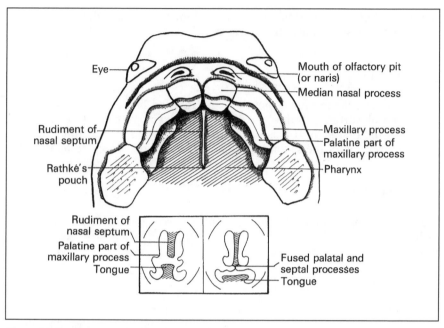

Figure 8.2 Development of palate (After His)

2. *Palatine processes.* Of the maxillary and palate bones, in the palatine processes of the maxillary mesoderm.

Formation of teeth

At about the sixth week of intrauterine life the *primary dental lamina* appears. This is a sheet of ectoderm, which grows into the mesoderm. It gives off a series of buds, which are called *tooth germs* and are responsible for causing the mesoderm to differentiate into the *dental papillae.* The ectoderm of the tooth buds is responsible for the enamel, the remainder of the tooth being mesodermal. From these first buds deciduous teeth are formed and at a later stage similar series of buds develop from the depth of the primary dental lamina to produce permanent teeth. When the tooth germs are well formed the primary dental lamina becomes absorbed but remnants of it always remain and are known as the *epithelial debris of Malassez.* It is these remnants that may subsequently give rise to cysts or certain dental tumours. Laterally there is another ingrowth of ectoderm, the *labiodental lamina,* which subsequently atrophies to form the labial sulcus.

DEVELOPMENT OF THE PARANASAL SINUSES

The paranasal sinuses develop as outpouchings of the mucous membrane of the nasal fossae. They begin to appear at about the third or fourth fetal month.

The sinuses grow during childhood and ultimately invade the surrounding developing bones. They are fully developed at about 20 years of age.

Maxillary sinus

Appears at about the fourth month of intrauterine life, as a shallow groove on the nasal surface of the maxilla, which develops from the maxillary process of the first arch. It exists at birth but does not reach its full size until after the eruption of the second (permanent) dentition of related teeth.

Ethmoidal sinuses

Begin to develop at about the fourth month. Two or three cells are present at birth.

Frontal sinus

Formed by invasion of the frontal bone by outpouchings of the mucous membrane of the anterior ethmoidal area. It is rudimentary or absent at birth, but is usually fairly well developed between the seventh and eighth years.

Sphenoidal sinus

As early as the third month of fetal life its future site may be indicated by an invagination of the sphenoethmoidal recess, and the sinus cavity can be recognized at birth. The sphenoid bone may be extensively invaded.

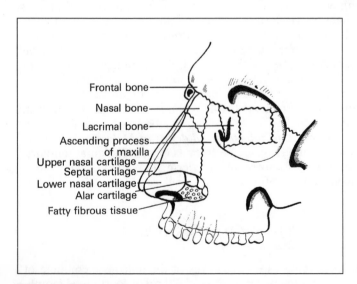

Figure 8.3 Skeleton of nose

ANATOMY OF THE NOSE AND PARANASAL SINUSES

External nose

The external nose is pyramidal in shape. Its shape is maintained by the skeletal framework (Figure 8.3).

Anterior nares

Situated in the base of the nose and open downwards. They are separated by the columella.

Bony constituents

Support the upper part of the external nose. They are:

1. *Nasal processes of the frontal bones*
2. *Nasal bones*
3. *Ascending processes of the maxillae*

Cartilaginous constituents

Support the lower part of the external nose. They are:

1. *Upper lateral cartilages*
2. *Alar cartilages*
3. *Quadrilateral cartilage of the nasal septum,* between the nasal cartilages of the two sides.

The cartilages are connected with each other and with the bones by continuous perichondrium and periosteum.

Skin. Thin over the upper part of the nose, thicker over the lower cartilaginous part, where it contains large sebaceous glands.

Vestibule is here included in the external nose because it is lined with skin and contains sebaceous glands and hairs (vibrissae).

It is limited above and behind by a curved ridge, the *limen nasi.*

Nasal fossae

The right and left nasal fossae (cavities) are separated by the nasal septum. The nasal fossa, as here described, includes only that part which is lined with mucous membrane. Each fossa communicates with:

1. *The paranasal sinuses,* through their ostia.
2. *The nasopharynx,* through the posterior choanae.

Each posterior choana is bounded by: body of sphenoid and ala of vomer, above; posterior margin of horizontal part of palatine bone, below; medial pterygoid plate of sphenoid bone, laterally; posterior free margin of vomer, medially. Branches of the sphenopalatine artery pass medially above the posterior choana from the sphenopalatine foramen to the septum.

Each nasal fossa is bounded by:

Floor is formed by:
1. *Palatine processes of maxillae,* in the anterior three-quarters.
2. *Horizontal parts of palatine bones,* in the posterior one-quarter.

Roof is very narrow and formed by:
1. *Nasal process of frontal bone,* anteriorly. This slopes downwards and forwards from the highest part of the fossa.
2. *Cribriform plate of ethmoid,* through which fibres of the olfactory nerve pass.
3. *Body of sphenoid bone,* posteriorly. This slopes downwards and backwards.

Medial wall. This is the nasal septum (Figure 8.4). The *nasal septum* lies in or near the midline. Crests and spurs are common. The three main constituents are:

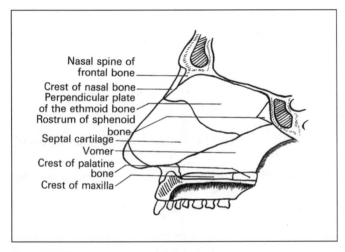

Nasal spine of
frontal bone
Crest of nasal bone
Perpendicular plate
of the ethmoid bone
Rostrum of sphenoid
bone
Septal cartilage
Vomer
Crest of palatine
bone
Crest of maxilla

Figure 8.4 Medial wall of nasal fossa (septum)

1. *Perpendicular plate of ethmoid,* above and behind.
2. *Vomer,* below and behind.
3. *Quadrilateral cartilage,* in the angle between 1 and 2. These articulate with other bones which contribute in a minor way to the formation of the septum. They are:

● Anterior nasal spines of maxillae.
● Nasal crests of maxillary and palatine bones.
● Rostrum and crest of sphenoid bone.
● Nasal spine of frontal bones.
● Crests of nasal bones.

Lateral wall is formed mainly by:
1. *Medial walls of maxilla.*
2. *Lateral mass of ethmoid and lacrimal bone.*

Other contributions are derived from:

1. Ascending process of maxilla, anteriorly.
2. Perpendicular part of palatine bone and, behind it, medial pterygoid process of sphenoid, posteriorly.

The main features of the lateral wall are (Figure 8.5):

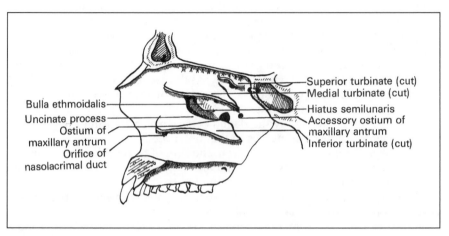

Figure 8.5 Lateral wall of nose

Three turbinates – superior, middle and inferior. The inferior turbinate is the largest.

Three meatus – named after the turbinates. Each meatus lies below and lateral to the corresponding turbinate.

Spheno-ethmoidal recess lies above the superior turbinate and receives the ostium of the sphenoidal sinus.

Superior meatus contains the ostia of the posterior ethmoidal cells.

Middle meatus is the most complex and by far the most important.

The ostia of the maxillary, anterior ethmoidal, and frontal sinuses open into it.

The *atrium* is a forward continuation of the middle meatus. The *agger nasi* is a curved ridge lying above the atrium. It passes downwards and forwards from the free anterior border of the middle turbinate and may contain 'agger cells'.

The *bulla ethmoidalis* is a smooth, rounded mass formed by the anterior ethmoidal cells. The ostia of these cells open on to the bulla or above it.

The *hiatus semilunaris* lies below and in front of the bulla and leads forwards into the *infundibulum*. It is bounded below by the *uncinate process of the ethmoid*.

Inferior meatus receives the nasal opening of the nasolacrimal duct.

Paranasal sinuses

These are air spaces within certain bones of the skull. There are four on each side: maxillary sinus; ethmoidal sinuses (labyrinth); frontal sinus; sphenoidal sinus. They are lined with a mucous membrane continuous with that of the corresponding nasal fossa through their ostia.

Maxillary sinus

Is pyramidal in shape and occupies the body of the maxilla. The base lies medially, the apex in the zygomatic portion of the maxilla. It is the largest of the sinuses, with an average capacity of about 15 ml in the adult.

Medial wall is the party wall between the sinus and the nasal fossa.

Apex may extend into the zygomatic process of the maxilla.

Roof is the thin floor of the orbit. It is grooved by the infraorbital nerve.

Floor is formed by the alveolar process and hard palate. In the child it lies at, or above, the level of the floor of the nasal fossa. In the adult it lies about 1.25cm below the floor of the fossa. The roots of several teeth may project into, or even perforate, the floor.

Posterior wall is pierced by the dental canals, which transmit the posterior superior dental vessels and nerves to the molar teeth.

Anterior wall separates the sinus from the skin of the cheek. It contains the anterior superior dental vessels and nerves (supplying the incisor and canine teeth), and the foramen for the infraorbital nerve.

Main ostium is situated high up between the medial wall and roof of the cavity. It opens into the hiatus semilunaris.

Accessory ostia are sometimes present, behind the main one. Both main and accessory ostia are surrounded by a wide area of mucous membrane unsupported by bone.

Relations

Orbit is separated from the antrum by the thin roof of the sinus which contains the infraorbital nerve.

Teeth may produce elevations in the floor of the sinus and the number of related teeth depends on the size of the antrum. The second premolar and first molar are usually related.

Middle meatus of nose is related to the upper part of the antrum. Hence the ethmoidal labyrinth can be approached through the antrum (Figure 8.6).

Inferior meatus of nose is separated from the middle part of its medial wall by bone, which is usually thick in front and below, thinner above and behind.

(Internal) maxillary artery is related to the posterior wall, where it occupies the pterygopalatine fossa. It may be approached through the antrum for ligature.

Maxillary division of the Vth cranial nerve also traverses the pterygopalatine fossa.

Nasolacrimal duct passes downwards, medial to the antrum, to open into the inferior meatus. Its lumen may be encroached upon by growths within the sinus.

Ethmoidal sinuses (labyrinths)

Consist of a number (approximately 7–15) of thin-walled cavities within the lateral masses of the ethmoid bones, and sometimes in the agger nasi and middle turbinate. The cells may invade any of the surrounding bones, including the frontal, sphenoid and maxillary bones. There are two groups of cells:

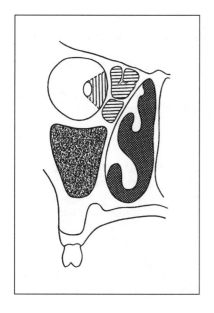

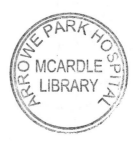

Figure 8.6 Coronal section of sinuses

1. *Anterior.* Usually small and numerous. They open into the upper part of the hiatus semilunaris or on to, or above, the bulla ethmoidalis. Secretions thus drain into the middle meatus.

2. *Posterior.* Usually large and few. They open into the superior meatus.

Relations

Anterior cranial fossa lies above the very thin roof of the upper ethmoidal cells.

Orbit is separated from the labyrinth by the orbital plate of the ethmoid bone. This is also thin (lamina papyracea) and may be absent in parts.

Lacrimal sac is related laterally to the anterior cells.

Optic nerve may be very close to the cells of the posterior group, especially when they invade the sphenoidal sinus.

Anterior and posterior ethmoidal vessels and nerves run from the orbit to the nasal fossa between the roof of the ethmoidal labyrinth and the under surface of the frontal bone.

Frontal sinus

Should be regarded as an upward extension of an anterior ethmoidal cell. It occupies a very variable extent of the frontal bone and may be partly loculated. Its average capacity is about 7 ml in the adult. The right and left sinuses are often asymmetrical. They are separated by a thin bony septum, which may be deficient in part. The sinus may invade the orbital plate of the frontal bone and occasionally it extends to the optic foramen. The *frontonasal duct* passes through the anterior part of the ethmoidal labyrinth. Its length and curvature vary considerably. Its lower end (ostium) usually opens into the infundibulum, less often independently above this level.

Relations
Anterior cranial fossa: separated from the sinus by the compact bone of its posterior wall.
   Orbit: lies below the floor of the sinus. This is also compact bone which may rarely be deficient.
   Skin and periosteum of forehead: cover the anterior wall, which is of diploic bone and is related to supraorbital and supratrochlear nerves.

Sphenoidal sinus

Lies behind the upper part of the nasal fossa. It occupies the body, and some-times the wings and pterygoid processes, of the sphenoid bone. The average capacity is about 7 ml in the adult. The right and left sinuses are rarely symmetrical. They are separated by a septum which may be deficient in part and is often oblique.
   The degree of pneumatization is very variable and is of three types:

1. *Conchal pneumatization* in which the sinus is rudimentary, having little depth or width. It is present in about 1% of the adult population of northern Europe and is a contraindication to trans-sphenoidal hypophysectomy.
2. *Pre-sphenoid pneumatization* in which the sinus is pneumatized as far as the anterior bony wall of the pituitary fossa. Present in about 40%.
3. *Post-sphenoidal and occipital pneumatization* in which pneumatization extends backwards below the pituitary fossa. In extreme cases it extends into the occipital bone. Present in about 60%.

   The *ostium* is situated in the upper part of the anterior wall of the sinus. It communicates with the superior meatus indirectly through the sphenoeth-moidal recess.
Relations
Cavernous sinus containing the IIIrd, IVth, Vth (ophthalmic and maxillary divisions) and VIth cranial nerves, lies laterally, with the *internal carotid artery* and *optic nerve.*
   Pituitary gland, optic chiasm, olfactory tract and *frontal lobe of brain* lie above the sinus. The pituitary gland may be approached surgically through the sinus.
   Vessels and nerves from sphenopalatine foramen lie in front of the lower part of the sphenoid face as they pass to the nasal septum.
   Vidian nerve (nerve of the pterygoid canal) runs forwards below its floor.
   Basilar artery and brainstem are related to its thick posterior wall (basisphenoid).
   The pterygopalatine fossa: a small pyramidal space between the posterior wall of the maxillary antrum anteriorly and pterygoid extension of the greater wing of the sphenoid posteriorly.
   It contains the third part of the maxillary artery and its terminal branches; the maxillary nerve; and the sphenopalatine ganglion and its branches.
   Surgically, the contents of the fossa are best approached by a transantral route, an opening being made in the (usually) thin posterior wall of the antrum. Through this window can be visualized the posterior (sphenoidal) wall of the fossa in which there are two foramina, the foramen rotundum and (8 or 9 mm below and medial to it) the entrance to the pterygoid canal.

Mucous membrane of nose and paranasal sinuses

The mucous membrane of the nose is of two types:

1. Respiratory

This lines the lower two-thirds of the nasal septum, the lateral wall of the nose below the superior turbinate and the floor of the nasal fossa.

It is pink in colour and is covered by a ciliated, columnar epithelium. This consists of tall ciliated cells which narrow in their deeper parts. Irregular basal cells fill the intervening spaces. Goblet cells, containing thick mucus, lie among the ciliated cells. Thin fluid comes from compound acinar secreting glands of two types, serous and mucinous. Both types of mucus are spread thin over the epithelium and propelled by cilia at a density of 5 million per square mm. Cilia move at 14 beats per second and in a healthy adult the mucociliary stream carries about a pint and a half of nasal mucus to the throat every 24 h.

A fibroelastic basement membrane separates the epithelium from the subepithelial connective tissue, which is loose and highly vascular and contains many mucous and serous glands. Its deeper portion is firmly blended with the underlying periosteum and perichondrium (Figure 8.7).

The respiratory membrane extends from the limen nasi throughout the nose and into the upper half of the nasopharynx. It also extends into the sinuses, through their ostia, and is thinner there. It is also continuous with the epithelia of the nasolacrimal duct and Eustachian tube. Above, it is continuous with the olfactory mucosa of the nose. Anteriorly at the limen nasi it becomes continuous with the skin of the nasal vestibule.

The *tubercle of the septum* is sometimes distinguished as a localized thickening of the respiratory mucous membrane of the septum opposite the anterior end of the middle turbinate.

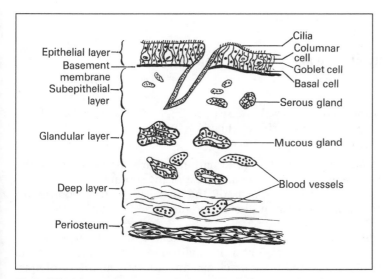

Figure 8.7 Mucus membrane of nose (respiratory)

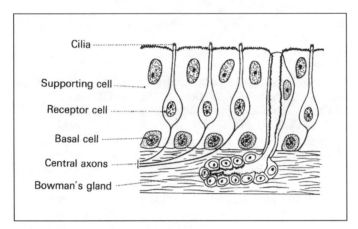

Figure 8.8 Olfactory mucus membrane

2. Olfactory

This (Schneiderian) membrane (Figure 8.8) lines the upper one-third of the nasal septum, the roof of the nose, and the lateral wall, above and including the superior turbinate. The olfactory epithelium is of non-ciliated columnar cells and is yellowish in colour. It contains the serous glands of Bowman. The cells are:

- *Olfactory.* Bipolar. The superficial process ends at the surface of the mucous membrane in a bulbous process which bears the olfactory hairs. The central process passes to the olfactory bulb through the cribriform plate.
- *Supporting.*
- *Basal.* Contain yellow pigment.

Blood supply of nose and paranasal sinuses

Arterial supply

The nasal fossae and paranasal sinuses are supplied by branches of the external and internal carotid arteries (Figure 8.9).

1. *Derivatives of external carotid artery*

- *Sphenopalatine artery:* via the (internal) maxillary artery supplies the turbinates and meatus of the nose and most of the septum.
- *Greater palatine artery:* a branch of the maxillary artery contributes branches to the lateral nasal wall and (via the incisive canal) to the anterior part of the septum.
- *Superior labial artery:* a branch of the facial artery. It sends branches to the tip of the septum and the alae nasi. Its anastomosis with a branch of the sphenopalatine artery and the greater palatine artery ('the artery of epistaxis') forms Kiesselbach's plexus, in Little's area.

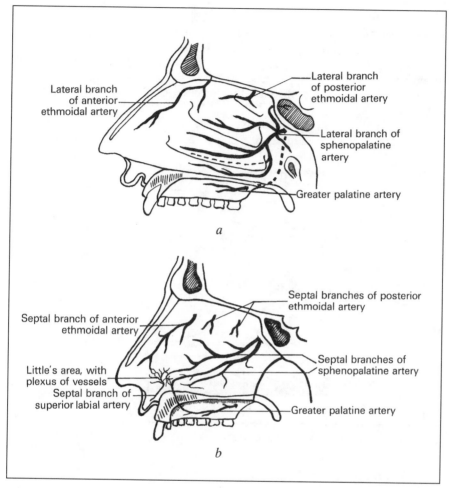

Figure 8.9 a, Blood supply of nose (lateral wall); b, blood supply of nose (medial wall – septum)

- *Infraorbital and superior dental arteries:* branches of the (internal) maxillary artery. They supply the maxillary antrum.
- *Pharyngeal branch of (internal) maxillary artery:* supplies the sphenoidal sinus.

2. *Branches of internal carotid artery*
- *Anterior and posterior ethmoidal arteries:* branches of the ophthalmic artery. They supply the roof of the nose, anterior parts of the septum and lateral wall of the nose, and the ethmoidal and frontal sinuses. Bleeding from these vessels is seen above the level of the middle turbinate.

Venous drainage

The veins form a cavernous plexus beneath the mucous membrane.

They open into:

1. *Sphenopalatine vein and anterior facial vein,* from the plexus.
2. *Ophthalmic veins,* from the ethmoidal veins.
3. *Veins on the orbital surface of the frontal lobe of the brain,* through foramina in the cribriform plate.
4. *Superior sagittal sinus,* through the foramen caecum (when the latter is present).

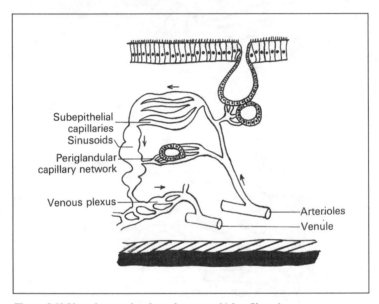

Figure 8.10 Vascular supply of nasal mucosa (After Slome)

Vascular arrangements of mucous membrane (Figure 8.10).

Arterioles lie in the deeper part of the subepithelial connective tissue. They are arranged in longitudinal rows.

Capillaries lie in networks under the epithelium and around the glands.

Sinusoids receive blood from the capillary networks.

Venous plexuses also lie in the deeper part of the subepithelial connective tissue. They drain the sinusoids.

Venules collect blood from the plexuses.

The *erectile tissue* formed by this vascular arrangement is most marked over the inferior turbinate, adjacent part of the septum, and the posterior part of the middle turbinate.

Autonomic nervous supply

This controls the vascular reactions of the nasal mucous membrane.

Sympathetic fibres. Postganglionic fibres pass from the superior cervical ganglion to the plexus around the internal carotid artery. They then form the deep petrosal nerve which, with the greater superficial petrosal nerve, becomes the nerve of the pterygoid canal (Vidian nerve). They are distributed without relay via the sphenopalatine ganglion. They maintain a constant tonic vasoconstrictor action. Section of the cervical sympathetic causes vasodilatation and a 'stuffy nose' is sometimes complained of.

Parasympathetic fibres. Preganglionic fibres are derived from the nervus intermedius and reach the sphenopalatine ganglion via the greater superficial petrosal and Vidian nerves. Postganglionic fibres are distributed to the mucosa. Stimulation of the Vidian nerve causes vasodilatation; section of the nerve causes vasoconstriction and diminution of nasal secretions.

Nerve supply of nose (Figure 8.11)

Nerves of common sensation are derived from:

1. Branches of the Vth cranial nerve

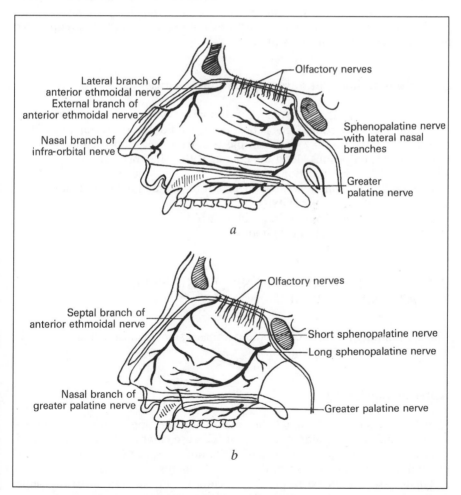

Figure 8.11 a, Nerve supply of nose – lateral wall; b, nerve supply of nose – sptum

- *Anterior ethmoidal nerve.* A branch of the ophthalmic (1st) division. It enters the nasal cavity through the anterior ethmoidal foramen and divides into:

(a) Medial branch, which supplies the anterior part of the septum.
(b) Lateral branch, which supplies the anterior part of the lateral wall of the nose, and the anterior parts of the middle and inferior turbinates.

2. Branches of sphenopalatine ganglion

- *Greater (anterior) palatine nerve.* Supplies most of the inferior turbinate and the middle and inferior meatus.
- *Short sphenopalatine (posterosuperior lateral nasal) nerves.* Supply the posterior parts of the superior and middle turbinates.
- *Long sphenopalatine (nasopalatine) nerve.* Supplies the remainder of the septum.

Olfactory nerves. The sense of smell is supplied by the 1st cranial nerve. Fibres arise from bipolar cells in the olfactory mucosa. They are non-medullated and pass through foramina in the cribriform plate. They enter the under-surface of the olfactory bulb.

Lymphatic drainage of nose and paranasal sinuses

The lymphatic vessels arise from a continuous network in the superficial part of the mucous membrane. This is best developed at the posterior end of the superior turbinate. They can be injected from the subarachnoid space, through communications along the course of the olfactory nerves which thus afford a pathway for infection.

Submandibular lymph nodes collect lymph from the external nose and anterior part of the nasal cavity.

Upper deep cervical nodes drain the rest of the nasal cavity, either directly or through the retropharyngeal nodes.

PHYSICAL EXAMINATION OF THE NOSE AND PARANASAL SINUSES

Clinical examination of the nose and paranasal sinuses must include an examination of the nasopharynx.

Anterior rhinoscopy

May be assisted by shrinking the mucosa by the application of vasoconstrictor solutions. In children, the tip of the nose can be turned upwards and backwards by the examiner's thumb. In adults, a speculum is used. By this method, it is possible to inspect the floor of the nose, the inferior and middle turbinates (with their corresponding meatus), and the septum to the same height. The superior turbinate and meatus are not seen.

Posterior rhinoscopy

The posterior ends of the middle and inferior turbinates (together with their corresponding meatus) can be seen, with the posterior edge of the septum and orifices of the Eustachian tubes. There are several methods:

1. Postnasal mirror

This may be fixed or movable (Michel). The posterior choanae, openings of the Eustachian tubes and roof of the nasopharynx are seen, and the nasopharyngeal tonsil if present. Under general anaesthetic the mirror is usefully combined with the operating microscope.

2. Fibrescope

Through the nostril a detailed view of the nasal cavities and nasopharynx is easily obtained.

3. Yankauer nasopharyngeal speculum

Can be used under general anaesthetic for examining the posterior wall of the nasopharynx and the fossae of Rosenmüller. It may be valuable for obtaining biopsy specimens but is of no use for examining the posterior choanae.

Palpation

1. *Digital examination* of the external nose and postnasal space may both give useful information. The latter should only be performed with general anaesthesia. Swelling or tenderness over the sinuses can also be elicited.
2. *Probing* of the nose provides further examination.

Ultrasound scanning

This is a simple outpatient procedure but at present is of very limited practical use.

Diagnostic lavage

This is described under Anatomical Principles of Sinus Surgery.

Examination of nasal airflow

This is described under Nasal Respiration

Examination of smell

This is described under Smell.

RADIOGRAPHIC EXAMINATION OF THE NOSE AND PARANASAL SINUSES

The nasal bones may be demonstrated by superoinferior and lateral views. Clinical examination and palpation are more informative and X-rays are not usually needed for nasal fractures.

Radiological examination of the sinuses is by far the most reliable adjunct to the clinical diagnosis of sinus disease.

Standard sinus views

1. Occipitomental

The slight backward tilt of the head throws the hard petrous shadow below the floor of the antrum, which is best seen in this view, which also shows the orbital margins. malar bones, and coronoid processes of mandible.

2. Occipitofrontal

The ethmoidal and sphenoidal sinuses are aligned one behind the other. The frontal sinuses are well shown.

3. Lateral

Determines the depth of the frontal sinuses and demonstrates the sphenoidal sinus. It also shows the profile of the jaws and facial bones.

4. Submentovertical

The ethmoidal and sphenoidal sinuses are seen from below.

5, 6. Right and left oblique

These views supply more details of the ethmoidal cells.

Radiopaque medium

A radiopaque medium may sometimes be introduced into the sinuses before exposure.

1. *By injection.* Through a cannula, usually into the antrum.
2. *By Proetz's displacement method.* Particularly into the sphenoidal and posterior ethmoidal sinuses. These methods have little advantage over good plain films of the standard views.

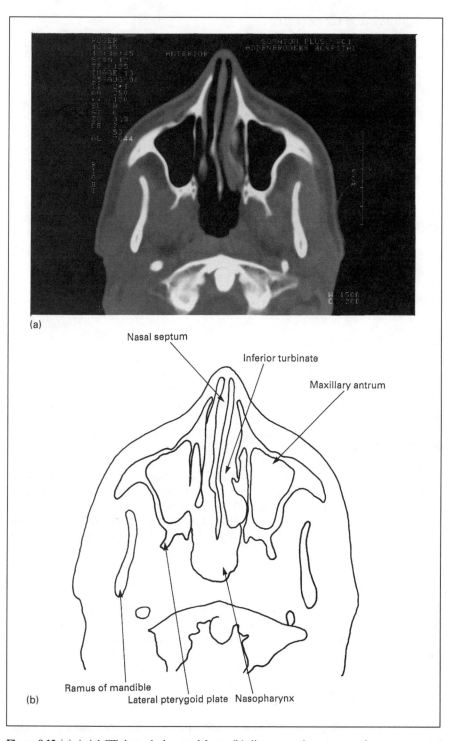

Figure 8.12 (a) Axial CT through the nasal fossa; (b) diagrammatic representation

Tomography and CT scanning

These may provide invaluable additional information (Figure 8.12). They are often the only way to demonstrate fractures or early destruction of the sinus walls, and to show foreign bodies or neoplasms in the sinuses or nasal fossae.

Magnetic resonance imaging

This modality has the advantage of being able to give information concerning the nature of soft tissues. In the case of sinus malignancy there is often associated infection, mucus-containing cysts and oedematous mucosa. This can create the impression on X-ray imaging that the tumour is larger than it is.

ANATOMICAL PRINCIPLES OF SINUS SURGERY

Anatomy of approach

Each of the sinuses may be approached by one of two routes:

1. Intranasal

Through the nose. Usually used for simple puncture and lavage for diagnostic purposes. It may also be used for permanent drainage operations, but its value is limited by the 'anatomical' dangers involved.

'Danger area' of nose. The area above and lateral to the attachment of the middle turbinate.

Orbit may be entered through the lamina papyracea, the thin outer wall of the ethmoidal labyrinth.

Optic nerve may be damaged as it enters the orbit through the optic foramen.

Meninges may be involved by spread of infection through the perineural lymphatics surrounding the olfactory nerve filaments. Damage to the cribriform plate and roof of the ethmoidal labyrinth will produce the same effect. Surgical emphysema, haematoma, cellulitis, or abscess of the orbit, blindness, and septic intracranial complications may follow accidental damage through the intranasal route.

2. External

Through incisions on the face or within the mouth. Direct visual access is gained by this approach which is therefore safer. This may include *lateral rhinotomy*, for removal of tumours in the nose and sinuses, or the transpalatal approach.

Diagnostic procedures

The sinuses may be punctured and washed out with normal saline for diagnostic purposes.

1. Maxillary sinus

- Through the inferior meatus by straight Lichtwitz trocar and cannula. The solution enters the sinus through the cannula and leaves it through the natural ostium in the middle meatus. If the ostium is completely obstructed a second cannula introduced through the inferior meatus will sometimes allow lavage.
- Through the middle meatus by curved (Watson–Williams) cannula. The mucosa covering the wide bony ostium is usually pierced, the true ostium itself rarely entered. In the latter event, the edges of the ostium may be damaged, with subsequent stenosis and interference with drainage. The orbit is more likely to be entered accidentally by this route which is now rarely used.
- Through the ostium or lateral wall of the nose by a fibrescope, permitting visual inspection of the sinus cavity.
- Through the inferior meatus or sublabially through the anterior sinus wall with a rigid endoscope which allows inspection and surgery to be performed.

2. Ethmoidal cells

Ethmoidal cells may be punctured through their thin medial bony walls with a straight, blunt-edged trocar and cannula. Suction is then applied through a syringe.

3. Frontal sinus

Frontal sinus can occasionally be entered by a curved frontal sinus cannula. Stenosis of the frontonasal duct may follow and the manoeuvre is rarely to be recommended.

4. Sphenoidal sinus

Sphenoidal sinus can be entered through its normal ostium. The blunt straight cannula is passed horizontally along the floor of the nose, until it touches the posterior pharyngeal wall. It now lies beneath the floor of the sinus.

By gradual withdrawal, the tip can be felt to slip upwards over the anterior wall. The ostium is situated on this surface and can sometimes be entered. If this is not possible the thin anterior wall may be pierced.

Radical surgery

These operations are most commonly undertaken for the relief of chronic infections in the sinuses, by drainage or obliteration; less commonly, for the excision of malignant neoplasms and for orbital decompression in thyrotoxic exophthalmos.

1. Maxillary sinus surgery

Antrostomy

A permanent drainage of the antrum. The opening is usually made into the inferior meatus of the nose and may facilitate gravitational drainage. It must be remembered that the cilia will continue to waft mucus towards the natural ostium. If it is made too far back, descending branches of the sphenopalatine or greater palatine arteries may be damaged, with severe haemorrhage. Two routes are used:

- *Intranasal.* Used for simple drainage of a chronic empyema.
- *Sublabial* (Caldwell–Luc). Through the canine fossa grossly diseased mucosa can be removed and the antrostomy created under direct vision through the antronasal wall into the inferior meatus. This approach may be extended through the posterior wall of the antrum to expose the contents of the sphenopalatine fossa, including the maxillary artery, and the Vidian and maxillary nerves.

2. Ethmoidectomy

An exenteration of the ethmoidal cells, usually for recurrent polypi. Three routes are used:

Intranasal

Must be used with great caution.

External

Through a skin incision in front of the inner margin of the orbit to enter the lamina papyracea.

Transantral (Horgan type)

The opening is made posteriorly at the junction of the roof and medial wall of the antrum which has been entered through the canine fossa. The anterior ethmoidal (agger) cells cannot be reached by this route.

3. Frontal sinus surgery

Drainage of frontal sinus

- *Trephining of the floor.* Provides temporary drainage for an acute empyema until the frontonasal duct regains its patency.
- *External frontoethmoid (Howarth) operation.* The floor of the sinus is removed in whole or in part, together with anterior ethmoidal cells and the frontonasal duct, to create a wide passage into the middle meatus.

Obliteration of frontal sinus

- *Removal of anterior wall and floor* allows the overlying soft tissues to become approximated to the denuded posterior wall. The depression can be filled in later with bone chips or fat.

- *Removal of mucosa of sinus and duct* is thought to result in obliteration of the sinus by fibrous tissue and/or bone (though regeneration of mucosa and stenosis will often lead to recurrence of infection). The best surgical exposure for this purpose is the forward reflection of a coronal scalp flap, with preservation and replacement of the anterior bony wall (Macbeth).

4. Sphenoidal sinus drainage

May be effected through several routes:

Intranasal

By partial removal of the anterior wall.

Transantral

By extension of the Horgan operation.

External

Via the ethmoidal cells (external sphenoethmoidectomy). This approach may also be used in hypophysectomy.

Transpalatal

By separation of the hard from the soft palate.

Trans-septal

By extension of submucous resection of the nasal septum. Also used in hypophysectomy.

5. Multiple sinus drainage

By a single external approach several sinuses may be drained simultaneously.

Fronto-ethmo-sphenoidectomy (Ferris Smith)

Performed by extension and modification of the Howarth operation. This operation may be combined with a sublabial approach to the antrum.

Ethmo-antrostomy (Patterson)

The antrum is entered through the floor of the orbit and the ethmoid through its outer wall by an incision in the nasojugal fold.

A separate sublabial approach to the antrum is more often used in combination with the Howarth type of operation.

6. Trans-sphenoidal hypophysectomy

Trans-sphenoidal removal of the pituitary gland may be achieved by either a trans-ethmoidal or a trans-septal approach, or by a combination of the two. It is contraindicated by poor pneumatization of the sphenoidal sinus.

7. Partial maxillectomy

This involves total removal of the hard palate of one side. It is a useful approach for the diathermic or cryosurgical removal of tumours confined to the palate and the cavity of the antrum. It creates a permanent portal for inspection of the cavity and can be closed by a prosthesis.

8. Lateral rhinotomy

Downward extension of the excision for external ethmoidectomy allows removal of nasal bone, frontal process of maxilla and lateral bony border of pyriform aperture. It gives a wide exposure of nasal and ethmoidal cavities.

9. Total maxillectomy

Indicated for some extensive tumours of the antrum and ethmoidal sinus. It is usually performed through a lateral rhinotomy with extension of the incision through the upper lip in the midline and may be extended to remove affected areas of skin or orbital contents (Ferguson).

10. Functional endoscopic sinus surgery

The advent of a range of rigid operating endoscopes has revitalized intranasal sinus surgery. The principle advantages of the technique are a reduced stay in hospital, avoidance of scars on the face and a reduction in unnecessary surgical trauma. Risks of entering the orbit or anterior cranial fossa are considerable compared to an open technique and consequently the trainee is advised to practise on cadaver material. As the operating field is narrow and magnified for the surgeon bleeding can be troublesome especially in polypectomy. An irrigation system helps to improve visual identification of important structures.

Argon or neodynium YAG laser light can be conducted through a fibre-optic delivery system. Pigmented lesions in the depths of the nose can therefore be treated endoscopically.

Chapter 9

Applied physiology of the nose and paranasal sinuses

NASAL RESPIRATION

The nose forms the uppermost part of the respiratory tract. So firmly established is the normal pattern of nasal respiration that infants unable to breathe through the nose have been known to asphyxiate. Mouth-breathing has to be learned. Nasal respiration also allows normal breathing to continue during mastication of food, although it is reflexly arrested during the act of swallowing. Further importance lies in the preparation of inspired air for the lower respiratory passages.

Nasal air currents (Figure 9.1)

Inspiratory air currents are determined by:

1. Direction of the anterior nares.
2. Narrowness of the limen nasi compared with the size of the posterior choanae. During quiet breathing, inspired air passes upwards, to curve below

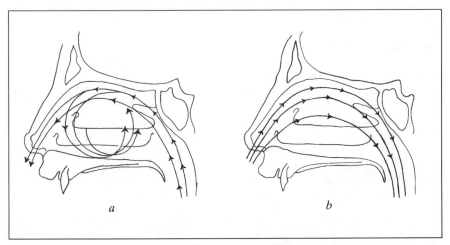

Figure 9.1 Respiratory air currents. a, Inspiratory; b, expiratory (After Proetz)

the roof of the nose (through the 'olfactory cleft') and continues downwards through the posterior choanae. The anterior end of the inferior turbinate is important in regulating the airflow.

Expiratory air currents pass in roughly the same parabolic curve as the inspiratory currents. Frictional resistance at the narrowed limen nasi allows only part of the expired air to reach the outside directly.

Eddies are formed by the remainder, partly under cover of the middle turbinate. In this way the sinus ostia are subjected only to air that has been conditioned by the methods to be described below.

Examination of nasal airflow

An impression of the degree of nasal airflow can be obtained by holding a cold mirror under the nose and observing the pattern of misting. This technique has been taken one step further by allowing the breath to impinge on a thermographic plate which can then be photographed.

Nasal resistance can be measured by rhinomanometry. Anterior active rhinomanometry has achieved some general acceptance in medicolegal work and research but as yet few surgeons use it routinely.

Nasal obstruction leads to hyponasality. The tonal quality of the speech can be recorded simultaneously by microphones placed one in front of the mouth and the other in front of the nose. The microphones are shielded from each other by a plate. The difference in tonal quality correlates with the degree of nasal obstruction. This method of assessing nasal airflow has obtained some favour in paediatric rhinology as it is better tolerated than rhinomanometry.

PROTECTIVE FUNCTIONS OF THE NOSE

The lower respiratory passages receive some protection by the nose through its treatment of the inspired air. The air is purified, warmed and moistened.

Purification

1. *Vibrissae.* These sift the coarser particles.
2. *Cilia.* The respiratory portion of the nose is lined in its entirety by a ciliated epithelium. The cilia are bathed in a viscous sheet of mucus. Fine particles (including bacteria) stick to the mucus, which is impelled as a continuous 'conveyor belt' into the nasopharynx, whence they are swallowed.

Cilia have an effective stroke and a recovery stroke and beat about 10 times per second. The movement is perpetual and is directed from before backwards. The complete sheet of mucus is cleared into the pharynx about twice an hour. Ciliary movement stops rapidly with drying.

3. *Lysozymes* are bacteriolytic enzymes found in the nasal mucus (and tears).
4. *Reflex sneezing* helps to expel inhaled foreign particles.
5. *Olfaction.* The breath is held if noxious smells are detected.

Warming

The rich vascular arrangements of the nasal mucosa allow the inspired air to be warmed in its passage through the nose. The extensive plexuses, especially in the inferior turbinates, provide an efficient radiating system.

Moistening

The inspired air is almost completely saturated in the nose. The moisture is derived from two sources:

1. Transudation of fluid through the epithelium, mainly.
2. Secretion from the mucosal glands and goblet cells, slightly.

The daily volume of nasal transudate and secretions is about 1 litre.

Therapeutic applications

Maintenance of ciliary activity. The normal functioning of the ciliary mechanism is of the greatest importance.

Moisture is essential. If the cilia are not working properly the sheet of mucus covering them cannot be moved efficiently and the self-cleansing functions of the nose are reduced or arrested.

Factors causing damage to cilia

1. *Drying* may result from:

- Constant exposure to dry air, as in excessive central heating or air conditioning.
- Localized deflections of the air currents. These cause an excessive concentration of dry air to fall upon localized areas of the mucous membrane. Local drying causes ciliary stasis, with crusting and secondary infection.

2. *Drugs:* decongestion is commonly required in nasal therapy. Many drugs will produce it but not all are safe to use.

- *Cocaine* is one of the most effective decongestants available but it reduces the activity of the cilia if allowed to remain in contact for too long.
- *Adrenaline* has similar effects to cocaine.

3. *Excessive heat or cold.*
4. *Hypertonic or hypotonic solutions.*
5. *Smoking.*
6. *Infective rhinitis of all kinds.*
7. *Exposure to noxious fumes.* This usually occurs in the working environment and may lead to litigation against an employer.

Tests of nasal mucociliary function

A history of keratosis obturans, Kartagener's syndrome, bronchiectasis or infertility should alert the surgeon to the possibility of congenital abnormality of ciliary structure or abnormally viscous mucus.

1. Saccharin test

This is a test of mucociliary clearance. A particle of saccharin is placed on the inferior turbinate 1 cm behind the anterior end. The time taken for the patient to taste the saccharin is noted. Ninety per cent of normal subjects should taste the saccharin within 20 minutes. If the patient has not tasted the saccharin after 40 minutes then an innate inability to taste saccharin should be excluded.

2. Ciliary beat frequency

A sample is taken with a cytology brush from the inferior turbinate. The specimen is mounted and placed on the warmed stage of a phase contrast microscope. Each beat of the cilium under observation breaks the light beam and this is detected by a photometer. The normal range is 10–15 Hz. The percentage of immotile cilia should also be noted.

3. Electron microscopy

This may reveal a structural abnormality.

4. Mucus viscosity

The actual viscosity of the mucus can be measured. A sweat test may be useful in identifying patients with cystic fibrosis.

Decongestant solutions for intranasal use

Must fulfil the following requirements:

1. They must cause vasoconstriction.
2. They must not damage the cilia.
3. They must be both isotonic and faintly alkaline.
4. They should not be followed by rebound congestion.

Ephedrine

Solutions in isotonic saline are widely used. In strengths of 0.5–2% they are in effect decongestants and do not damage the cilia.

Proprietory synthetic vasoconstrictors

In the form of drops or spray. The long-term use of any topical vasoconstrictor applications in the nose may produce a chronic hypertrophic rhinitis ('rhinitis medicamentosa').

Solution for moistening the nose

'AGS' solution (Proetz). When the mucosa is dry:

Alcohol 3%
Glycerin 6% in distilled water.
Sodium chloride 09%

SMELL

The process by which an odorous substance stimulates the olfactory end-organ is not entirely known. Recent evidence indicates that the odour of a substance is related to the shape of its molecules, and to some extent to its molecular vibrations.

Olfactory mucosa

Is described on p. 180

Disturbances of smell

Anosmia

The complete loss of the sense of smell. It must be bilateral before it is noticeable. Loss of olfaction is often described as a loss of 'taste' as flavours are largely perceived through the olfactory apparatus. Medicolegally, tests of smell are important. Being subjective, they may be difficult to interpret. Test solutions, such as lemon, peppermint and cloves, must not be stale. Quantitative tests (Elsberg, Douek) have been described. Ammonia, which stimulates the Vth cranial nerve, may be used when a psychogenic cause is suspected.

Hyposmia

This is a partial loss. It may be qualitative or quantitative, or both. There are several causes:

1. *Nasal obstruction* from polypi, enlarged turbinates, or gross deflections and swellings of the septum. There must be sufficient obstruction to prevent the passage of odours through the 'olfactory cleft'. The oedema and rhinorrhoea of the common cold and in some cases of allergic or vasomotor rhinitis cause temporary anosmia.
2. *'Vasomotor rhinitis'* causes permanent anosmia quite commonly, even in the absence of mechanical obstruction.
3. *Peripheral neuritis* particularly from influenza, in which the symptom is usually permanent.
4. *Atrophic rhinitis* is a degenerative lesion of the nasal mucosa which may involve the olfactory area.

5. *Trauma* especially in basal skull fractures involving the anterior cranial fossa, with tearing of the olfactory filaments. This is likely to be permanent unless recovery has begun within three months of the injury.
6. *Intracranial lesions* may cause compression of the olfactory tracts. They include abscess, tumour and meningitis.
7. *Exposure to noxious gases* e.g. bromine.

Cacosmia

The perception of a bad smell due to some intrinsic cause. Common causes are:

1. Maxillary sinusitis, usually of dental origin.
2. Foreign bodies in the nose.
3. The presence of foetid pus in chronic infections of the middle ear cleft.

Parosmia

A perversion of the sensation of smell or a subjective sensation of non-existent smells. It may be:

1. Functional
2. Organic
● Of central origin, due to:
   (a) Influenzal neuritis.
   (b) Epileptic aura.
   (c) 'Uncinate fits'. In lesions of the temporal lobe of the brain.
   (d) Drugs, e.g. streptomycin, arsphenamine.
● Of peripheral origin, due to:
   (a) Nasal disease, as in the causes of anosmia, above.
   (b) Drugs, e.g. topical applications of tyrothricin.

Theories of smell

Several observers have tried to define different types of olfactory receptors for a limited number of primary odours (e.g. ethereal, camphoraceous, musty, floral, pungent, putrid), and have suggested that all smells can be accounted for by permutations of these primary receptors stimulated to varying degrees. However, this theory has not been substantiated.
Theories of smell can be grouped into two main divisions:

1. Receptor site configuration

Unlikely as there is insufficient variation in site shape to account for the wide range of odours. There is a lack of structural similarity between some substances that smell the same.

2. Molecular vibration

There is a similarity in smell between substances with a close frequency of vibration.

3. *Adsorption*

The molecule is adsorbed onto the receptor membrane which it then penetrates. This penetration causes a local depolarization of a rate, amplitude and duration dependant on the molecular structure of the trigger substance.

It is known that smell is a complex process starting with the stimulation of the olfactory epithelium by air-borne odoriferous molecules. This sets up a transmitted electrophysiological impulse along the olfactory pathways. However, no wholly acceptable theory has yet emerged.

Tests of smell

Test by asking the subject to sniff from simple smell bottles (e.g. coal tar, concentrated essences of coffee or lemon) and to name them if he can. Quantification of the sense of smell – 'olfactory spectrometry' – has a diagnostic potential as yet unrealized in practical clinical work.

Scratch cards are commercially available. These emit an odour when scratched.

Cortical evoked response olfactometry is in development.

FUNCTIONS OF THE PARANASAL SINUSES

The functions of the sinuses are uncertain. There are several theories:

1. *Result of facial development*

After birth the facial skeleton grows at a greater rate than the overlying cranium to allow for increased respiration and mastication.

In certain bones this is attained by the formation of air spaces.

2. *Air conditioning*

The sinuses have been thought to increase the surface area for warming and moistening of the inspired air. There is, however, little air exchange in the sinuses, which also lack 'erectile' tissue in the mucosa.

3. *Lightening of skull*

This is insignificant.

4. *Resonance of voice*

The sinuses are now thought to play little or no part in resonance.

Chapter 10

Diseases of the nose and paranasal sinuses

CONGENITAL MALFORMATIONS

Facial clefts

Deformities result from genetic or teratogenic factors operating in the second month of fetal life. They commonly involve the lip, nose and palate.

Cleft lip

Results from failure of fusion of the maxillary process on one side with the median nasal process. A fissure is present between the philtrum and the lateral part of the upper lip. It may be bilateral so that the philtrum is isolated.

Flattening of the nostril may occur on the side of a unilateral cleft lip, and may be gross in bilateral defects.

Cleft palate

Due to failure of the palatine processes to fuse with each other and with the nasal septum.

Inferior free border of septum may be exposed in severe degrees of cleft palate. The septum is often thickened.

Bifid uvula and submucous cleft represent minor degrees of failure of palatal fusion.

Median cleft of mandible

Occurs occasionally in the midline and may vary from a cleft lower lip to one involving the whole of the mandible and floor of the mouth.

Transverse facial cleft (macrostomia)

May take the form of a crease or fissure and appears on the cheek between the developmental areas of the maxillary and mandibular processes.

Lateral nasal furrow

Occurs rarely, when the maxillary process fails to fuse with the lateral nasal process.

Congenital fistula of the lip

A rare condition in which two fistulae are present, one on each side of the midline in the lower lip.

Hemihypoplasia and hemihyperplasia of face and jaws

Rare developmental abnormalities affecting one side of the face, mouth, and jaws in varying degrees.

Bifid nose

Rarely a midline cleft runs through the tip, bridge, and columella of the nose and divides it into two halves.

Hypertelorism

Crouzon's disease is associated with wide separation of the eyes and may be corrected by craniofacial osteotomy.

Dermoid cysts and sinuses

These are found in the midline, rarely at other sites of fusion.
    Slight swelling only may be present on the bridge of the nose.
    Gross deformity is seen in extreme cases. A fistula is often present.

Treatment

By complete excision by dissection, after excluding a meningocele at this site.

Aplasia of sinuses

Aetiology

Failure of pneumatization, often of frontal sinus, less commonly in sphenoid and maxilla.

Clinical features

Seen radiologically. Antrum impossible to enter with trocar and cannula.

Atresia and stenosis of anterior nares

Aetiology

Atresia is caused by the non-canalization of an epithelial plug between the median and lateral nasal processes. The condition is rare.

Treatment

The web must be excised.

Atresia of posterior nares (congenital choanal atresia)

Aetiology

Said to be due to persistence of the primitive bucconasal membrane.

Types

There are three types:

1. Bony, most commonly.
2. Membranous.
3. Partly bony, partly membranous.

Degrees

1. Complete unilateral atresia, most commonly.
2. Complete bilateral atresia.
3. Incomplete unilateral atresia (choanal folds).
4. Incomplete bilateral atresia.

Pathology

The partition is attached to:

1. Basisphenoid, above.
2. Medial pterygoid plate of sphenoid, on the outer side.
3. Vomer, on the inner side.
4. Hard palate, below.

   Both faces of the partition are covered with mucous membrane. Its thickness may vary from 1 to 10 mm.

   A *central dimple* may be present on the posterior surface of the partition, especially in bilateral cases. Females are more commonly affected than males.

Clinical features

Unilateral atresia

1. Nasal obstruction may not be noticed for some years.
2. Excessive nasal discharge. Characteristically tenacious and 'glue-like' in consistency.

Bilateral atresia

This will usually make itself evident at, or soon after, birth. The symptoms may be urgent and cause death from asphyxia.

1. *Asphyxia.* Two types are described:

- *Cyclical.* Consists of a quiescent period, followed by one of asphyxia. This is relieved by opening the mouth but recurs when it is closed.
- *Suckling.* Symptoms come only when the mouth is closed in suckling.

2. *Nasal discharge*
3. *Delayed symptoms*

- Mouth-breathing.
- Failure to develop taste and smell. These symptoms are noticed in bilateral cases which have survived the earlier dangers without recognition or treatment.

Diagnosis

Can be confirmed by:

1. *Total absence of nasal airflow* ('mirror' test). No condensation occurs on a cold metal surface held close to the nostrils.
2. *Plastic catheter or probe.* Cannot be passed through the nose into the nasopharynx.
3. *Air blown into the nostril* through a closely fitting tube is not heard to enter the pharynx.
4. *CT scan.* The thickness of a bony atresia is seen.
5. *Contrast radiography.* A radiopaque substance instilled into the nose does not reach the nasopharynx.

Treatment

Transpalatal excision

Preferred in all cases, except in the acute emergency of the newborn. It is best performed after early childhood.

The palate is opened by a transverse incision just in front of the posterior edge of the hard palate. The *posterior edge of the vomer* must be removed. *Plastic tubing* is placed through the new opening and left in situ for 6 weeks. *Bouginage may be necessary, at lengthened intervals.*

Transnasal perforation

Simple perforation, with gouge or burr or other perforating instruments, may be required as an emergency procedure in infants, particularly with cyclical asphyxia. A 3 mm endotracheal tube may be modified by two transverse incisions to enter both nasal fossae astride the columella. The ends of the tube lie just in the nasopharynx and are secured by a nylon suture which runs in through the left tube lumen and out through the right tube lumen to form a complete circle. In this way there is an airway and path for suction and the tubes cannot come out until the suture is cut at 6 weeks.

Tracheostomy

To be avoided if possible but may be urgently required: skilled nursing is imperative.

TRAUMA TO NOSE, PARANASAL SINUSES AND JAWS

Patients with maxillofacial injuries may be suffering from other injuries and diseases and thorough general medical examination is essential. Signs of shock and cerebral damage must be sought. It must be remembered that a fractured base of skull coexists not uncommonly with a fractured maxilla. The most important consideration in maxillofacial injuries is the *maintenance of an airway*. All foreign bodies, e.g. broken dentures and teeth, must be removed from the mouth and great care must be taken to see that the patient is not laid on his back, when the tongue may fall back and asphyxiate him. Dentures may later be useful as splints, even if they are broken, and they should therefore not be thrown away.

Fractures of the nose

Aetiology

Usually caused by blows to the front or side of the nose, occasionally by penetrating wounds. The nasal bones may be involved in more extensive injuries of the facial bones and base of skull. The commonest causes are, personal assault, sports injuries, road traffic accident and personal accident.

Classification

Type 1

Due to a frontal or frontolateral blow. There is a vertical fracture of the nasal septum (Chevallet fracture). The thin distal portion of the nasal bone is depressed or displaced.

Type 2

Nearly always due to lateral trauma. The nasal bones are displaced laterally but there is no gross depression. There is a 'C'-shaped fracture of the perpendicular plate of the ethmoid and the quadrilateral cartilage (Figure 10.1). The frontal processes of the maxillae may be fractured.

Type 3

This requires a major blow as the fracture has extended to involve the ethmoid complex (Figure 10.2). There is a marked depression. The perpendicular plate of the ethmoid rotates backwards and the septum collapses into the face turning up the tip of the nose and revealing the nostrils.

Clinical features

1. Deformity

External swelling. Follows quickly. It may be so severe as to obscure the bony deformity.

'Black eye'. Common. The ecchymosis is periorbital and subconjunctival.

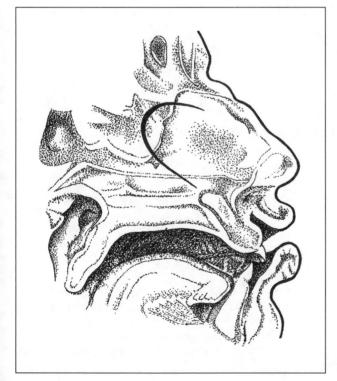

Figure 10.1 Type 2 nasal fracture

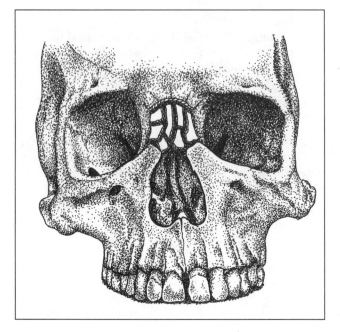

Figure 10.2 Type 3 nasal fracture

2. Pain

Not usually severe after the initial impact but there is marked tenderness.

3. Epistaxis

Frequent.

4. Nasal obstruction

Due to dislocation or haematoma of the septum.

Diagnosis

Radiograph. Important medicolegally, but is of little value clinically.

Treatment

1. Early

If the patient is seen very early, before swelling appears, *reduce immediately*. Local analgesia is often sufficient. Elevation with a pair of closed Spencer Wells forceps under the nasal bones, combined with laterally applied digital pressure, is usually effective in achieving disimpaction and realignment. Walsham's forceps, one blade in the nasal cavity and the other outside, may be needed for disimpaction.

2. Intermediate

When the swelling is marked and the landmarks lost, *leave* until the swelling has subsided.

3. Late (7–14 days)

Probably the most satisfactory time to treat is as soon as the swelling has subsided.

When the swelling has subsided reduction can be undertaken under local or general anaesthesia. The fragments are mobilized with Walsham's forceps when necessary. In many cases they can be replaced by an elevator in the nose.

An external splint may not be required at this stage as the haematoma surrounding the fragments is organizing and forms an internal splint.

In Type 2 fractures there may be difficulty in reduction of the bones due to overlapping of the fractured ends of the quadrilateral cartilage and the perpendicular plate of the ethmoid. If this is the case the septal fracture may need to be excised via a Killian's incision.

In a Type 3 fracture the nasal bones will require elevation. This frequently requires an open reduction and wiring. The septal deformity nearly always requires a septal exploration.

4. Malunion

Requires *rhinoplasty*. This procedure involves refracture of the nasal bones and their separation from the ascending processes of the maxillae and the nasal septum. Bone, cartilage or synthetic implants may also be necessary.

Fractures of the middle third of the face

Definition

Fractures involving that part of the face between the supraorbital ridge and the upper teeth (Figure 10.3).

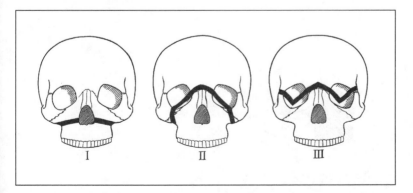

Figure 10.3 Middle-third face fractures. Le Fort's lines of weakness. I is Guérin's fracture. Any of the three types may be unilateral or bilateral

Types

There are two principal types but variations and combinations are encountered.

1. Central (fractures of the nasomaxillary complex)

The fracture line crosses the nasal arch and runs outwards across the medial walls and floors of the orbits and then passes down the anterolateral walls of the maxillae to the pterygoid fossae. This type is due to direct anteroposterior force applied by heavy blows, as in head-on crashes.

Clinical features
- *Collapse of nasal bridge* is usually accompanied by:
- *'Step' deformity* of the infraorbital margin (Le Fort II)
- *Malocclusion.* Floating palate (Le Fort I) or anterior open bite (Le Fort II and III).
- *Soft-tissue swelling* is usually severe and may mask the bony deformities. The eyelids are usually completely closed. Subconjunctival haemorrhage, which may be unilateral or bilateral, produces 'black eye'.
- *Epistaxis* is sometimes accompanied by cerebrospinal rhinorrhoea.
- *Numbness of the cheek* is due to involvement of the infraorbital nerve.
- *Diplopia* is usually transient when it is caused by extravasation of blood into the orbit. Gross misalignment of the bony orbital floor may produce permanent diplopia.
- *Nasal obstruction*
- *'Dish-face'* deformity of the face when the soft-tissue swelling has subsided.

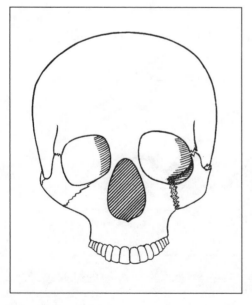

Figure 10.4 Lateral-third face fracture – the malar-maxillary complex

- *Concussion* often accompanies these injuries.
- *Anosmia* is common.
- *Epiphora* occurs when the nasolacrimal duct is involved.

Diagnosis
Radiographs will show the fracture lines. An opaque antrum usually indicates the presence of blood and is not an indication for antral puncture.

Treatment
Reduction is difficult. The displaced bones must be brought forwards with lion forceps and tilted in such a way that the lower rim of the orbit becomes continuous and the bite is normal. In late cases an osteotome may be required to open up the fracture lines for disimpaction.

Splinting is necessary to maintain the position of the replaced fragments. *Dental cap splints* hold together the teeth of the upper and lower jaws. *Metal bars,* attached to the head with a plaster-of-Paris cap, or 'halo', or box-frame with pin fixation to keep the bones forward. *Continuous traction* may be effected by elastic bands or weights suitably attached. This may suffice to effect reduction in some cases.

2. Lateral

Otherwise known as the malar-maxillary complex fracture. This type is due to blows struck from the side. They fracture the malar bone and force it backwards and downwards into the antrum (Figure 10.4).

Clinical features
- *Flattening of malar eminence* may be seen in very early stages.
- *External swelling* soon masks the flattening.
- *'Step' deformity of infraorbital margin* may be palpated.
- *Diplopia* is present in some cases.
- *Trismus* may be due to obstruction to the forward movement of the coronoid process by a zygomatic fragment.
- *Anaesthesia of cheek.*
- *Proptosis.*
- *Diminished visual acuity.*
- *Haematoma of buccal sulcus.*

Treatment
Should be undertaken within 10 days of the injury.
1. In minor cases. The zygomatic arch may usually be elevated through a small vertical incision, through skin and then temporal fascia, above the zygoma. It may also be elevated and the fracture reduced by an intra-oral incision in the buccal sulcus over the tuberosity. This is an excellent method in skilled hands as it allows one not only to elevate the arch but also to see the fracture and, if necessary, to wire it.
2. In severe cases. Reduction is effected by opening the antrum through a sublabial incision and elevating the orbital floor. This is combined with zygomatic elevation. The reduced fragments are kept in position by gauze packing or inflatable balloon in the antrum after creation of an antrostomy.

Fractures involving paranasal sinuses

Maxillary sinus

Involved in the central and lateral fractures of the middle-third of the face described above. May also be involved by a horizontal fracture line which separates the upper alveolus from both maxillae (Guerin's fracture, Figure 10.3).

Occasionally a blow on the eyeball will fracture the orbital floor which then opens into the antrum like a trap door – *burst orbit* or *blow-out* fracture of orbit. The closing trap grips the inferior rectus muscle as the globe rises again into the orbit so as to prevent the upward rotation of the eyeball. Other movements are unimpaired. X-ray tomography helps to confirm the diagnosis. Treatment is to free the caught muscle as soon as possible, and repair the orbital floor.

Ethmoidal labyrinth

Involved in:

1. Fractures of the nasal bones, sometimes.
2. Fractures of the anterior cranial fossa passing through the cribriform plate and/or roof of the labyrinth. *Cerebrospinal rhinorrhoea* follows if the dura is torn. *Meningitis* is the danger if infection follows. *Surgical emphysema* may follow nose-blowing when the lamina papyracea is fractured. *Aerocele* may occur if the dura is torn.

Treatment
consists of:

1. *Systemic antibiotics* to prevent meningitis.
2. *Avoidance of nose-blowing* to prevent surgical emphysema.
3. *Fascial graft* to the site of any dural tear, later, if cerebrospinal rhinorrhoea persists.

Frontal sinus

May be injured by direct violence or by extension of a skull fracture line.

Treatment

1. If the anterior wall is involved alone and there is no deformity, no treatment is required other than systemic antibiotics.
2. If the anterior wall is involved and deformity is present, the fragment must be elevated through a small incision under the eyebrow.
3. If the posterior wall is involved and an intracranial aerocoele is present, a fascial graft must be applied as soon as possible via craniotomy.
4. If the posterior wall is involved and no aerocele is present, it should be left alone.
5. If both anterior and posterior walls are involved and an aerocele is present, it may be necessary to remove both walls and obliterate the sinus.

(Mandibular fractures are discussed on pp. 377–378.)

Cerebrospinal rhinorrhoea

Definition

A flow of cerebrospinal fluid from the nose.

Aetiology

1. *Traumatic* from fractured base of skull involving the anterior cranial fossa, with tearing of the dura mater.
2. *Spontaneous* from destructive lesions involving the floor of the anterior cranial fossa. These are rare causes.

Clinical features

Watery fluid. Drips from the nose. This is the most prominent symptom and sometimes the only one. The fluid contains practically no mucus or albumin and dries soft on a handkerchief. It contains glucose.
Meningitis may supervene and may first bring the condition to notice.

Investigation

The site of the CSF leak is identifiable by radioactive tracer injected into the lumbar CSF followed by wool pledgets placed in the roof of both nasal cavities under general anaesthetic. Each pledget is subsequently measured for radioactivity and the most active pledget indicates the anatomical location. Gamma camera scanning of the head may give an indication as to the site.

A simpler method is placement of "Dextro-stix' in the various sites to look for the glucose in CSF.

Treatment

Immediate

Avoid meningeal infection by:

1. Systemic antibiotics.
2. Avoidance of nose-blowing.
3. Avoidance of any local treatment to the nose, e.g. packing.

Delayed

1. Lumboperitoneal shunt (to reduce CSF pressure) if leak persists for more than 4 weeks.
2. Craniotomy and fascial graft if this fails.
3. Treatment of any causative tumour.

Oro-antral fistula

Definition

A fistula through which the antral cavity communicates with the oral cavity.

Aetiology

The condition may follow:

1. *Dental extraction.* When the fistula forms through the tooth socket. This is an *alveolar fistula.*
2. *Sublabial (Caldwell–Luc or similar) operations.* In which the incision fails to heal. This is a *sublabial fistula.*
3. *Erosion by malignant disease.* Usually from the antrum.
4. *Penetrating wounds of the upper jaw.* Extent of damage proportional to size and velocity of missile.

Clinical features

1. *Discharge in the mouth.* Pus from an infected antrum may be detected in the mouth. In the case of dental infections particularly, this may lead to a complaint of a bad taste in the mouth.
2. *Regurgitation of food particles and air into the nose,* particularly fluids. The playing of wind instruments is rendered impossible.
3. *Symptoms of maxillary sinusitis* occur frequently.
4. *A probe* can be passed into the antrum from the mouth.
5. *Prolapse of antral lining* may occur.

Treatment

1. With a very *small alveolar fistula,* the epithelial lining of the fistula is scraped away with a burr, curette, or cautery as first line of treatment, but it often fails. When a fistula is recognized at the time of dental extraction an immediate suturing of the gum over the fistula often heals by first intention under antibiotic cover. If the root lies in the antrum it must be removed by a Caldwell–Luc operation, or through the tooth socket.
2. With a *sublabial fistula,* the rim of the fistula must be excised. The mucosal edges are then undercut and stitched carefully.
3. With a *larger alveolar fistula,* the opening may be closed with a flap from the palate or buccal mucosa after excision of the fistula and adequate reduction of the bony alveolus. The tooth socket fistula is a rigid bony track. At least the outer half of its circumference may need reduction (unless the buccal flap is generous) to allow the tissues of the alveolus to fall in and obliterate it in late cases. The making of a naso-antral opening (antrostomy) allows drainage into the nose and permits lavage. It is preferable to have a dental plate ready for immediate postoperative use, to protect the suture line.
4. Penetrating wounds. Residual defects with fistula, after emergency surgery, may be repaired together with facial reconstruction, using skin grafts.

Bullet wounds

Missiles may cause any or all of the above injuries. A cavity many times the missile diameter forms when the velocity is high. Shock waves cause damage distant from the path, passing along and ploughing up the intima of the carotid artery for example. Suction draws in organisms from the skin.

Principles of treatment

1. Establish airway.
2. Ligate major vessels, excise devitalized tissue.
3. Fix facial skeletal elements in a position of function.
4. Close by primary suture where possible or graft. (Delayed closure is advocated in other sites, but the blood supply of the face is so good that delay is not needed.)

Barotraumatic sinusitis

Definition

Pathological changes in the sinus mucosa due to lowering of the pressure within the sinus compared with that of the surrounding atmosphere.

Aetiology

The usual cause is descent in non-pressurized aircraft in the presence of valvular obstruction of the sinus ostium. Flying with an upper respiratory infection predisposes.

Pathology

1. Congestion and inflammation of the lining membrane.
2. Oedema and effusion.
3. Mucosal or submucosal haemorrhages.

Clinical features

Pain is felt during descent (sometimes ascent) in aircraft. It may be severe in either:

1. Frontal region.
2. Cheek.

Treatment

Preventive

Avoidance of flying with upper respiratory infections or obstruction, particularly by polypi. Septal deviation may be a relevant factor and require operation.

Symptomatic

1. Analgesics and sedatives.
2. Decongestant nasal drops to free the ostium.
3. Treatment of allergies or infections and their products, e.g. polypi.

Septal deflections and spurs

General considerations

Few adults have a completely straight septum. Only gross deflections causing mechanical obstruction give symptoms or require correction.

Aetiology

Trauma is by far the commonest cause of a septal deformity requiring surgical correction. Compression of the nose during birth may initiate it in some cases.

Errors of development produce either bending or spurs. The position of the fetus in utero may have an influence on these deformities. The developing septum buckles because it grows faster than its surrounding skeletal framework. The condition is often seen in conjunction with a high-arched palate. This narrows the floor of the nasal fossa transversely, thereby increasing the obstruction.

Pathology

Deflections may involve cartilage and/or bone.

1. *Simple.* A single curve to one side, usually involving the cartilage only.
2. *Sigmoid.* A double bend.

Spurs are isolated thickenings, often found at the junction of bone and cartilage. These are sometimes elongated. Drainage may be impeded by deflections or spurs so predisposing to sinusitis and maintaining it. Spurs may also predispose to epistaxis from vessels on their convex surfaces.

Thickening is frequently seen in cases due to trauma, when overriding of dislocated fragments results in reduplication of the cartilaginous layers.

Clinical features

Nasal obstruction is the presenting symptom.

External deformity results in some cases.

Pressure headaches possibly result from contact of the deflected septum with structures of the lateral wall of the nasal fossa.

Nose bleeding may occur, especially from a prominent vessel over a bony spur.

Treatment

1. *No treatment* is needed in minor degrees of deflection without obstruction.
2. *Submucous resection (SMR)* is usually performed in adults. Very satisfactory results are obtained when the symptoms are those of a purely mechanical obstruction. It consists of the removal of deflections or spurs of cartilage or

bone from between the two coverings of mucoperichondrium and/or mucoperiosteum. Pieces of the cartilage may be replaced between the flaps, to give
stiffness, when a large amount has been removed.
3. *Septoplasty.* A more elaborate technique to remodel the septum, conserving,
but straightening the cartilage and bones. This may be combined with rhinoplasty (septorhinoplasty). The conservative principles of septoplasty are especially appropriate for septal deformities demanding correction in children.

Haematoma of septum

Definition

A collection of blood beneath the mucoperichondrium or mucoperiosteum
of the septum.

Aetiology

The condition is nearly always traumatic in origin. It may be due to:

1. Direct blows or falls on the nose, especially in children.
2. Operations on the nose, e.g. after SMR.
3. Blood dyscrasias, rarely.

Clinical features

Nasal obstruction is usually bilateral and often complete.
Septal swelling is soft and sometimes red.

Complications

1. *Septal abscess and cartilage necrosis* are due to secondary infection.
External deformity such as saddling results.
2. *Permanent thickening of the septum* may be caused by fibrosis.

Treatment

1. *Simple aspiration* may suffice when the haematoma is small. It may have
to be repeated.
2. *Incision and drainage.* Drainage can be maintained by inserting a drainage-
tube or by excising a small 'square' of mucoperichondrium on one side.
3. *Nasal packing* will prevent further oozing of blood beneath the mucoperichondrium.
4. *Systemic antibiotics* to prevent secondary infection.

Abscess of septum

Aetiology

Traumatic. An abscess is usually secondary to haematoma.

Spontaneous. May follow measles or scarlet fever, and may complicate nasal furunculosis.

Clinical features

Pain may be severe and throbbing.
Nasal obstruction is often complete.
Pyrexia will usually distinguish abscess from haematoma.
Symmetrical swelling of septum. This is commonly of a dull purplish colour. It is tender.

Complications

1. *External deformity* may result from cartilage necrosis.
2. *Perforation of septum* follows sloughing of the mucous membrane and cartilage.
3. *Meningitis and cavernous sinus thrombosis* are rare.

Treatment

1. *Incision and drainage* as for haematoma, urgently.
2. *Systemic antibiotics.*
3. *Plastic surgical correction of deformities* may be required later.

Perforation of septum

Aetiology

Traumatic

This is the commoner type.
1. *Septal operations* may be followed by perforation, if there are openings in the mucoperichondrium of both sides opposite to one another. Repeated cauterization can also result in perforation.
2. *'Pick ulcer'* results from picking off an ulcerated area of the septum, in the young and the old.
3. *'Chrome perforation'* is an occupational condition, seen in some chromium-platers. It is caused by erosion by acid fumes. Certain chrome salts are known to be carcinogenic.
4. *'Snuff-taker's perforation'* may occur in tobacco or in cocaine addiction.
5. Foreign bodies, safety pins, ornaments, etc., placed deliberately through the septum.

Pathological

This may be due to:
1. *Lupus.* The perforation is surrounded by thick, pale granulations. Lesions are usually present on the face.
2. *Syphilis.* Now rare. Involves the bony septum particularly. Other manifestations are present.

3. *Haematoma or abscess of septum.*
4. *Malignant (non-healing) granuloma and periarteritis nodosa (Wegener's granulomatosis).* Must always be suspected in absence of an overt cause.
5. *Rhinitis sicca and rhinitis caseosa* are rare causes.
6. *Pressure* of neglected nasal polypi, foreign bodies, or rhinoliths.

Idiopathic

The perforation may be discovered by chance without any history of trauma or previous disease.

Clinical features

Irritation in the nose is commonly the first, often the only, symptom.
Crusts may be blown away or picked off from the exposed cartilage in the unhealed edges of the perforation.
Epistaxis follows separation of the crusts.
Whistling is sometimes caused by smaller perforations.
Pain and foetor are present in the active stage of a gumma.
Site of perforation. The perforation is usually in the bony part of the septum in syphilitic cases, in the cartilaginous part in all other cases.

Investigations

Should include biopsy, serological tests for syphilis, and sedimentation rate or plasma viscosity.

Treatment

In many cases, no treatment is required.
   Alkaline douche and narist. Glucose 25% in glycerine. Will often loosen the crusts and make their expulsion easier.
   Chlorhexidine cream 0.5% may be applied after separation of crusts.
   Fused silver nitrate may be applied to bleeding granulations.
   Closure may be effected in smaller perforations. Sliding mucoperichondrial flaps are used for these plastic procedures.
   Removal of exposed cartilage allows healing of the marginal mucosa in larger perforations.

Foreign bodies in nose

Aetiology

Foreign bodies are much more common in children. They may enter the nose by several routes:
1. Through the anterior nares, most commonly.
2. Through the posterior choanae. Food may enter during an attack of vomiting.
3. Through penetrating wounds.

Pathology

Anything small enough to pass the anterior nares may be pushed into the nose. Foreign bodies may be organic or inorganic. Paper, beads, buttons and pebbles are common. Swabs or cotton-wool pledgets may be left accidentally. Bony sequestra may be found, particularly in syphilitic disease or neoplasm. An inflammatory reaction quickly follows impaction and is accompanied by a discharge.

Clinical features

A history of the introduction of a foreign body may not be obtained, especially in very young children.

1. *Unilateral nasal discharge,* usually foul-smelling, is the characteristic symptom. Foreign bodies are rarely bilateral.
2. *Nose bleeding* may occur.
3. *Pain* may occur soon after introduction but usually subsides quickly.
4. *Sneezing* may follow the immediate irritation and may expel the foreign body.
5. *Foreign body* is commonly found on, or near, the floor of the nasal fossa. It is often obscured by inflammatory exudate and may remain hidden for many years. A radiograph will confirm if the foreign body is radiopaque.

Treatment

Removal is the only treatment. Forcible nose-blowing may expel the foreign body. If this fails, it must be removed under direct vision through the anterior nares. This should be done under general anaesthesia in young children, with a pack in the nasopharynx. It is sometimes necessary to push it into the nasopharynx before retrieval.

Rhinoliths

Definition

Nasal concretions formed around a foreign body, blood, or mucus.

Aetiology

1. *Foreign bodies.* The commonest cause (exogenous).
2. *Blood clot or inspissated pus.* May become surrounded by concretions (endogenous).

Pathology

Rhinoliths may be friable or hard, and are sometimes multiple. They are greyish, brown or black in colour. The concretion is formed of phosphates and carbonates of calcium and magnesium, often arranged in concentric layers.

Clinical features

1. *Nasal discharge.* Usually unilateral. It may be mucoid or mucopurulent and is commonly foetid. It may also be bloodstained.
2. *Nasal obstruction.* Usual.
3. *Rhinolith.* Commonly lies on, or near, the floor of the nasal fossa. It is radiopaque and can be detected by a probe.

Treatment

Removal. Through the anterior nares under general anaesthetic. It may be necessary to break a rhinolith and remove it piecemeal. Rarely, a lateral rhinotomy may be required.

INFLAMMATIONS OF THE NOSE

Acute and chronic nasal inflammation result from:

1. *Infection,* both viral and bacterial.
2. *Allergy and vasomotor rhinitis.*
3. *Physical and chemical trauma* including rhinitis medicamentosa (iatrogenic).

These aetiological factors are frequently combined and the clinical picture is coloured accordingly. Only those caused predominantly by infection are considered in this chapter.

Inflammations of the external nose

The skin covering the external nose is subject to those inflammations affecting the skin elsewhere.

1. Furunculosis

Furunculosis of the nasal vestibule is an acute staphylococcal infection of a pilosebaceous follicle in the vestibule.

Clinical features

1. *Pain.* As the inflammation spreads into the subcutaneous tissues an intensely painful indurated swelling presents in the vestibule and usually at the tip of the nose. This becomes tender, red and unsightly.
2. *Headache* may be present.
3. *Evacuation of pus* normally occurs spontaneously in 4 or 5 days. the furuncle pointing in the vestibule in most cases.

Treatment

Systemic antibiotics. Flucloxacillin, erythromycin or cephalexin are 'first-choice' drugs.

Complications

1. *Cavernous sinus thrombosis.* Resulting from spreading thrombophlebitis, via the angular and superior ophthalmic veins.
2. *Cellulitis of upper lip* (and sometimes abscess of the septum): Particularly if the furuncle is in the floor or inner wall of the vestibule.

2. Non-specific infective nasal vestibulitis

This is a dermatitis in the nasal vestibule, secondary to a nasal discharge. It may be acute or chronic.

Aetiology

In the presence of infection. the following are aetiological factors:

1. *Irritation and maceration:* Produced by the rhinorrhoea.
2. *Trauma:* From picking with the finger or rubbing with a handkerchief.

Clinical features

1. Induration, excoriation, and painful fissures affect the nasal vestibule in the acute form. Painful fissures persist in the chronic form.
2. The upper lip may be similarly involved.

Treatment

Treatment is that of the cause of the nasal discharge. A simple ointment, e.g. petroleum jelly, may act as a protective barrier. A cream containing chlorhexidine and neomycin is useful to eliminate local infection. 'Naseptin' or chlorhexidine cream is helpful in staphylococcal carriers.

3. Erysipelas

Erysipelas is an acute spreading streptococcal dermatitis.

Clinical features

1. A red swollen area' with irregular but sharply defined margins. The inflammation tends to spread outwards on to the face and the eyelids become oedematous.
2. Congested, haemorrhagic, nasal mucosa.
3. Pyrexia.
4. Lymphadenitis.
5. Marked constitutional disturbance.

Treatment

1. Systemic penicillin.
2. Ichthammol dressings. May relieve the pain.

4. Impetigo

This is an acute contagious staphylococcal dermatitis which forms crusts. These may extend into the vestibules. This condition, common in children, is unaccompanied by constitutional upset. Treatment is by systemic or local antibiotic.

5. Rhinitis

Acute or chronic specific forms of rhinitis may involve the external nose.

6. Miscellaneous conditions affecting the external nose

1. *Eczematous and seborrhoeic dermatitis* as in the corresponding conditions of the external ear, a secondary infection may obscure the underlying pathology. The treatment is similar to that of the aural condition.
2. *Acne rosacea* which may progress to rhinophyma.
3. *Lupus erythematosus,* with a characteristic 'butterfly wing' extension on to the cheeks.
4. *Pernio* (chilblain) of the nasal tip.
5. *Sycosis barbae* spreading from the upper lip.
6. *Herpetic lesions* due to herpes simplex or herpes zoster of the fifth cranial nerve.
7. *Pemphigus*
8. *Sarcoidosis, syphilis and lupus vulgaris.* See pp. 228–233.

Inflammations of the nasal cavities

The term *rhinitis* implies an inflammation of the mucosa of the nasal fossae. Owing to the continuity of the mucosa of the nasal fossae with that of the sinuses, some degree of inflammation is often present in the latter at the same time, so constituting a *rhinosinusitis.* When the inflammation of the sinus is primary or overshadows that in the nasal fossae the condition is termed *sinusitis.*

Acute rhinitis

1. The common cold (coryza)

Aetiology

A virus infection, which is conveyed by contact or airborne droplets. Usually complicated by a secondary bacterial infection.

Pathology

Transient ischaemia of the mucosa is followed by *swelling, hyperaemia* and *profuse secretion* of clear seromucinous fluid. The rhinorrhoea becomes mucopurulent later, owing to the rapid growth of the resident flora of the nose, which appear to be activated by the virus infection. The *organisms* found include:

Streptococcus haemolyticus
Pneumococcus
Staphylococcus
Haemophilus influenzae
Klebsiella pneumoniae
Branhamella catarrhalis

The pathogenic respiratory viruses include:

1. Influenza viruses.
2. 'Picorna' viruses comprising:

- Coxsackie virus.
- Reovirus.
- ECHO virus.
- Rhinovirus – most frequent cause of common cold.

3. Respiratory syncytial viruses (bronchitis in children only).
4. Para-influenza viruses (mainly in children).
5. Adenoviruses (mainly affecting pharynx).

Clinical features

Vary greatly. Four stages may be distinguished:

1. *Ischaemic stage.* After an incubation period of 1–3 days, a *burning sensation* is experienced in the nasopharynx. The nasal mucosa irritates, *sneezing* occurs, and the patient feels chilled (*shivering*). Sense of smell is altered or lost.
2. *Hyperaemic stage.* In a few hours, *profuse rhinorrhoea* and varying degrees of *nasal obstruction* ensue. *Pyrexia* is common.
3. *Stage of secondary infection.* As secondary infection and leucocytic invasion occur, the *discharge* becomes *yellow* or *green*. It also thickens, owing to a high mucin content, and will stiffen a handkerchief.
4. *Stage of resolution.* Resolution occurs in 5–10 days.

Differential diagnosis

1. *Allergic rhinitis and vasomotor rhinitis* are often described by the patient as a 'cold', but the rhinorrhoea is characteristically spasmodic and the condition is apyrexial.
   The discharge remains clear, does not stiffen a handkerchief, and may contain an excess of eosinophils unless secondarily infected.
2. *Influenzal rhinitis* in which the constitutional symptoms are much more severe.

Complications

Secondary infection may spread throughout the mucosa and lymphatic tissues of the whole respiratory tract, including the middle ear cleft.

Treatment

1. *Prophylactic.* Contact with known cases must be avoided. Vaccines for prevention have not been widely effective.
2. *Therapeutic*
General treatment consists of:

- Rest and warmth. Ideally the patient should stay in bed.
- Analgesics. Codeine, aspirin and alcohol are of value.
- Pseudo-ephedrine by mouth relieves congestion.
- Antihistamines and vitamin C are of doubtful value.
- Antibiotics should be reserved for the treatment of secondary infective complications.

Local treatment consists of:

- Inhalation of steam. Comforting. Tinct. Benzoin Co. or menthol may be added but is not essential.
- Vasoconstrictors. In the form of drops or sprays, give quick but temporary relief from the nasal obstruction. They should not be abused.

2. Acute rhinitis associated with influenza and the exanthemata

This differs little from that of a common cold, except for the presence of the associated disease, of which it is usually a prodromal feature. It may, however, be very severe and even purulent. Complications are apt to follow and may be serious.

3. Special forms of acute infective rhinitis

These are rarely seen.

1. *Diphtheria.* Sometimes causes a *membranous rhinitis,* which occurs either primarily or secondarily to the disease in the throat. In some cases the symptoms may be so slight that the patient is not treated and becomes a carrier.
2. *Erysipelas.* May extend from the external nose to infect the mucosa.
3. *Rare acute infections.* Include glanders, anthrax and accidental vaccinial inoculation.

Chronic rhinitis

1. Non-specific chronic infective rhinitis

Several types are described:

(a) Simple chronic rhinitis

Aetiology
Attacks of acute rhinitis in rapid succession, and the maintenance of the acute inflammatory condition by one or more of the many predisposing and contributory factors. These include:

- *Neighbouring infections* such as: sinusitis, chronic tonsillitis, adenoids.
- *Vasomotor rhinitis.* The resultant obstruction predisposes to chronic infection.
- *Chronic irritation* as from dust, smoke, tobacco, snuff and the abuse of therapeutic vasoconstrictors. Polluted atmosphere, as by overcrowding. Sudden and extreme changes of temperature. Excessive dryness or humidity.
- *Nasal obstruction* leading to retention of discharge, e.g. deviations of the septum and intranasal adhesions.
- *Metabolic factors* which include imbalance of diet, as by excess of carbohydrate and by deficiency of vitamins. Endocrine disorders, especially of the thyroid. Lack of exercise and sunlight, alcoholic overindulgence, or gout.

Pathology

- *Chronic hyperaemia* of the nasal mucosa, accompanied by inflammatory cellular infiltration and sometimes chronic oedema.
- *Swelling of inferior turbinates* due to engorgement of the cavernous spaces (sinusoids) in the submucosa. The epithelium tends to lose its cilia and the goblet cells increase.
These changes are reversible.

Clinical features

- *Nasal obstruction.* Marked, variable and usually alternates from side to side. On change of posture the dependent side blocks as the inferior turbinate swells.
- *'Postnasal drip.'* A clear, viscid secretion trickles into the nasopharynx, to descend into the pharynx. This tends to become mucopurulent as infection increases.
- *Nose-blowing and hawking*
- *A blocked or heavy feeling in the nose.* Common, with mild headache and mental apathy.
- *Transient anosmia*
- *The mucosa.* Red if infection is active, mauve when venous stasis is marked, pale and oedematous at other times. Strands of mucus stretch across the nasal fossae, especially from the inferior turbinates.

Diagnosis
A history of recurrent attacks of acute rhinitis and the presence of predisposing factors are suggestive. The soft, swollen mucosa over the inferior turbinates pits with a probe and shrinks with a 5% solution of cocaine. If morning sneezing is frequent the condition is likely to be associated with vasomotor rhinitis. An excess of eosinophils in the mucus suggests nasal allergy. Chronic infective sinusitis must be excluded by radiographs.

Treatment
- *General.* Correction of any predisposing factors, where possible, e.g. tobacco, alcohol or contact with persons suffering from colds. Change of habitat.

● *Local.* A slightly alkaline nasal douche used night and morning to remove sticky mucus.

Mild vasoconstrictors, used as sprays, paints or drops, usually of 1–2% ephedrine preparations, to which an antibiotic may be added. Such treatment must not be prolonged. Topical steroids, as spray or drops will help in some cases.

Treatment of any sinusitis or other adjacent infection.

(b) Hypertrophic rhinitis

Aetiology
The condition represents an advanced stage of simple chronic rhinitis, in which permanent hypertrophic changes have followed. The causes are similar, but it is frequently seen also in patients who have used topical decongestants in large quantities and/or for long periods ('rhinitis medicamentosa').

Pathology
● *Permanent hypertrophic changes* accompany the inflammatory oedema and cellular infiltration in all the constituent parts of the mucosa, i.e. stroma, glands, blood vessels, and lymphatic tissues. The epithelium loses cilia and shows a tendency to squamous metaplasia. The mucosa becomes thick and nodular, especially at the extremities and free border of the inferior turbinate. At the posterior end a *mulberry-like enlargement* may occupy the posterior choana.
● *Fibrosis* can cause venous and lymphatic obstruction. If the resulting passive oedema occurs in a situation where the mucosal stroma is loose, *polypi* may form. Nasal polyposis, however, usually indicates an allergic or vasomotor origin of the rhinitis, in which the polyposis results from increased capillary permeability.

Clinical features
Similar to those of simple chronic rhinitis but are unremitting in character. Pitting of the firm mucosa with a probe and shrinkage with cocaine are less marked than in simple chronic rhinitis.

Treatment
As for simple chronic rhinitis, with the addition of *limited reduction of the hypertrophied inferior turbinates and removal of any polypi.* Topical decongestant preparations must be discouraged or discontinued. Reduction is achieved by:

● Electrocoagulation, by submucosal diathermy or linear cauterization by galvanocautery.
● Cryosurgical probe.
● Surgical trimming of the hypertrophied free border. Reduction of the anterior ends is sometimes sufficient. Amputation of an enlarged posterior end may be necessary. Avulsion or total removal of the inferior turbinate may be performed, but a persistent crusting can result.

(c) Atrophic rhinitis

Definition
A chronic inflammation of the nasal mucosa, in which its various constituents undergo atrophy as a result of periarterial fibrosis and endarteritis of the terminal arterioles.

Aetiology
The exact aetiology is not fully known but its incidence has markedly decreased in Western Europe. Besides infection, other factors such as *undue patency of the nasal airway* and possibly *endocrine or vitamin disturbances* may play apart.

Types
1. *Primary atrophic rhinitis* (ozaena). Possibly the sequel of a rhinitis associated with an exanthema in childhood. The process may have passed through a hypertrophic stage before becoming atrophic, perhaps after a long interval. A familial variety has been described.

Pathology
Degeneration of the ciliated epithelium and seromucinous glands causes the formation of thick adherent crusts in the nose. These become secondarily infected with saprophytic organisms. The bony structures of the turbinates atrophy and the airway is widened. The sinuses may be small due to arrested pneumatization but are often normal. There appears to be a tendency to spontaneous recovery in later life in some cases.

Clinical features
The condition, now seldom seen, is bilateral and more common in females. It appears about puberty. The *foul stench* is not noticed by the patient, who is anosmic.
Epistaxis may follow separation of the crusts.
   A *sensation of obstruction* is experienced, despite the unduly wide airway. Similar atrophic changes may be seen in the pharynx and larynx.

Differential diagnosis
Crusting from sinus suppuration is accompanied by other features of sinusitis. In secondary atrophic rhinitis, evidence of the causal condition is present. Syphilis must be excluded.

Treatment
Removal of the crusts is best achieved by syringing with warm isotonic solutions.
   Glucose 25% in glycerin drops prevent adherence of fresh crusts and inhibit saprophytic infection.
   Local or systemic antibiotics can be used initially, as indicated by the sensitivity of the organisms isolated.
   Several measures have been used in an attempt to increase the glandular activity and blood supply of the atrophic mucosa and to narrow the airway. These include *potassium iodide* therapy, *endocrine preparations* (such as stilboestrol locally or systemically), *surgical measures* to reduce the calibre of the airway (by submucosal insertion of grafts, Teflon paste submucosal

injections) and to form adhesions between the septum and the infractured lateral nasal walls; *moistening of the mucosa* has been attempted, by diverting Stensen's duct into the antrum.

Complete surgical closure of the nostrils for periods of several months has given striking improvement in the state of the mucous membranes.

2. *Secondary atrophic rhinitis.* Destruction of the nasal mucosa and subsequent healing are associated with fibrosis of the submucosa and metaplasia of the ciliated epithelium. These changes occur as a result of:

- *Deviated septum,* when severe, may be responsible for atrophic rhinitis in the wider nasal fossa.
- *Syphilis.*
- *Lupus*
- *Excessive operative procedures.* Especially on the inferior turbinates.

(d) Rhinitis sicca

A rather ill-defined crusting condition, affecting the anterior third of the nasal cavities of patients who work in dusty surroundings.

Periglandular fibrosis and *metaplasia* of the ciliated epithelium result in a viscid and stagnant mucus blanket which forms *crusts.* These are not foetid but are sometimes bloodstained and may lead to a *septal perforation.*

There is no generalized atrophic change or any increase in calibre of the airway.

Treatment is by correction of occupational surroundings and lubrication by sprays, paints, or ointments, applied to the affected area.

(e) Rhinitis caseosa

A rare condition in which cheesy material enters the nose from a sinus, usually the maxillary antrum. It possibly results from failure of resolution of a sinusitis, when contents inspissate and the lining mucosa becomes granulomatous. The bony wall of the sinus becomes eroded and the *foul cheesy debris* is extruded into the nose. The cranial cavity may be invaded from the sphenoid. A foreign body may initiate the process.

Treatment
By *removal of the mass of debris and granulation tissue,* with free *drainage* of the affected sinus. Biopsy of the granulations is essential, to exclude malignant disease.

(f) Wegener's granulomatosis

An autoimmune disease involving areas in the lungs, subglottic region, kidneys, sclera, nasal cavity and ears. In this form periarteritis nodosa and giant-cell formation are seen in the granulation tissue.

Other features include splinter haemorrhages, flitting arthritis and granulomas in the skin. There is a high plasma viscosity and in many cases the antipolymorpholeucocytic antibody test is positive.

Treatment

Large doses of steroids which are later reduced as the clinical condition improves and as the very high sedimentation rate subsides. High dose cyclophosphamide given intravenously has been used with good results. Oral cyclophosphamide or azathioprine can be used for maintenance therapy. Antibiotics for the secondary infection. Secondary complications such as renal failure are treated expectantly.

Prognosis

This has been much improved by the administration of steroids, and high dose cytotoxic therapy holds additional promise.

(g) Gangosa

A slow and painless ulceration, clinically resembling yaws, but of unknown aetiology. The geographical distribution includes the Pacific Islands, Equatorial Africa and Sri Lanka. Serological tests are negative. Starting on the palate to perforate the nose, it sometimes destroys much of the face. Though not responding to antibiotic therapy, it is not usually fatal.

(h) 'Malignant granuloma' (Lethal midline granuloma, Stewart's granuloma)

Rare. Originally thought to be a granulomatous disease this has now been classified as a histiocytic lymphoma. It causes rapid localized destruction of the nose and facial tissue. Treated by radiation and chemotherapy.

2. Specific chronic infective rhinitis

(a) Syphilis

Two forms:

Congenital

Two forms are distinguished:
1. *Early form.* Up to the third month.
   'Snuffles' is the name given to the commonest nasal manifestation. This is a rhinitis which rapidly becomes purulent.
   Fissuring and crusting of the vestibule and lips are caused by the irritating discharge, so that suckling may be prevented. Occasionally necrosis of bone and cartilage occurs.
2. *Late form* (third year to puberty). *Deformities* similar to those in the tertiary stage of acquired syphilis result from gummatous infiltration of the nasal mucosa and subsequent destruction of the nasal framework. Other stigmata affecting the eyes, teeth, and ears may be present.

Acquired

Three stages are distinguished:

1. *Primary stage.* Onset 3–6 weeks after contagion.

Chancre. Rare in the nose and appears as a hard painless papule in the vestibule or on the adjacent septum. It soon ulcerates to form a 'sore' which has been likened to a painless furuncle. The submaxillary and preauricular glands are disproportionately enlarged but painless.

2. *Secondary stage.* Onset 6–9 weeks after contagion.

Persistent coryza. The presenting symptom in the nose. Mucous patches are rarely distinguishable on the nasal mucosa, but they may be seen in the mouth and pharynx. A generalized lymphadenitis and a roseolate rash are usual accompaniments.

3. *Tertiary stage.* Onset usually 1–5 years after contagion. A *gumma* of the nose is the commonest nasal manifestation of syphilis. Usually starting in the periosteum of the septum, it soon causes a *perforation.* When the nasal bones are involved, the bridge sinks *('saddleback' deformity).* Less often the nasal floor may be perforated by a gumma, while the lateral walls are rarely affected. The external nose may also be attacked, when the alae, columella and adjacent upper lip are destroyed.

Nasal obstruction and headache, the latter worse at night, are the earliest symptoms.

Before ulceration, a nasal gumma presents as a non-pitting rubbery swelling, which is reddish-purple in colour. May be diffuse or localized, and is accompanied by a *mucoid rhinorrhoea.*

After ulceration, there is *crusting* and a foul bloodstained discharge. The ulcer has a sloughy ('washleather') base in which dead bone or fragments of necrotic cartilage may be detected. The overlying soft tissues of the face may become swollen and tender and even break down in advanced cases.

Diagnosis

Confirmation depends upon identification of *Treponema pallidum* in smears from primary and secondary lesions. Serological tests are negative in the primary stage but positive in 90% of others. Biopsy. Trial therapy.

Treatment

General antisyphilitic treatment by systemic penicillin. Nasal toilet, as by irrigation with warm hydrogen peroxide (10 vol). In 'snuffles', suction followed by instillation of 1% ephedrine solution may render suckling possible.

Sequelae

Healing may result in vestibular stenosis, secondary atrophic rhinitis, perforations of the palate and septum, and deformities of the external nose.

(b) Yaws (framboesia)

Possibly a form of syphilis, as it also exhibits three stages and is caused by a treponema indistinguishable from *T. pallidum* and has similar serological reactions. Occurs in the tropics and is conveyed by extragenital cross-infection in childhood. Nasal lesions are not common. Treatment is that for syphilis, though the bilateral swellings caused by chronic osteitis of the nasal bones *(goundou)* should be excised.

(c) Lupus vulgaris

Aetiology
Caused by the inoculation of tubercle bacilli of low virulence, probably as the result of nose-picking. The source of infection is frequently a member of the family suffering from pulmonary tuberculosis.

Pathology
Large mononuclear ('epithelioid') cells of the reticulo-endothelial system mass round the bacilli and fuse to become multinucleated *'giant' cells.*

Collections of these form a *'tubercle'.* These tubercles appear as nodules, which ulcerate and become covered by crusts. Being avascular, they undergo coagulative necrosis in their centres *(caseation).*

Clinical features
Chronic unilateral vestibulitis is the presenting picture. It is more common in young women.

'Apple-jelly' nodules are seen through a glass slide pressed on the skin lesions. May also be demonstrated on the mucosa by spraying it with cocaine solution.

Ulceration may involve any part of the nose, also the pharynx; the lacrimal apparatus is liable to be infected.

Perforation of the septum in its cartilaginous part. The face is often involved and may be primary to the nasal infection.

Diagnosis
Biopsy confirms the diagnosis.

Treatment
Calciferol (vitamin D2) 150 000 units daily, for 3–6 months. This is usually combined with a course of antituberculous drugs (rifampicin, ethambutol, INAH, streptomycin, and PAS in planned schedules for long-term therapy). Healing is by fibrosis so that deformities occur and these may require plastic surgical procedures.

(d) Tuberculosis

Aetiology
1. *Miliary spread,* from a focus in the lungs.
2. *Fingernail inoculation,* in the predisposed tuberculous patient.

Clinical features
1. *Tuberculoma* occurs on the cartilaginous portion of the septum.
2. *Ulceration and perforation of the septum* follow, and spread to the nasal floor and inferior turbinates. Nasal tuberculosis is much rarer than laryngeal tuberculosis.

Treatment
Treatment is that of the lung condition, and includes the use of long-term antituberculous drugs (rifampicin, ethambutol, INAH, streptomycin, PAS).

(e) Sarcoidosis

Histological appearances are similar to tuberculosis, except for the absence of caseation. Mantoux test is negative. Kveim test is sometimes positive.

The disease may be widely distributed in the body–lungs, salivary and lymphatic glands, skin and uveal tract being often affected. In the nose it presents as *nodules* on the *septum* and in the *vestibules*. Spontaneous recovery is usual. Tuberculosis of the lungs has been known to follow in some cases.

(f) Chronic diphtheritic rhinitis

A fibrinous chronic rhinitis due to *Corynebacterium diphtheriae*. Seen very occasionally in debilitated children. Toxaemic and paralytic symptoms are absent. Treatment is by systemic antibiotics and nasal toilet. Antitoxin is unnecessary. Isolation should be enforced.

(g) Scleroma

A chronic infection of the respiratory tract, especially of the nose. Thought to be due to *Klebsiella rhinoscleroma*, an organism similar to *Klebsiella pneumoniae*. Mode of infection is unknown. Occurs mainly in Central and Eastern Europe and in Central and South America. Greatly increased travel facilities, however, have resulted in a few isolated cases being seen in the UK.

Pathology
Granulomatous tissue infiltrates the submucosa and is characterized by the presence of:

1. Large foam cells *(Mikulicz cells),* containing bacilli in the vacuoles.
2. *Russell bodies.* Plasma cells with eosinophil-staining cytoplasm and prominent nuclei.

Infiltration starts at the vestibulonasal junction, to encircle the nasal fossae and spread posteriorly.
Atrophic degeneration follows. After a massive proliferation the granuloma slowly undergoes dense fibrosis, leading to stenosis or atresia.
Adhesions may form, but ulceration occurs only with secondary infection.

Clinical features
Young adults are principally affected. Lymphadenitis and constitutional signs are absent. Three stages are distinguished:

1. *Atrophic stage.* There is nasal obstruction, associated with crusting, discharge and some adhesions.
2. *Tumefactive stage.* With formation of soft, red, tumour-like masses in the nasal fossae. The external nose and lip may become bulbous by subdermal extension.
3. *Cicatrizing stage.* An unyielding concentric stenosis of the fossae takes place over the years, and nose is dry.

Treatment
Streptomycin and the tetracyclines, combined with steroid drugs, have given good results after several month's administration.

Prognosis
Good for life, but plastic repair may be necessary.

(h) Leprosy

An extremely chronic tropical infection due to *Mycobacterium leprae*. Occurs in Asia, Africa and in Central and South America.

Pathology
M. leprae are conveyed to the septum by the fingernail. Initial coryza causes sneezing and discharge teeming with *M. leprae*. This is the infectious stage of the disease.

After an interval of up to 10 years, a nodular thickening develops at first on the septum. The nodules show a perivascular cellular infiltration of the tissues which includes vacuolated giant cells and bacilli in parallel bundles.

Untreated progressive ulceration goes on with subsequent destruction of the nose. Palate and larynx may be involved.

Ulceration of the skin is painless because of nerve involvement causing analgesia.

Treatment
By rifampicin, clofazimine and dapsone for long periods.

(i) Rhinosporidiosis

An infection by a sporozoön, *Rhinosporidium kinealyi or Rh. seeberi*. It occurs in India, Sri Lanka and Africa.

Clinical features
A *bleeding raspberry-like polypus* of the nasal mucosa is the presenting sign.

Pathology
The sporangia are scattered in the vascular, fibromyxomatous tissue of the polypus. These are oval or round chitinous cysts, full of spores, which burst through the germinal pore of the cyst.

Treatment
Radical removal of the polypus and diathermy to the area.

(j) Nasopharyngeal leishmaniasis

A granuloma occurring in South America. The parasite is transferred to exposed parts by the sandfly and a nodule develops which ulcerates and then heals with scarring. Years later other ulcers appear about the mouth and nose and spread to destroy the face, though the bones escape, leading to death if untreated. The parasite is found in the discharge. Treatment is by intravenous antimonials.

(k) Aspergillosis

Occurs very rarely in the nasal fossa compared with the ear.

Clinical features
A *black or grey membrane* lines the nasal cavities. A *musty-smelling discharge* is present. Infections of the sinuses and bronchi have been recorded.

Treatment
The condition yields to repeated cleaning and local application of 1% aqueous solution of gentian violet. Amphotericin B may be given systemically if absolutely necessary.

(l) Actinomycosis and blastomycosis

These are very rare.

(m) Candidiasis (thrush)

The presence of *Candida albicans* is rare in the nose compared with the mouth. It is predisposed to by debility in the very young and very old but is more common as a sequela of antibiotic therapy. A *white plaque* is surrounded by a *red areola*. It is removable. Applications of 1% aqueous solution of gentian violet or nystatin may be made locally; alternatively, amphotericin B may be given systemically in severe cases.

(n) Histoplasmosis and sporotrichosis

Rarely encountered in the nose.

INFLAMMATIONS OF THE PARANASAL SINUSES

Inflammations may be restricted to a single sinus or may be present in several (multisinusitis) or in all of one or both sides (pansinusitis, unilateral or bilateral). Acute and chronic non-specific infections occur with the production of either suppurative or non-suppurative forms. A sinusitis is said to be 'closed' if the contained inflammatory exudate cannot escape, either through the viscosity of the exudate or through closure of the ostium by oedema. It is said to be 'open' if ciliary action and overflow permit escape of the exudate. Specific infections are rare.

Acute non-specific infective sinusitis

Aetiology

1. *Acute infective rhinitis* generally due to a 'cold' or influenza. The infection spreads to the sinuses by way of the submucosal lymphatics and/or surface spread through the ostium, assisted by sneezing and nose-blowing. The discharge from one sinus can infect another in the same way. Rhinitis is the commonest cause of acute sinusitis.
2. *Swimming and diving* may similarly cause direct spread through the ostium.
3. *Dental extraction or infection* may cause infection to enter the maxillary antrum from a dental root.

4. *Fractures involving the sinuses* may be followed by sinusitis either through direct spread of infection through the fractured bony walls or through infection of a blood clot in the sinus.

5. *Barotraumatic sinusitis* may occasionally become secondarily infected.

6. *Predisposing factors* include:

(a) Local
- *Nasal obstruction* from any cause.
- *Obstruction of the sinus ostium* especially by nasal polypi, vasomotor and allergic swellings, rarely by a tumour.
- *Neighbouring infection,* e.g. tonsillitis and adenoids.
- *Previous infection* in the same sinus.

(b) General
- *Debilitation.*
- *Mucociliary disorders.*
- *Immunodeficiency.*
- *Irritating atmospheric conditions.*

Bacteriology

The causative organisms, in order of frequency, are: Pneumococcus, Streptococcus, Staphylococcus, *Haemophilus influenzae, Klebsiella pneumonae.*

The latter two organisms are sometimes found in pure culture in epidemics.

E. coli and anaerobic streptococci are associated with sinusitis of dental origin.

Pathology

The inflammatory changes in the mucosa of the affected sinuses include:

1. *Hyperaemia.*
2. *Oedema.*
3. *Cellular infiltration.*
4. *Increased mucus production.*
5. *Exudation* is *serous* at first but, with increasing intensity of the infection, it becomes purulent, so that an empyema results. Sometimes resolution occurs before suppuration whilst other cases proceed to a state of chronicity. A sinusitis may progress even though the initiating nasal infection is subsiding.

Acute maxillary sinusitis

Maxillary sinusitis is the commonest of all sinus infections to present as a single *clinical* entity (though not necessarily as a pathological one). The origin of the infection may be either nasal (90%) or dental (10%).

Acute maxillary sinusitis of nasal origin

Diagnosis
Pain in the cheek. It is frequently referred to the region of the frontal sinus, temporal region, or upper teeth.

Tenderness also over the cheek. It is not present over the orbital roof unless a frontal sinusitis coexists.

Oedema of cheek is rare, except in children.

Discharge in the middle meatus or postnasal space in 'open' sinusitis may be evident only after cocainization. Spontaneous evacuation of the sinus contents into the nose may occur suddenly, especially on bending down.

Radiographs are helpful They will usually show an opacity or a fluid level, and also supply additional information about the other sinuses.

Constitutional symptoms include pyrexia, malaise and mental depression.

Special local treatment. The sinus is irrigated, by puncture through the inferior meatus, with isotonic saline, after the invasive stage has passed, if response to medical treatment is tardy. This is repeated as necessary.

Intranasal antrostomy. Needed urgently in closed infections failing to respond to antibiotics.

Acute maxillary sinusitis of dental origin (Figure 10.5)

There are three types:
1. *Following dental extraction.* The sinus may be opened during extraction of the premolar or molar teeth or their root stumps. The bone between the socket and the sinus can be so thin that it inevitably comes away on the apex of the root. The tooth or root stump may sometimes be pushed into, and

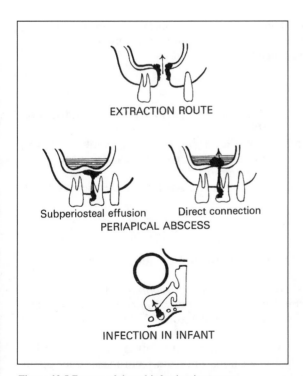

Figure 10.5 Routes of dental infection in antrum

retained in, the sinus. There is no history of a preceding rhinitis but one of dental extractions.

2. *Following apical abscess.* Of the premolar or molar teeth. This may cause an inflammation of the overlying sinus mucosa so that effusion and suppuration follow. Caries of the intervening bone may provide direct communication between the abscess and the sinus. The toothache due to an apical abscess may be slight. A root-filled or dead tooth with abscess can be painless.

The *pus* in these two types is characteristically *malodorous,* owing to the anaerobic and saprophytic organisms associated with dental disease. *Cacosmia* is usual.

Treatment is by irrigation of the sinus and general therapy, as in suppuration of nasal origin. A tooth or root retained in the sinus should be removed as soon as convenient, by a sublabial approach. This must be combined with intranasal drainage. If perforation without retention of the root is noted during extraction, immediate suture of the gum and systemic antibiotics usually suffice.

3. *In acute dental sac infection in infancy.* This rare condition is probably preceded by injury. An osteomyelitis of the upper jaw occurs, with swelling of the alveolus and hard palate. Empyema of the maxillary sinus follows. Treatment is by systemic disinfection and drainage of any collection of pus. Sequestra or dead tooth buds are removed later.

Acute frontal sinusitis

Usually associated with an infection of the homolateral anterior ethmoidal cells, and often of the maxillary sinus. The tortuous front nasal duct is easily obstructed by oedema of the mucosa.

Special clinical features

1. *Frontal headache* may be severe. It is usually periodic, in that it starts soon after waking and subsides in the afternoon.
2. *Extreme tenderness* to pressure on the orbital roof, at a point internal to the supraorbital notch. Percussion of the anterior sinus wall is painful.
3. *Oedema of the upper lid* is not uncommon.
4. *Discharge* is seen in the high anterior portion of the middle meatus, when the infection is 'open'.

Special local treatment

Concomitant maxillary sinusitis must be treated by antral lavage. This may avoid the need for a frontal trephine.

In severe cases, the sinus cavity is entered by *trephining* the orbital roof, just internal to the supraorbital notch, after confirmatory radiography. The sinus mucosa, and especially that of the frontonasal duct, is undisturbed except at the point of entry.

The insertion of a small plastic tube allows intermittent irrigation with a 0.1% ephedrine solution in isotonic saline, until the frontonasal duct opens and the solution appears in the nose clear of pus.

Catheterization of the duct is difficult and may cause trauma to the duct. It is not recommended.

Acute ethmoiditis

Though very commonly involved with other sinuses an infection of the ethmoidal labyrinth seldom produces a separate clinical entity in the adult.

Special clinical features

1. *Pain between the eyes.* Accompanied by frontal headache.
2. *Discharge.* In the middle and superior meatus, from the ostia of the anterior and posterior group of cells respectively.

Special local treatment

Usually none is necessary. The treatment of any acute infection in the larger sinuses commonly procures resolution in the ethmoids.

Acute sphenoiditis

Though usually occurring as part of a pansinusitis, it is particularly associated with infection of the posterior ethmoidal cells. It is rare.

Headache may be vertical, frontal, occipital, or central, or it may be referred to the temporal region, when it simulates the pain of a mastoiditis.

Discharge is not seen by anterior rhinoscopy. Posterior rhinoscopy discloses the discharge on the superomedial surface and posterior end of the middle turbinate; it also streams down the roof and posterior wall of the nasopharynx.

Special local treatment

Lavage of a coexisting antral infection may clear the sphenoidal infection. *Catheterization of the ostium* may be needed in severe cases for aspiration and lavage. If the ostium is not found easily, the face of the sphenoid may be punctured.

Differential diagnosis of acute sinusitis

1. *Pain of dental origin.*
2. *Migraine.*
3. *Trigeminal neuralgia.*
4. *Neoplasms of the sinuses.*
5. *Erysipelas.*
6. *Temporal arteritis, angioneurotic oedema and insect bite.*
7. *Herpes zoster.*

Principles of treatment of acute sinusitis

1. *Treatment of the infection.* Systemic penicillin is nearly always effective. A sample must be sent. In severe infections, while awaiting sensitivities,

ampicillin and flucloxacillin will cover most organisms. In infection of dental origin metronidazole should be added.

2. *Treatment of the pain:*

● *Analgesics.* Such as Tab. Codeine Co. or paracetamol.
● *Local heat.* As by radiant heat, hot water bottle, or steam. Short-wave diathermy may hasten resolution in the subsiding stage and is often comforting. It must not be used in the acute stage.

3. *Establishment of drainage* may be effected by:

● *Decongestant solutions.* Such as 0.5 or 1% ephedrine in normal saline, used either as drops or spray.

A solution of 5% cocaine (with adrenaline 1 in 10 000) is a powerful vaso-constrictor but should not be used repeatedly.

These solutions aim at reducing the swelling of the nasal mucosa, especially in the region of the sinus ostium.

● *Irrigation* of the acutely infected sinus, preferably after the invasive stage. General anaesthetic is usually advisable. The local application of antibiotics into the sinus cavity appears to have no advantage.

Simple chronic non-specific suppurative sinusitis

Aetiology

Follows single or repeated attacks of acute sinusitis without other complicating disorders of the nasal mucosa of an intrinsic nature. It is a diagnosis of exclusion in which nasal allergy, vasomotor rhinitis,and hormonal dysfunction have been ruled out.

Pathology

Every stage from a hypertrophic change (even including polypus formation) to one of an atrophic character may be found at one and the same time.
The pathological processes include:

Oedema, which ranges from slight thickening of sinus mucosa to gross polyposis.
Chronic inflammatory cellular infiltration.
Fibrosis of the submucosal stroma supervenes on the inflammatory changes of the acute infection. Venous and lymphatic compression augment oedema.
Multiple small abscesses in the thickened mucosa.
Epithelial metaplasia and glandular hypertrophy are frequent.
True cyst formation may also occur from fibrotic compression of the glands.
Ulceration of the epithelium results in the production of true granulation tissue.

Bacteriology

The organisms are usually mixed, streptococci, often including some anaerobic ones, being commonest. Pneumococci may also be found. *B. proteus, Ps. pyocyanea,* and *E. coli* are often secondary invaders.

Clinical features

The clinical features of chronic suppurative infections of the various sinuses are similar to those of the acute forms which they follow, but are of a lesser degree. Acute exacerbations are apt to occur, but in the intervals the symptoms may be reduced merely to the presence of a nasal or postnasal discharge. *Postnasal or nasal discharge* is usual and may be frankly purulent or merely mucoid (clinically non-suppurative).

Nasal obstruction of varying degrees.

Headache is caused by obstruction to drainage or exacerbations of the infection. It is often described as a heavy feeling in the head, or as merely a dull ache over the sinus affected.

Anosmia may be present, or even a marked *cacosmia,* especially in infections of dental origin.

Constitutional disturbances are usually mild, but may include malaise, anorexia and mental apathy. Sore throat, cough, and eustachian tube dysfunction are common secondary effects.

Principles of treatment

Decongestants. Long term use of topical decongestants should be avoided. Oral decongestants may be of value.

Systemic antibiotics. With particular regard to the mixed nature of the infection. Local disinfection of the nose or even direct instillation into the sinus has no advantage over systemic therapy.

Chronic maxillary sinusitis

Special local treatment

1. *Irrigation by repeated puncture.* Through the inferior meatus. An indwelling tube may be useful in a child for intermittent irrigation but holds no advantages in the cooperative adult.
2. *Intranasal antrostomy* is effective if the case is of short duration and has failed to resolve after several irrigations.
3. *Sublabial antrostomy* (Caldwell–Luc operation) is indicated in long-standing cases or where the above methods have failed.

The sublabial approach allows free removal of grossly diseased mucosa and the making of an opening into the inferior meatus under direct vision.

Chronic frontal sinusitis

Some cases can be controlled without resorting to surgery on the frontal sinus itself, provided that any coexisting infection in the maxillary sinus is eradicated. In the event of failure of these measures, an operation is required to establish adequate drainage or to obliterate the sinus. Minor procedures, such as reduction or in-fracture of the middle turbinate, are of doubtful value. Intranasal operations on the frontonasal duct may be dangerous, and postoperative cicatrization often makes them insufficient. Thus an external approach to the frontal sinus is preferred.

Special local treatment

1. Operations to provide drainage include:

● *Howarth's operation.* The incision curves round the inner margin of the orbit.

The floor of the sinus is removed and the ethmoidal cells and frontonasal duct are exenterated, so that a wide opening replaces the duct. Diseased membrane only is removed. Loculations in the sinus are laid open, including any horizontal extensions over the orbit, and a search is made for a perforation in the intersinus septum or posterior wall.

The passage into the nose is maintained for several weeks postoperatively by a wide-bore drainage tube placed between the sinus and nasal cavities before closure of the incision.

● *Patterson's operation.* The incision is made about one finger's-breadth *below* the inferior orbital margin. In most cases this approach enables the maxillary sinus to be dealt with at the same time as the frontal and the ethmoidal sinuses.

2. Operations to obliterate the sinus

● Mucosal stripping. If Howarth's operation is combined with scrupulously complete removal of every vestige of mucosa from the sinus and duct, it is possible for them to become obliterated by the formation of fibrous tissue and new bone.
● *Removal of anterior wall and floor.* More frequently the operation is extended to remove the anterior sinus wall and allow the soft tissue to come into contact with the posterior sinus wall after the mucosa has been removed. The resulting deformity may be corrected 6 months later by subcutaneous inserts of bone, cartilage, or fat.
● *Osteoplastic flap.* The anterior bony wall of both frontal sinuses is lifted as an osteoplastic flap. The outlines of the sinuses are marked by superimposing an X-ray film and the sinus is entered along these limits. A coronal forehead incision is used and the bony flap is fractured at the supraorbital rim. The virtues of this approach are its cosmetic advantage, both frontal sinuses can be inspected simultaneously, and supratrochlear and supraorbital nerves are not endangered by the incision.

Chronic ethmoiditis

Special local treatment

1. *Intranasal exenteration of ethmoidal labyrinth.* Dangerous because of a poorly visualized operational field and the proximity of the cribriform plate and optic nerve.

2. *Horgan's operation.* Via the maxillary sinus. The posterior cells are easy of access, but a supplementary intranasal approach is often necessary to ensure opening of the anterior cells. Infected anterior ethmoidal cells often escape attention.

3. *Ferris Smith's operation.* Via the inner wall of the orbit (lamina papyracea and lacrimal bone) as part of an external fronto-spheno-ethmoidectomy

4. *Patterson's operation.* An approach which starts at the inner part of the orbital floor, to enter the antrum, after identification of the nasolacrimal duct, and then extends inwards to the ethmoidal cells and (if necessary) upwards to the frontal sinus.

Chronic sphenoiditis

Operations on the sphenoidal sinus are usually part of a combined operation for a multisinusitis.

Special local treatment

1. *Via the maxillary sinus.* As an extension of the Horgan operation. The posterior ethmoidal cells are traversed to reach the sphenoid.

2. *Via an external ethmoidectomy.* Through the inner orbital wall. This is to be preferred if the frontal sinus is involved.

3. *Direct intranasal attack.* On the sphenoidal face, or an intraseptal approach as an extension of submucous resection of the septum. These operations are rarely used.

Complex infective chronic sinusitis

Aetiology

Secondary infection results from chronic obstruction of the ostium. The bacteriology is the same as in the simple chronic infective form. In addition there is at least one of the factors listed below.

1. Smoking.
2. Vasomotor and allergic rhinitis.
3. Nasal polyposis.
4. Myxoedema or other endocrine disorder.
5. A congenital or inherited mucociliary disorder.

Pathology

The condition represents a combination of the changes due to simple chronic infection upon a chronic vasomotor or allergic state. It is commonly a bilateral pansinusitis.

Mucosal oedema is caused by increased capillary permeability, which leads to gross thickening of the mucous membrane.

Polypi are often present.

Turgescence of erectile tissue, particularly of the inferior turbinates.

An excess of eosinophils occurs in the mucous membrane and in the discharge when allergy is present, but may be masked by the polymorphonuclear leucocytes caused by infection.

There is a degranulation of mast cells due to the presence of infection and allergic mechanisms.

False cysts are sometimes formed by distension of the intracellular spaces in the submucosa. They may be large enough to fill a whole sinus cavity (cystic polypus).

Clinical features

The onset is usually insidious but may be dated by the patient from an acute sinusitis. The condition is usually bilateral and tends to affect all the sinuses, but the antra and ethmoids are those whose symptoms usually predominate.

Nasal and postnasal discharge varies in character and amount. It may be clear and mucoid (as when infection is minimal) or frankly purulent.

Anosmia is common due to obstruction.

Asthma, eczema and hayfever may be found in the personal or family history. Skin prick tests and nasal smears looking for eosinophils are suggestive of allergy when positive, but a negative result does not exclude a hypersensitivity. Response to trial therapy with antihistamines may point to an allergic origin.

Principles of treatment

Treatment of the infection. As for simple chronic sinusitis.
   Treatment of the vasomotor or allergic state by:

1. Avoidance of precipitating factors, where possible.
2. Antihistamine therapy.
3. Topical steroid drops or sprays.
4. Desensitization when applicable. Anaphylaxis may occur.
5. Correction of any endogenous corticosteroid or thyroxine deficiency.

Indications for surgery

1. *To control the infection* by removing chronically infected tissue and by providing efficient drainage.
2. *To remove polypi* from the nose and from their sites of origin in the sinuses. Removal of the entire polypus-bearing area (most commonly in the ethmoids) ensures a greater chance of their permanent elimination.
3. *To remove other manifestations of vasomotor or allergic component* in the sinuses, if producing symptoms. These include:

● Recurrent cysts.
● Collections of thick, gluey, mucoid material which may completely fill the sinuses.

Operative procedures

Minimal surgery for the provision of an adequate airway, as by removing polypi and reducing enlarged turbinates, or by SMR when the septum is deflected.

Radical surgery such as fronto-ethmo-spehoidectomy with a Caldwell–Luc procedure. Indicated for gross infection, especially in cases of previous operative failure, or for excessive and recurrent polypi. The infective and allergic factors must each be assessed and provided for in planning treatment.

Prognosis

The vasomotor or the allergic factor often renders treatment by surgery unsatisfactory. Other manifestations (e.g. asthma) may continue or appear subsequently.

Specific infections of the paranasal sinuses

These are rare. The treatment is as for similar specific infections of the nose.

Tuberculous and syphilitic infections

These involve the sinuses only as a direct extension of nasal disease.

Fungal infections

Particularly those due to aspergilli in the maxillary sinuses, only common in immunosuppressed patients, i.e. receiving cytotoxic therapy or whole body radiation with marrow replacement. They may be treated with evacuation and drainage operations and antifungal packs or irrigations. Amphotericin B and 5-fluorocytosine systemically are used. Actinomycosis requires massive penicillin therapy. Craniofacial mucor mycosis is usually terminal in the immunodeficient.

SINUSITIS IN CHILDREN

Aetiology

1. Systemic factors

(a) Allergy.
(b) Antibody deficiency (rare).
(c) Endocrine factors.
(d) Mucociliary dysfunction such as mucoviscidosis or Kartagener's syndrome.
(e) Heredity.

2. Environmental factors

(a) Dietary deficiency.
(b) Social deprivation.
(c) Lack of ventilation.

3. Local causes

May be classified as:

(a) Intranatal. By infection contracted during passage through the birth canal.
(b) Neonatal. Due to infection from the mother or others at a time of physiological antibody deficiency.
(c) In older children. Viruses play an important role but are hard to find in
chronic cases. The bacteriology shows a mixed infection, but a pneumococcus
is usually present.

4. Clinical causes

These include:

(a) Repeated colds. The commonest cause. They usually result from contagion at school, but a primary allergic or vasomotor basis with secondary
infection is frequent.
(b) Influenza, whooping-cough, scarlet fever and measles are other causes.
(c) Swimming may initiate it in older children.
(d) Dental sac infections, though rare, may lead to maxillary sinusitis in
infants.
(e) Adenoids commonly maintain a sinus infection in a state of chronicity.

Pathology

The maxillary and ethmoidal sinuses are the usual sites, the frontal sinus
being poorly developed before the fifth year. After 10 years of age the condition is similar to that in the adult. Non-suppurative cases are more common
than suppurative

Clinical features

1. *Acute sinusitis.* The general and local features tend to be more pronounced
than in the adult. Oedema of the eyelids and cheeks is not uncommon.
2. *Chronic sinusitis.* Chronic nasal obstruction is associated with a discharge
(usually mucopurulent), mouth-breathing, snoring, and coughing and sometimes early morning vomiting. Pain is unusual. The child is frequently
apathetic and dull.

Diagnosis

Radiography and proof-puncture (under general anaesthesia) will confirm
the diagnosis. A nasal foreign body must be excluded.

Treatment

1. *Acute sinusitis.* Will usually respond to non-operative treatment, but irrigation of the maxillary sinus is occasionally required.
2. *Chronic sinusitis.* General treatment (including anti-allergic measures if
required) will usually suffice, together with decongestant nasal drops.

Attention to general hygiene is of paramount importance. In the absence of complications no surgery may be necessary. In other cases the introduction of a polythene tube into the maxillary sinus by means of a cannula, for intermittent irrigation can be helpful. Infected tonsils and/or adenoids should be removed. Dental causes must be treated.

COMPLICATIONS OF SUPPURATIVE SINUSITIS

Spread of infection beyond the bony walls of the sinuses is uncommon. It is most frequently seen during an acute exacerbation of a chronic suppurative infection.

Modes of spread of infection

Direct spread

Through the bony wall, by:

1. *Osteitis.* In compact bone (caries).
2. *Osteomyelitis.* In diploic bone.
3. *Osteoporosis.* Ethmoidal polypi may cause dehiscences in the lamina papyracea or the floor of the anterior cranial fossa.
4. *Accidental or surgical trauma.* Via fracture lines, from a sinus infected before or after the injury.

Venous spread

By way of:

1. *Septic venous thrombosis.* This occurs in the diploic veins during an osteomyelitis.
2. *Thrombosis in minute veins in sinus mucosa.* Spreads to the small veins in the periosteal layer of the dura mater and so leads to the production of meningitis, thrombosis of intracranial venous sinuses, and infection of the brain.
3. *Septicaemia and pyaemia.* Represent further stages of venous spread.

Lymphatic spread

Perivascular lymphatics convey the infection through the vascular foramina to form subperiosteal abscesses.

Spread via perineural spaces

Of the olfactory nerves, to the subarachnoid space.

Complications

Osteomyelitis

Aetiology

Infection of the frontal sinus is the usual cause of this (now) uncommon condition. It rarely follows infection of the other sinuses. Streptococci and staphylococci are the organisms most commonly responsible. They may be anaerobic. It is most frequent in young adults.

Pathology

Entry of infection into the marrow spaces occurs by direct or venous spread. It is often precipitated by trauma or operation on the anterior wall of the frontal sinus especially in the absence of prophylactic systemic antibiotics.

Spreading thrombosis occurs in the diploic veins. The larger veins (of Brechet) may explain the apparently isolated areas of the disease found in the frontal bone.

Subperiosteal abscesses form extracranially and *extradural abscesses* form intracranially. *Sequestration* occurs later. Thrombosis of venules crossing the suture line allows the whole calvarium to be affected.

Clinical features

1. *Dull local pain and headache* occur at the onset, which is insidious.
2. *An oedematous area* arises on the forehead, often a short distance above the upper limit of the frontal sinus. This is a *Pott's puffy tumour.*
3. Spread to other areas is either continuous or intermittent. Toxaemia and intracranial complications are common.

Diagnosis

Radiographs show loss of bone pattern after a week or two, but a spreading area of necrosis with sequestration can be seen later, usually above the frontal sinus. The bony sinus wall may be seen to be breached.

Treatment

1. *Prophylaxis* is by *antibiotic cover* at operations, particularly on the frontal sinus.
2. *Treatment of early cases.* When associated with an acute frontal sinusitis, these cases can often be controlled by intense and appropriate *systemic antibiotics.*

No operation is needed, other than *irrigation of the maxillary sinus* and possibly simple *trephining of the frontal sinus floor.* In cases associated with chronic sinusitis, the offending sinus can be opened and drained whilst a trial of antibiotic therapy is given.

3. *Radical surgery* is indicated if improvement is tardy or unsatisfactory, if sequestration is present, or if intracranial complications threaten.

A coronal incision from ear to ear allows the frontal sinuses to be approached from above. Infected bone and sequestra are removed and careful inspection is made of the underlying dura mater. The resultant deformity may require correction by plastic surgery. In young patients the bone defect may regenerate spontaneously and rapidly.

Orbital complications

Aetiology

All the sinuses enter into the boundaries of the orbit. Here the walls are thin and are liable to be eroded by an osteitis. Orbital infection is uncommon but is seen most frequently in children as a result of *ethmoiditis.*

Pathology

Caries of the lamina papyracea or the floor of the frontal sinus causes an orbital *cellulitis,* with or without the formation of a subperiosteal *abscess.* Pus easily lifts the periosteum from the bone in an anterior direction and points through the lids. The periosteum is a strong barrier but, if penetrated, the globe may be destroyed. Thrombophlebitis of veins between the sinus and the orbit forms an alternative route of infection. Further spread to the cavernous sinus is a possibility.

Clinical features

1. *Pain referred to the eye* may be only slight but is aggravated by eye movements.
2. *Chemosis* may close the lids.
3. *Proptosis* may result from oedema of the orbital contents even without orbital abscess.
4. *Diplopia* results from displacement of the globe by the expanding subperiosteal abscess or oedema. Eye movements may be restricted.
5. *Fluctuation* is difficult to elicit.
6. *Engorgement of the retinal veins* is the only change seen in the fundus.

Differential diagnosis

1. *Dacryocystitis.* Presents as a swelling deep to the medial palpebral ligament, in the absence of a sinusitis. Pus leaks through the canaliculus.
2. *Cavernous sinus thrombosis.* There is early paralysis of the eye muscles and marked fundus changes. It tends to be bilateral.
3. *Mucocele.* There is a long history of a painless swelling and an absence of acute symptoms. The swelling is fluctuant after erosion of the bone. 'Eggshell cracking' may be felt.
4. *Simple intra-orbital cyst.* Slow growing and painless.
5. *Osteoma.* Which is hard, painless, and of long duration. The radiological appearances are characteristic.

6. *Malignant orbital tumours.* When rapidly growing, may cause difficulty. These tumours are painless. Radiography and biopsy are required to establish the diagnosis.

7. *Erysipelas of the eyelids.* Distinguished by the characteristic appearance of the skin lesions, the absence of sinusitis, and the tendency to a bilateral distribution.

Treatment

Antral lavage is imperative. Further action may be required for:

1. *Cellulitis* which will usually respond to intensive systemic antibiotics. Failure suggests abscess formation.

2. *Subperiosteal abscess.*

- In children, an orbital abscess due to ethmoiditis is difficult to distinguish from cellulitis. An emergency CT scan will show if pus has formed. Drainage is then essential and performed through the inner part of the upper lid.
- When the abscess arises from an acute frontal sinusitis, both sinus and abscess should be drained by supraorbital incision.
- Orbital abscess or oedema from chronic sinusitis requires radical operation on the sinus.

Prognosis

Complete recovery of eye function is to be expected. Retrobulbar neuritis is very rarely, if ever, attributable to sinus suppuration except in association with cavernous sinus thrombosis.

Intracranial complications

These are all described under Neurological Diseases (see p. 545). They include:

1. *Pachymeningitis,* with or without *extradural* or *subdural abscesses.*
2. Leptomeningitis: serous or purulent, localized or diffuse.
3. *Thrombophlebitis* of the cavernous sinus, sagittal sinus, and frontal cortical veins.
4. *Brain lesions:* note that infections of the individual sinuses show a tendency to be associated frequently with particular intracranial lesions.

- *Frontal sinusitis* leads to frontal lobe abscess, via an osteitis of the posterior sinus wall (adhesions may protect the subarachnoid space) or to cortical vein thrombosis, via spreading thrombosis of venules crossing the subarachnoid space.
- *Ethmoidal sinusitis* can cause diffuse suppurative meningitis, via a perforation near the cribriform plate.
- *Sphenoidal sinusitis* can cause diffuse suppurative meningitis, and thrombosis of the cavernous and other venous sinuses. Both of these occur via thrombophlebitis of the diploic venules in the sinus wall.
- *Maxillary sinusitis* rarely causes any intracranial lesion. When spread does occur it is via the venous route from the pterygoid plexus.

Secondary effects of suppurative sinusitis

1. *Infection in the nasopharynx.* May cause or aggravate:

- *Lateral pharyngitis and tonsillitis,* sometimes limited to the side of a single infected sinus.
- *Otitis media,* both acute and chronic.
- *Laryngotracheitis.*
- *Bronchitis,* especially common in children with sinusitis.

2. *Association with bronchiectasis.* The relationship between bronchiectasis and sinusitis is not fully understood but there is a common cilial fault in Kartagener's syndrome and a mucus one in cystic fibrosis. One certainly aggravates the other. Irrigation of the sinuses should precede any chest operation.

3. *Association with asthma.* When asthma is associated with chronic infective-allergic sinusitis, a radical sinus operation may improve the asthma temporarily, but recurrence is common.

Asthma may be 'triggered off' for the first time after operation as part of the natural progress of the allergic state. In the absence of gross infection, surgery should be limited to the removal of obstructing polypi.

4. *Focus of infection.* A chronic sinus infection may occasionally act as a focus of infection at distant sites, but such a relationship is much more doubtful than was previously supposed. There are, however, a few conditions which do sometimes respond to the elimination of a suppurative sinusitis. These include infective polyarthritis, tenosynovitis and 'fibrositis', and certain skin diseases.

TUMOURS AND CYSTS OF THE NOSE, PARANASAL SINUSES AND JAWS

Benign tumours

These are all fairly common. They may arise from epithelial, connective, or neural tissue.

Epithelial-tissue tumours

Papilloma

1. *In the nasal vestibule.* Singly as a small sessile or pedunculated 'wart' or in the multiple form. After excision, the base should be treated with cautery or diathermy, to prevent recurrence. Carcinoma must be excluded by histological examination.

2. *In the nasal fossae and paranasal sinuses.* Epithelial papillomatous tumours (transitional cell or inverted papilloma). Gross thickening of the epithelial surface leads to infolding but the basement membrane remains intact. In the same tumour there can be areas of columnar, squamous, or

transitional types of epithelium. A malignant change occurs in about 3% of cases. It is a rare tumour and usually occurs in men over 50. The commonest site is on the lateral wall of the nasal cavity and/or in the antrum and ethmoids. It may be multicentric. Obstruction is the presenting symptom. The tumour should be removed *in toto* – this usually requires a lateral rhinotomy. Recurrence suggests malignancy.

Adenoma

Rare. Remains encapsulated and is frequently symptomless, but it may cause nasal obstruction. May become malignant (as an adenocarcinoma) and can be compared clinically with mixed salivary tumours (pleomorphic adenoma).

Odontome

See p. 260.

Connective-tissue tumours

Fibroma

Rare. The *turbinates* and *septum* are the commonest sites. Usually remain small and cause no symptoms other than slight *nasal obstruction* and occasional slight *epistaxis*.

Osteoma

There are two main types:

1. *Localized compact osteoma* occurs most commonly in the *frontal sinuses*. Probably arises from periosteal tissue and may be sessile or pedunculated. It is ivory-hard in consistency but may have a small area of cancellous bone in the centre.

Clinical features
Symptoms become evident most often in young adults, but many of these tumours remain small and symptomless and are only discovered on radiographic examination. *Displacement of the eye* is sometimes caused by expansion of the affected sinus by the tumour. *Empyema* or *mucocele of the sinus* results from obstruction of the frontonasal duct. Pressure atrophy of the wall of the anterior cranial fossa predisposes to cerebrospinal rhinorrhoea and intracranial infections. *A dense bony mass with well-defined edges* is seen on radiography. A large osteoma may completely fill the sinus.

Treatment
Removal is required only if symptoms develop. The approach to an osteoma in the frontal sinus may be through the floor of the sinus or by way of a cranial approach with an osteoplastic flap if a portion lies in the anterior cranial fossa, in which case a fascial graft will be required to obviate leakage of cerebrospinal fluid.

2. *Localized cancellous osteoma* occurs most commonly in the maxillary and *ethmoidal sinuses*. It is usually slow-growing but may increase rapidly in size

in the younger patient. Osteoid tissue is frequently found in fibromas and chondromas.

Fibrous dysplasia

Pathology
May not be a true neoplasm. The swelling consists of irregular *spongy subperiosteal bone with a thin cortex* and an ill-defined edge, unlike that of a true benign neoplasm. The lesions may be monostotic or polyostotic. The mandible and maxilla may both be involved in polyostotic lesions, but they are more commonly the site of monostotic lesions. There are two forms involving the sinuses:

1. *Diffuse.* Involving several of the facial and cranial bones. This must be distinguished from Paget's disease which occurs in older persons and always involves the cranial and/or long bones as well as those of the face.
2. *Localized.* Involving the maxillary and ethmoidal bones. This type may be difficult to distinguish from other bony tumours without a biopsy. A small swelling may be confused with a fibroid epulis, a nasopalatine cyst, or an adamantinoma. *Hyperostosis frontalis interna* is a form of localized dysplasia limited to the inner table of the frontal bone and occurring mainly in elderly females.

Clinical features
Apart from hyperostosis frontalis interna, these dysplasias occur mainly in *adolescents. Deformity* due to swelling is the main symptom and is usually limited to one side. Growth is slow, but continues after somatic growth has stopped.

Polyostotic fibrous dysplasia associated with endocrine disorders and cutaneous pigmentation is called *Albright's syndrome.*

Headaches occur in hyperostosis frontalis interna.

Treatment
Best avoided, but *partial removal* of the affected bony tissues may occasionally be undertaken after puberty for cosmetic reasons.

'Angioma'

There are two types of so-called 'angioma':

1. *Capillary* is the commonest type and is associated with varying amounts of fibrous stroma. The commonest site is the nasal septum, when the condition is erroneously called a *'bleeding polypus of the septum'. Epistaxis* is the usual symptom. The tumour may become large and ulcerated, when it resembles a malignant tumour clinically. *Treatment* is by *excision.* Recurrence is inhibited by application of diathermy cautery, or the cryoprobe to the site of origin.
2. *Cavernous* may develop to involve the whole tip of the nose.

Benign reparative giant-cell granuloma (osteoclastoma)

Rare. Usually affects the ends of long bones. Can occur in the maxilla and ethmoid. Slow growing tumour with a firm cortex and friable light brown substance. Radiograph shows a circumscribed tumour with 'soap bubble' trabeculation. Treatment is by radical excision.

Chondroma

Rare, but cartilaginous tissue is found in many tumours.

Chordoma

More often seen in the nasopharynx but has been known to occur in the septum and in the sinuses, especially in the sphenoidal and ethmoidal sinuses. Arises from notochordal remnants. This contains large vacuolated ('foam') cells, but the histology is highly variable. It may simulate a benign cartilaginous tumour but it erodes bone extensively. It is radioresistant. Metastases are rare so that palliative surgery is of value.

Craniopharyngioma

Probably derived from the remnants of Rathke's pouch. There is an intracranial portion which can cause raised intracranial pressure, and endocrine dysfunction. The extracranial portion can occupy the sphenoid sinus and erode into the post nasal space. There is no capsule and it consists of cystic spaces and septa. A combined subfrontal and transpalatal approach may be required.

Rhinophyma

Not strictly a neoplasm. It is caused by a fibrosis and hyperplasia of the sebaceous tissue of the skin of the nose, usually as a result of acne rosacea. *Swelling of the nasal tip and nostrils results. Treatment* consists in shaving off the excess tissue. A covering skin-graft is rarely necessary.

Torus palatinus

Not strictly a neoplasm but an exostosis found in the midline of the hard palate. Sucking sweets against it or ill fitting dentures can cause ulceration of the overlying mucosa.

Malignant tumours

Pathology

1. Epithelial tumours (excluding odontogenic)

Carcinoma

- *Squamous-cell carcinoma* is the commonest malignant tumour in the nose and paranasal sinuses. All degrees of differentiation are found but many are anaplastic. The tumour infiltrates the soft tissues, destroys bone, and ulcerates into the mouth, pharynx and even the skin of the face. Lymphatic metastasis to the upper deep cervical glands and retropharyngeal glands occurs but is uncommon. Haematogenous metastasis is rare. It used to be seen in the nickel industry. The incidence has declined since modifications in the industry.

- *Lymphoepithelioma* (Polygonal-cell carcinoma) found more often in the nasopharynx than in the nose or sinuses.
- *Adenocarcinoma* arises from the glands of the upper respiratory mucous membrane, particularly in the maxillary antra. The rate of growth is relatively slow but relentless, sometimes crossing the midline, and metastases are late. Long industrial exposure to hard-wood dust is an aetiological factor.
- *Adenoid cystic carcinoma* (cylindroma). Columns of cells cut in cross section resemble a series of tubes. There is no stellate reticulum. They appear as firm, round, localized, encapsulated tumours especially on the alveolus, hard palate, antral floor, wherever there are minor salivary glands. They tend to recur locally, spread intracranially by following the course of cranial nerves and are regarded as malignant. Rarely metastases to regional lymph nodes or lungs occur but a patient may live for several years with such disease. They are generally radioresistant.
- *Olfactory neuroblastoma.* Derived from neuroectoderm. Rare. may present as a nasal or ethmoidal tumour as well as a lesion of the anterior cranial fossa. May produce vasoactive hormones. Treatment by craniofacial resection and radiotherapy.
- *Malignant melanoma.* Rare tumour which may present as a sessile mass on the septum or lateral nasal walls or as a polypus. They may appear as pale or dark polypoid masses. Surgery can control macroscopic disease. Radiotherapy and chemotherapy appear to have little influence on the long-term outcome which probably depends more on the patient's own immune system.

2. *Connective-tissue tumours*

- *Sarcoma* is rare. Fibrosarcoma, osteosarcoma and lymphosarcoma occur. The latter may be considered as a form of reticulosis of the lymphoid type and is usually associated with multiple foci elsewhere. A relatively benign form of myxochondrosarcoma is reported, very similar to a mixed salivary tumour. Treatment is by chemotherapy and radiotherapy.
- *Nasal lymphoma* (Stewart's lethal midline granuloma.) Originally thought to be a non-healing granuloma, now there is strong evidence to support that this lesion is a T-cell lymphoma. It presents as a slow progressive destruction of the midface without much in the way of systemic disturbance. Treatment is by radiotherapy. An accepted effective cytotoxic regimen has yet to be reported.
- *Malignant lymphoma* (Burkitt tumour) is strongly associated with the Epstein-Barr virus. Occurs in tropical Africa mostly affecting children between the ages of 4 and 8. Cases have occurred outside Africa. Usually attacks the upper jaw but often both upper and lower jaw of same side simultaneously as a massive swelling of the face and palate. The teeth fall

out and there are large areas of bone destruction. It is highly sensitive to cytotoxic agents; usually cyclophosphamide and vincristine are given with prednisolone.

3. Metastases from other primary sites

Rare, but those from the breast, prostate and thyroid have been known to simulate primary growths of the sinuses, even many years after apparent cure of the primary.

Sites of malignant tumours

Eighty per cent of malignant tumours of the nose and paranasal sinuses are squamous cell carcinomas. Approximately 60% of tumours arise in the antrum, 30% in the nasal cavities and 10% in the ethmoids. Tumours of the frontal and sphenoid sinuses are rare. Palpable metastases are present in about 15% of patients at the time of diagnosis.

No classification system has been universally accepted. There are problems in assessing tumour size, however, these are being overcome with more wide spread use of CT and MR scanning. The principal system used for classification of nasal and paranasal sinus growths is that proposed by the American Joint Committee on Cancer which incorporates the Lederman system.

Clinical features

Differ according to the site of origin.

1. *Unilateral nasal obstruction* may be due to:

- *The growth itself*
- *The presence of polypi.* Of two types:
  (a) Oedematous mucosa, caused by the reaction in the mucosa peripheral to the growth.
  (b) Polypoid neoplasm. Usually in cases of squamous cell carcinoma or rarely of melanoma.
- *Thickening of the nasal walls due to infiltration,* with or without ulceration.

2. *Bleeding and discharge from the nose* may occur separately and the amount of each varies considerably. When unilateral these symptoms are always very suspicious.
3. *Swelling* of the cheek, alveolar margin, nasal bridge or palate.
4. *Loosening of teeth* may occur, or they may even fall out. This can be a presenting feature.
5. *Unilateral proptosis* can arise at an early stage by compression of the orbital veins following extension of the tumour into the pterygoid region from a small primary in the sphenoidal or posterior ethmoidal sinuses. More commonly but later the orbital contents may be displaced by destruction of the bony walls of the affected sinus and invasion by growth.
6. *Involvement of facial skin* occurs in the later stages.
7. *Ulceration of the palate* by extension of an antral neoplasm. This may be the presenting sign.
8. *Pain* is a relatively late feature. Commonest in the superolateral group of

antral tumours, where the maxillary nerve is involved early with facial pains, earache, or toothache. Involvement of the alveolus itself causes little toothache, as the dental nerves are destroyed early.

9. *Facial paraesthesia* may precede the pain.

10. *Severe headache* is a late symptom in the superomedial group of antral tumours and is due to involvement of the dura mater.

11. *Epiphora.* Results from involvement of the nasolacrimal duct.

12. *Other features* include diplopia, trismus and limitation of jaw movement, loss of sensation on the palate, anosmia, optic atrophy and frontonasal duct obstruction leading to maxillary and frontal sinusitis.

13. *Metastases*

- *Lymph nodes.* The deep cervical and perhaps the retropharyngeal nodes are involved (10–15%) but later and less commonly than in growths of the nasopharynx. The medial groups of growths metastasize earlier than the lateral. Squamous-cell carcinoma invades the nodes more often than other types.
- *Other organs* are not often involved, but widespread carcinomatosis is seen occasionally.

Diagnosis

1. *Radiography.* Cysts and benign tumours give well-defined shadows; malignant tumours dense and ill-defined shadows, often with neighbouring areas of bone erosion. CT scan will define the macroscopic extent of the tumour. MRI gives better tissue differentiation.

2. *Biopsy.* All encapsulated tumours should, after complete removal, be subjected to microscopy to exclude malignancy. Large friable masses must have an adequate portion removed for examination. A negative biopsy of a suspicious polypoid mass does not exclude underlying malignancy. Likewise frozen sections and aspirations of antral contents are of value only when positive. Discovery of a squamous-cell carcinoma in a cervical node biopsy must always direct attention to the paranasal sinuses.

Treatment

A flexible combination of irradiation and various degrees of excision is likely to produce the best results. Cytotoxic therapy is really only of value in tumours of mesodermal origin.

1. *Irradiation.* Megavoltage radiation is used before radical surgery in most cases. However, early alveolar or palatal tumours which are easily excised, and larger tumours involving the malar bone which shields the antrum, are preferably given irradiation postoperatively. Intracavity irradiation is applied to residual disease after external irradiation or radical surgery.

2. *Surgical procedures.* Various types of procedures are used, singly or in combination and extended as required.

- *Sublabial antrostomy* is used for biopsy of suspected neoplasms of the antrum. It may be extended as a partial maxillectomy for limited neoplasms in the alveolar and palatal regions.

- *Lateral rhinotomy* may be used as an approach to localized growths in the region of the lateral nasal wall and ethmoid.
- *Partial maxillectomy.* Usually comprises an extended 'palatal fenestration', the removal of half the hard palate and the upper alveolus (including, if necessary, the maxillary tuberosity). Suitable for limited growths of palate, alveolus and floor of antrum. A modified denture with occluding obturator is fitted. The surgical cavity allows easy regular follow-up inspection for detection and treatment of recurrences.
- *Total excision of upper jaw.* Performed through an incision starting in the inner third of the eyebrow and continuing along the nasojugal fold to divide the upper lip in the midline. Besides allowing excision of the maxilla this approach also permits exploration and exenteration of all the homolateral sinuses. The septum and hard palate of the opposite side may also be removed. If necessary the eye and orbital contents are removed *en bloc* with the maxilla. An extended sublabial incision will allow per-oral excision of the maxilla but access is restricted. It can be used for the removal of growths from the septum and nasal fossae. Split-skin grafting to line the operative cavity and the use of a dental prosthesis prevent contraction of the facial soft tissues. Orbital excision may be disguised by a prosthesis carried on spectacles or secured to the skull by osseo-integrated titanium bolts.
- *Transcranial ethmoidectomy.* Growths invading the cribriform plate can be encompassed surgically by combining lateral rhinotomy and maxillectomy techniques with anterior craniotomy. The frontal lobes of the brain are retracted to expose the cribriform plate from above. Clearance of otherwise inoperable growths is thus achieved. The cranial floor is reconstructed by fascia and cartilage grafts.

3. *Cytotoxic therapy.* Cytotoxic drugs in a combination regimen are effective in producing a long-term survival in many patients with sarcoma and lymphoma. All are potentially hazardous and should only be administered by those experienced in their use. Careful consideration must be given to blood count levels, and impaired renal, cardiac and respiratory function can all contribute to a fatal result when these drugs are given by inexperienced practitioners.

Recent studies on single agent and combination chemotherapy in squamous cell carcinoma of the head and neck have shown little benefit in long term survival rates. Chemotherapy may have a role in controlling pain in selected cases. Chemotherapy in combination with surgery and radiotherapy as firstline treatment has not been fully evaluated.

Prognosis

The results of treatment have not changed in the past decade, and only 25–35% of 5-year cures are obtained in most clinics.

Pituitary tumours – hypophysectomy

Sellar, as opposed to suprasellar, tumours tend to expand into the airspace of the sphenoidal sinuses. They are accessible for removal by combined trans-septal and transethmoidal exposure. The technique avoids some of the hazards of craniotomy, including danger to the optic chiasma. Acidophil adenoma causing acromegaly is particularly suitable for this approach, but Cushing's syndrome also may be so treated. Tumours within the gland may be removed by microdissection. The operation is said to be more difficult if the tumour has been previously treated by radioactive implants. Hypophysectomy for hormone dependent cancers is now rarely performed due to advances in drug treatment.

Cysts

Pathological types

1. Cysts associated with fusion of embryological elements forming the maxilla (Figure 10.6)

May be separated into:

(a) Medial group in which there are three forms:

- *Median alveolar cyst* (Figure 10.6c) which separates the upper central incisor teeth.
- *Median palatal cyst* (Figure 10.6e) which lies between the palatine processes of the developing maxillae.

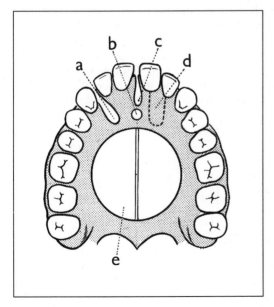

Figure 10.6 Cysts associated with fusion of embryological elements forming the maxilla. a, Lateral alveolar cyst; b, nasopalatine (incisive canal) cyst; c, median alveolar cyst; d, naso alveolar cyst; e, median palatal cyst

- *Nasopalatine cyst* (Figure 10.6b) arising from tissue in the incisive canal or nests in the papilla palatina and present either on the palate or on the nasal floor.

(b) Lateral group. There are two forms:

- *Lateral alveolar cysts* (Figure 10.6a): sited at the line of fusion of maxillary and premaxillary elements of the palate, so as to cause separation of canine and lateral incisor teeth.
- *Naso-alveolar cysts* (Figure 10.6d): occur in the lateral half of the nasal floor, anterior to the inferior turbinate. They enlarge to splay the nostril and to cause a fullness of the upper lip. Because they are developed from the nasal mucosa they are lined by columnar (respiratory) epithelium, but may show metaplasia to squamous epithelium in the presence of infection. When large they cause nasal obstruction and may thin the bony nasal floor. They are sometimes mistakenly incised as furuncles, only to recur later.

2. Cysts of dental origin (Figure 10.7)

These are derived from the epithelium that has been connected with the development of the tooth concerned.

(a) Primordial cysts arise from the epithelium of the enamel organ before the formation of the dental tissue. They occur in young people and the most common site is in the third molar region of the mandible.

(b) Cysts of eruption arise over a tooth that has not erupted from the remains of the dental lamina. Occur in young people and may appear over a deciduous or permanent molar tooth, appearing as small bluish swellings.

(c) Dentigerous (follicular) cysts (Figure 10.7a) usually arise from the follicle around an unerupted tooth. The tooth projects into the cavity.

(d) Dental (radicular) cysts (Figure 10.7b) arise from epithelial remains in the periodontal membrane and are the most common cysts that occur in the jaws. Chronically infected dead teeth or roots produce a granulomatous reaction at the apex. This granuloma contains epithelium and it is this epithelium that proliferates initially to produce the cyst lining. Therefore, the dead tooth or

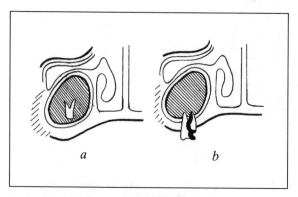

Figure 10.7 Cysts of dental origin. a, Follicular; b, radicular

root is usually seen in conjunction with such a cyst although it must be remembered that teeth or roots might have been removed, the cyst remaining (residual cyst). Any of these cysts may be thin walled and histologically show keratinization. Such cysts have a tendency to recur.

3. Dermoid cysts

Found at the surface lines of embryonic fusion. They may occur in the midline of the nose, and these may extend into the septum; others may occur at the inner and outer parts of the orbital margins, viz. internal and external angular dermoids. Dermoid cysts form external swellings, with or without fistula.

4. Mucoceles of the paranasal sinuses

May be caused by:

(a) Blockage of a mucous gland duct.
(b) Cystic formation of the mucosa undergoing polyposis.
(c) Atresia or stenosis of a sinus ostium. Mucoceles occur most commonly in the frontal sinus and enlarge to bulge into the orbit.

5. Haemorrhagic bone cysts

Found in the mandible and it is thought that the cause is related to trauma which may have occurred several years previously. It is probable that an intraosseous haemorrhage leads to excessive osteoclastic activity which slowly regresses, leaving the cyst behind.

Clinical features

All cysts tend to expand gradually without pain unless infected. The deformity depends upon the position of the cyst.
'Egg-shell crackling' can be elicited when the bone is thin.

Radiographic appearances

Usually diagnostic in showing a *clear outline* in typical positions. When the outline is not clear or there is a multiple appearance, hyperparathyroidism should be excluded by serum electrolyte studies.
1. *Median palatal cysts* show a complete central dehiscence of the palate.
2. *Incisive canal cysts* cause an expansion of the canal.
3. *Naso-alveolar cysts* cause a thinning of the nasal floor.
4. *Follicular cysts* usually have a tooth follicle present within them.
5. *Radicular cysts* have an infected dental root below them.

Differential diagnosis

Diagnosis is from any lesion which can produce a clearly defined radiolucent area in the bone (e.g. osteoclastoma, haemangioma, eosinophilic granuloma, myeloma, etc.).

Treatment

Complete removal or marsupialization.

Odontomes – odontogenic tumours

General considerations

These tumours are derived from the cells concerned in tooth development. While some are true neoplasms, others are developmental anomalies. They may arise from the epithelial remains, from the mesoderm, or from a mixture of both tissues.

1. Ameloblastoma

Sometimes called adamantinoma, or multilocular cyst. However, this tumour does not contain enamel, is not necessarily multiloculated, and may not be cystic. It may arise from any part of the epithelium responsible for tooth formation.

Pathology

The tumour increases in size slowly and invades the bone, which may eventually become completely resorbed. It may progress to a large mass and may be monocystic or polycystic. Some tumours may remain solid. Microscopically here are masses of cells arranged in palisaded groups separated by a connective-tissue stroma. It is in the solid mass of cells that cystic degeneration may occur. Many specimens appear very similar to a basal-cell carcinoma. Several different types of ameloblastoma have been described.

Clinical features

These tumours occur more commonly in young adults and the mandible is more frequently affected than the maxilla. In the first instance they appear as a *slow expansion of the jaw,* but when the bone has been destroyed the tumour feels firm. The teeth in the region of the lesion become loosened and as the tumour increases in size it may become ulcerated.

Radiographic appearance

The radiographic appearance is that of a multilocular cyst (most commonly) or a unilocular cyst. Resorption of tooth roots may be seen.

Treatment

These tumours must be regarded as locally malignant. *Radical excision* is therefore necessary. When the mandible is affected, partial excision may have to be followed by bone-grafting.

2. Composite odontoma

Several different types of these odontomas have been described and they arise from the epithelial and mesenchymal parts of the tooth germ. They consist of a mixture of the dental tissues in varying degrees: some appear very nearly like normal teeth; others, at the opposite extreme, consist of calcified masses or a number of tooth-like structures surrounded by a capsule or cyst.

Clinical features

Composite odontomas are most commonly seen in children or young adults, and one or even two teeth are sometimes missing.

A *smooth hard swelling* is noticed in the jaw, its size depending upon the odontoma. They rarely give rise to pain unless secondary infection has occurred.

Radiographic examination

In this, the most common type of odontoma where calcification has taken place, the odontoma can be clearly seen and an associated cyst may be present.

Treatment

Surgical removal.

MISCELLANEOUS CONDITIONS OF THE NOSE AND PARANASAL SINUSES

Epistaxis

Aetiology

1. Local causes

- 'Idiopathic'. Spontaneous arterial bleeding from the nasal septum especially in Little's area is the commonest. In young people venous bleeding from the retrocolumellar vein is also frequent. This type may be initiated by slight trauma or by atmospheric drying leading to crusting (*see* Environmental below).
- *Traumatic.* With abrasion of the nasal mucosa from a direct blow on the nose, often trivial.

Compound (internal) fractures of the bones or cartilage of the nasal cavity and sinuses and fractures of the base of the skull are more serious causes. Blood may be mixed with cerebrospinal fluid in the latter.

Foreign bodies, animate or inanimate, may cause bleeding. They include rhinoliths. Bleeding may be reactionary or secondary after nasal operations. Nose-picking is a frequent cause, especially in childhood and old age.

Epistaxis is not uncommonly associated with septal spurs.

- *Inflammatory.* In acute or chronic rhinitis of bacterial or viral origin. Rhinitis sicca and atrophic rhinitis are uncommon causes, but mild bleeding may occur in sinusitis.
- *Neoplastic.* Benign or malignant tumours in the nose, sinuses, or nasopharynx may present with epistaxis.
- *Environmental.* High altitudes have a drying effect and also lower the atmospheric pressure. Air-conditioned rooms may cause drying. Industrial exposure to caustic fumes and dusts such as chrome salts.

2. General causes

- Hypertension does not cause epistaxis. However, epistaxis in hypertensive individuals is more severe and prolonged and therefore more likely to lead to a hospital admission.
- Raised venous pressure. As in cardiac and pulmonary disorders including whooping-cough and pneumonia. This is associated with venous bleeding from the retrocolumellar vein.
- *Diseases of blood and blood vessels.* Such as leukaemia, especially the acute lymphatic and myelogenous types; haemophilia; Christmas disease (lack of Factor IX); purpura; sickle-cell anaemia; deficiencies of vitamins C and K; severe liver disease; von Willebrand's disease; and familial haemorrhagic telangiectasia (Osler–Rendu disease). These diseases of the blood and blood vessels may be diagnosed by complete blood count (red and white cells and platelets), estimation of antihaemophilic globulin (AHG) and of the prothrombin time. Bleeding and clotting times are unreliable as they may be below or at the upper limit of normal in less severe degrees of dyscrasias.

Sites of bleeding

1. Nasal septum

Little's area (Kiesselbach's plexus) is the commonest site. Between 75% and 90% of all cases of epistaxis seen in hospitals come from the septum. A single vessel may be seen, or a leash of them. Some run up from the floor; some are very near the mucocutaneous junction. The 'bleeding polypus' (an inflammatory granuloma) of the septum arises in this area. Bleeding may also occur from other parts of the septum besides Little's area, often behind a spur.

2. Inferior turbinate and nasal floor

These are other sites of simple bleeding.

3. Above the middle turbinate

Bleeding comes from the anterior ethmoidal vessels, usually in cases of hypertension.

4. The middle meatus

A rare site. Spontaneous bleeding from a polypoid swelling must always lead to suspicion of a neoplasm.

5. The sinuses

Rarely there is spontaneous bleeding from the vessels of the antrum or ethmoidal sinuses.

Blood vessels involved

The main vessels are: anterior ethmoidal, posterior ethmoidal, greater palatine, sphenopalatine and superior labial. The origins of the first two are from the internal carotid artery, the others arise from the external carotid system. The retrocolumellar vein is a common site in young people. In middle and old age there is a progressive replacement of the tunica media by collagen. The loss of the muscle reduces the ability of the artery to contract down and so bleeding may persist.

Age incidence

Adolescents and old persons form the predominant groups.

Clinical features

Bleeding. Varies greatly in degree, from trivial to lethal. It usually occurs from the anterior nares. It may, however, flow back into the pharynx at the same time, and often appears in the opposite nostril. Sometimes the bleeding may be entirely into the pharynx, when the 'concealed' source in the nose is not obvious. Such blood is occasionally inhaled or swallowed, to be produced later as a suspected *haemoptysis, haematemesis* or *melaena.* Familial multiple telangiectases (Osler's disease) often cause very severe bleeding.

Treatment

1. Immediate

- *Pressure on the nostrils.* From outside, compresses the vessels on the septum in the common cases of bleeding from Little's area. The patient is instructed to breathe quietly through the mouth with the head leant forward.
- *Ice or cold packs.* Applied to the bridge of the nose may be helpful. Ice held against the roof of the mouth constricts terminal branches of the palatal artery passing through the incisive foramen.
- *Packing of the nose*
  (a) Gauze or cotton-wool. Impregnated with paraffin or BIPP (Bismuth iodoform paraffin paste), or haemostatic alginate wool or gauze.
  (b) Inflatable bag, or soft nasal splint.

- *Sedatives.* Must be administered if the patient is uncomfortable. Opiates should be used only with very great caution. The fear associated with the nose bleed may lead to a raised blood pressure which prolongs the epistaxis. Mild sedation will calm the patient along with bed rest. Excessive sedation may lead to hypostatic pneumonia.
- *Packing of the postnasal space.* Rarely necessary but may be life-saving. Inflatable (e.g. Foley's) catheters are passed through the nostrils and their balloons are expanded with 3–7 ml of air. Traction is required to impact each balloon into the posterior nasal cavity. Care is necessary to avoid pressure ulceration of the alar skin.
- *Systemic antibiotics.* To prevent secondary infection when packing is retained for more than 24 hours.

2. Curative and preventive

These measures are needed when immediate treatment fails or repeated bleeding occurs.

- *Cauterization of the bleeding-point* is most effectively done with the galvanocautery. Fused (solid) silver nitrate is a useful chemical caustic in controlling bleeding. Liquid acids may cause visible burns and scars. They are not recommended. If the bleeding vessels are near the cutaneous margin, an injection of lignocaine must supplement the mucosal surface analgesia produced by cocaine or one of its substitutes. Cauterization may have to be repeated. In children a general anaesthetic is frequently necessary. A submucous resection may occasionally have to be performed to provide access to the bleeding point or to insert an effective pack.
- *Examination under general anaesthetic* may become necessary (even in adults) if the above measures fail, to allow better identification of the bleeding site, more effective cautery, and/or more effective anterior and postnasal packing.
- *Arterial ligature* is indicated only on the rare occasions when the haemorrhage is not controlled by packing and cautery.
  (a) External carotid artery is ligated distal to the lingual branch.
  (b) Ligation or 'clipping' of the maxillary artery in the pterygomaxillary fossa may be preferable, but the transantral approach can be difficult in some cases.
  (c) Ethmoidal arteries. For bleeding from the upper part of the nose, above the middle turbinate. These arteries can be reached through an external incision near the inner canthus. The orbital periosteum is pushed laterally and the vessels occluded by silver clips.
  (d) Blood transfusion. Absolutely essential when blood loss has been severe. A normal haemoglobin percentage is found in the early stages of haemorrhage because dilution of the blood by tissue fluids is only gradual. In blood dyscrasias replacement therapy is necessary.
  (e) Embolization. A fine catheter is placed in the maxillary artery via the femoral artery with the aid of screening radiography. Absorbable emboli e.g. gel foam are injected. If emboli reflux back into the internal carotid artery there is a risk of a stroke. There is a risk of a neurological deficit in about 2% of patients.

(f) Vitamins C and K. May be given in large doses. Calcium can be added to the diet.

(g) Injection of haemostatics. Various preparations are available, but none is yet truly proven. Lignocaine is reported as useful in arteriosclerotic patients. Aminocaproic acid has value in cases where bleeding is due to increased fibrinolysis.

(h) Treatment of causative conditions, whether local or general.

3. Special situations

● *Clotting abnormalities.* Instrumentation of the nose will only make matters worse by provoking bleeding into the tissues. Gauze packing should be avoided. The deficiency should be corrected by the administration of the appropriate blood product.

Often the bleeding is a continuous slow ooze. Cocaine spray can be of advantage after clots have been gently washed from the nose. If this is unsuccessful then a roll of alginate gauze can be gently inserted. A few millilitres of cryoprecipitate can then be dropped on the gauze followed by a few millilitres of thrombin.

● *Hereditary haemorrhagic telangiectasia.* This is an hereditary disorder characterized by the formation of multiple telangiectases in the mucous membranes and skin especially of the head. The first signs of the disease usually start in early adult life. Arteriovenous malformations may arise in the lungs, liver and gut. Haemorrhage can be severe. In later life these patients start to develop the complications associated with repeated blood transfusions such as antibody development.

(a) Oestrogen therapy. This is suitable for women with this disorder. It induces a metaplasia of the nasal mucous membrane which reduces the bleeding.

(b) Septodermaplasty. Mucous membrane that repeatedly bleeds can be excised and replaced by spit skin grafts. However, within a few years telangiectases develop in the grafts.

(c) Radiation. As a last resort bleeding areas of mucosa can be irradiated.

(d) Laser therapy. The argon laser can be used with a fibreoptic delivery system to treat telangiectases in the nose and upper respiratory tract.

Vasomotor rhinitis (VMR)

Definition

This term denotes a combination of nasal obstruction, watery rhinorrhoea and sneezing of unknown aetiology. It appears to mean different things to different people and is probably best considered as a 'dustbin' term for a group of ill understood conditions. The symptoms appear to be due to a predominance of parasympathetic activity.

Aetiology

Predisposing factors

1. *Heredity.* Plays a significant part in some families.
2. *Infection.* A preceding history of bacterial or viral infection leading to hyper-reactivity is common.
3. *Psychological and emotional factors.* The symptom may be in the nature of a 'stress phenomenon'. Fear produces a vasoconstriction whereas humiliation, frustration and anxiety lead to engorgement of the mucous membranes. Rhinitis may be part of the polysymptomatic presentation of an affective disorder.
4. *Endocrine influences.* May be even more important than in allergic rhinitis. VMR is particularly common at puberty; during menstruation and pregnancy; with sexual excitement ('honeymoon rhinitis'), and in old age (senile rhinitis; commonest in men).
   Myxoedema leads to nasal mucosal congestion.
5. *Sensitive loci.* Small areas on septum and inferior turbinates (Francis).
6. *Drugs.* Hypotensive drugs (adrenergic blocking agents, methyl dopa and reserpine) cause oedema of nasal mucosa in some patients.
   Aspirin intolerance may present with chronic rhinitis, nasal polyposis as well as asthma and urticaria.
   Anticholinesterases such as neostigmine.
   Oral contraceptives high in oestrogen.
7. *Overuse of local applications.* Tends to produce 'rhinitis medicamentosa' from 'rebound' mucosal congestion. Applications tend to be habit forming.

Precipitating factors

Usually act as a 'trigger' on a hyper-reactive mucosa.

1. *Atmospheric conditions.* Changes in humidity and temperature may cause attacks. These may give the impression of seasonal allergy.
2. *Fumes, dust and alcohol.* May provoke a non-allergic hypersensitivity.
3. *Reflex.* The sneezing on waking or getting out of bed on to a cold floor may be of this nature. Exercise may act as a factor.

Pathology

The nasal mucosa may sometimes be normal in colour and texture but is generally hyperaemic and hypertrophic.
   Polypi. Occur, contrary to previous views, more commonly than in true allergy. They contain eosinophils especially in cases of aspirin intolerance.
   Hypertrophy of the inferior turbinates. The commonest change. The anterior ends are more commonly affected, but the posterior ends may be very bulky and pale. Hypersensitive areas may be present on the septum or turbinates.

Age incidence

Any age.

Clinical features

Similar to those of allergic rhinitis. The chief complaints are:

1. Sneezing which is paroxysmal.
2. Rhinorrhoea which is spasmodic, profuse and watery.
3. Nasal obstruction, which is often variable and may alternate from side to side, especially with positional changes.
4. Postnasal discharge ('drip').
5. 'Nasal tip dew-drop' in elderly persons.

All of these complaints are summarized by the lay patient as 'catarrh'.

Differential diagnosis

From:

1. Allergy.
2. Infection.
3. Foreign bodies, adenoids in children.

Treatment

1. *Avoidance.* May be practicable with some patients, when precipitating factors are known, e.g. drugs.
2. *Antihistamines* are useful in many cases, especially for patients with rhinorrhoea and sneezing. Given by mouth.
3. *Nasal medicaments.* Topical steroids as drops, spray or aerosol may be effective (betamethasone, beclomethasone dipropionate). Sodium cromoglycate insufflation (Rynacrom) or drops (Lomusol) also deserves trial. Ipratropium bromide is useful especially for watery rhinorrhoea.
4. *Cryosurgery* or *hot wire cauterization* to the surface of interior turbinates reduces the population of mucus glands. Scarring produced can improve the airway. The effect is short lived.
5. *Submucosal diathermy* to swollen inferior turbinates reduces the bulk of the submucosa. The effect lasts for about 6 months. Trimming of the inferior turbinates is effective but if the airway is increased excessively especially when combined with intranasal antrostomies, atrophic rhinitis can result. Before considering turbinate surgery it is important to ascertain that the patient has true obstruction. It is not uncommon to find patients who complain of nasal stuffiness with what appears to be a perfectly adequate airway.
6. *Removal of polypi* if large and obstructive.
7. *Correction of septal deflections of spurs* should be considered, to relieve an obstructed airway.
8. *Vidian neurectomy* rarely may be justified in severe cases where sneezing and rhinorrhoea are the chief complaints. Symptoms frequently return within 2 years. Various techniques such as clipping the ends of the cut nerve, introducing silastic sheets into the pterygopalatine fossa have been tried to prevent reinnervation but without long-term success.
9. *Psychological adjustment* is a very important line of treatment in many cases. Sedatives and/or tranquillizers, may be needed.

Nasal allergy

Allergy is an abnormal reaction of the tissues to certain substances. The causal substances are called *'allergens'*. They may be known or only presumed. They are antigens, capable of making the body produce antibodies. In allergic subjects, in addition to these normal antibodies, a special form of antibody (IgE, reagin) is produced. These reaginic antibodies easily fix on tissue cells, including those of the nasal and bronchial mucosae or the skin. Similar reactions can be produced by non-specific and non-allergic factors (*see* Vasomotor rhinitis) thereby causing confusion.

Aetiology

Mechanism of allergy

There are three main phases:

1. IgE is formed by lymphocytes. In normal individuals there is an IgE suppressor factor which keeps IgE synthesis in check. In allergic individuals there is an IgE helper factor which appears to promote production at times of exposure to an allergen.
2. IgE is bound to mast and basophil cells. An interaction between the cell-bound IgE and the allergen initiates the secretion of pharmacologically active substances such as histamine that lead to the clinical manifestations.
3. Changes occur as in acute inflammation, capillaries become permeable, the ground substance viscosity is reduced by enzymes such as hyaluronidase and oedema occurs. Eosinophils infiltrate the tissues and are easily detected in the secretions. Serous alveolar glands are stimulated either directly or via an autonomic reflex nervous patterning to produce excess watery secretion.

Predisposing factors

These are very important. Many may coexist.

1. *Hereditary.* A family history of similar or allied complaints is common. No exact genetic basis has been established. The term *'atopy'* is used to define the inherited tendency.
2. *Physical.* Changes in the humidity and content of the inspired air sometimes render the nasal mucosa more susceptible.
3. *Infection.* From viruses and bacteria, may alter the permeability of the tissue to allergens.

Precipitating factors

Allergens may be grouped as:
1. *Exogenous.* Coming from outside the body.

- *Inhalants* form the biggest group and are especially important in adults. A very large number have been recorded and they include dusts, pollens, animal emanations, feathers, and fungal spores and the house-dust mite (*Dermatophagoides*).

- *Ingestants (foods)* are especially important in children. There may be one obvious substance such as eggs, strawberries, nuts or fish; but in nasal allergy it is more common to have a less obvious cause such as milk or wheat.
- *Contacts to skin or nasal mucosa* are uncommon causes of nasal allergy but inquiry must be made to exclude a coexisting dermatitis. Face powders, and hair from electric razors, must be excluded. Nasal drops or sprays used for the relief of symptoms may produce an adverse reaction, as also may penicillin and sulpha drugs when used locally.
- *Drugs:* it can be difficult clinically to differentiate from true allergic rhinitis and vasomotor rhinitis due to drug effects on the autonomic nervous system. Penicillin allergy usually manifests with an allergic skin reaction or asthma; nasal symptoms may be part of a more generalized allergic response.
- *Infection:* bacterial allergy has been suspected but never proved. Fungi and parasites may produce the same effect.

2. *Endogenous.* Coming from within the body. These include tissue proteins (from injured tissues, transudates and exudates).

Pathology

The reaction of the upper respiratory mucosa bears some relationship to the 'weal' reactions of the skin.

1. Local mucosal changes

- *Oedema.* From intercellular transudation of tissue fluid. Due to damage to capillary endothelium, and loosening of cellular cement.
- *Infiltration with eosinophils and plasma cells*
- *Thin watery discharge.* From increased activity of the seromucinous glands. The mucin content is reduced; the fluid is sterile and contains eosinophils and is more alkaline than normal.
- *Vascular dilatation.* Occurs, and when stasis is predominant, it leads to a purplish discoloration. This affects particularly the inferior turbinates, which may become enormously enlarged, especially at their anterior and posterior ends.
- *Polypi.* Pedunculated portions of oedematous mucosa. Eosinophils are present. Polypi may be single or multiple. Usually develop in the ethmoidal cells, less often from the middle turbinates or antral lining.
- *Superadded infection.* Common. The mucosa is reddish in colour and the secretions are more viscid (jelly-like) before becoming frankly purulent. After each attack resolution occurs, but fibrosis follows with each ensuing attack. There is eventually a permanent fibrous thickening.

2. Involvement of the sinuses. Tends to occur as the condition progresses. The commonest pathological changes are:

- *Generalized thickening of the lining mucosa.*
- *Polypi in the sinuses.* Single (usually on the floor) or multiple. They increase the liability to superadded infection. More common in vasomotor rhinitis.

● *Fluid effusion into the sinuses.* The fluid is sterile and clear but may become thick and gum-like in some chronic cases.

Clinical types

1. *Seasonal ('hay-fever': pollinosis).*
2. *Non-seasonal (perennial).*

Age incidence

Nasal allergy often becomes manifest in children of school age. A common sequence is eczema in infancy, then rhinitis followed by asthma. Nasal allergy is less common after 50 years of age.

Differential diagnosis

1. Vasomotor rhinitis.
2. Irritant rhinitis. Industrial fumes, tobacco, dust and toxic gases are the commonest.
3. *Eosinophilic non-allergic rhinitis.* These patients have the typical picture of perennial allergic rhinitis. However, skin prick tests are negative, negative serum radioallergosorbent tests (RAST), and negative metacholine provocation challenges are found on investigation. Nasal biopsies reveal eosinophilia, inactivated cilia and damaged epithelium. There is an oedematous submucosa infiltrated with plasma cells, eosinophils, lymphocytes and neutrophils with some mast cells. The condition may be exacerbated by the ingestion of non-steroidal anti-inflammatory drugs. It does not respond to Rynacrom.

Clinical features

Vary in severity from day to day, or even from hour to hour.

1. *Nasal obstruction.* Due to venous stasis of the inferior turbinates and/or mucosal oedema. This is usually bilateral. Obstruction from polypi tends to be constant, but they occur less commonly in allergic than in vasomotor rhinitis.
2. *Rhinorrhoea.* A clear, watery discharge may be extraordinarily profuse. A postnasal 'drip' may occur, though less often than in infective rhinitis.
3. *Sneezing.* Commonly occurs in paroxysms. Some patients are never afflicted, others are exhausted by it.
4. *Nasal irritation.* A 'tickling' sensation may be present without sneezing.
5. *Anosmia.* Sometimes complained of intermittently or continuously, even in the absence of obstruction.

Diagnosis

1. *Careful history.* The most important aid to a correct diagnosis. Evaluation of family and personal records is essential. A record of infantile eczema is common. Symptoms of asthma are sometimes a feature. Occupations such as hairdressing and fur trading are noted.

2. *Clinical examination.* May give immediate diagnostic aid but because of the paroxysmal nature of the complaint can be very indeterminate. There is no 'typical allergic nose'.

3. *Eosinophils.* May be found in great numbers in the nasal secretions or on microscopical examination of the nasal mucosa or polypi. The eosinophil count of the blood is raised, especially in the morning, and always in the presence of an extrinsic allergen. The count may be normal in hayfever sufferers out of the season.

4. *Skin tests.* These are confirmatory. They may show single or multiple sensitivities. Positive results are obtained in less than 50% of cases clinically suggestive of a non-seasonal allergy. Nearly all patients with seasonal symptoms will give confirmatory positive skin responses. In highly sensitive patients great care must be taken with test solutions to avoid widespread reaction, even anaphylaxis.

5. *Intranasal test.* A drop of test solution may promote rhinorrhoea and sometimes lacrimation – so-called 'nasal provocation' test.

6. *Elimination tests.* Can occasionally be helpful, especially in suspected food allergies.

Treatment

1. *Avoidance of precipitating factors.* The most important principle. It may be easy or virtually impossible. Dust elimination and similar prophylaxis should be endeavoured. The use of vasoconstrictor nose-drops and sprays must be condemned.

2. *Desensitization.* This is indicated, except in the very young, if the allergen cannot be avoided and medical treatment has failed. It is really only of value in those patients who are sensitive to only one or two allergens. Significant risk of anaphylaxis exists. Desensitization injections must be given only where resuscitation equipment and staff are available for 2 hours after injection.

● *Specific extracts.* Contain minute doses of known causal factor or factors. They are applicable to inhalants chiefly. In the seasonal type, pre-seasonal injections are given.

3. *Antihistamine drugs.* These have afforded the biggest advance in therapy. They are best given by mouth. A very large variety is available, and difficulties arise in choosing the best for each individual as effects differ considerably. Some have marked sedative side-effects.

4. *Endocrine therapy*

● Topical steroids. Spray, drops and aerosols are safe and effective with few side-effects when used only in the nose. Patients who are on high doses of inhaled steroids for asthma as well as topical nasal steroids can develop adrenal suppression.

● *Depot steroids.* Triamcinolone acetonide 40 mg by intramuscular injection in seasonal rhinitis is helpful where symptoms interfere with special events, e.g. school examinations.

Systemic steroids by mouth are dangerous both to continue and withdraw. A 2-week course of prednisolone 60 mg/day reducing by 5 mg/day is occasionally justified after unavoidable airway surgery in a very allergic nose.

- *Oestrogens* can be given by mouth if the history suggests an association with the menopause.

5. *Sodium cromoglycate.* Often effective in controlling symptoms, used either as powder by insufflation, or as an aqueous spray.
6. *Psychotherapy.* May be indicated in some cases.
7. *Surgical methods.* Operations on the nose and throat should be avoided whenever possible in cases of nasal allergy. Surgery may be necessary, however, for the relief of gross obstruction or for the drainage or removal of infected material.

- *Removal of polypi.* If obstructive.
- *SMR.* May be indicated when a marked septal deflection is present, to improve the airway.
- *Reduction of inferior turbinates.* Cauterization is largely superseded by submucosal diathermy. The cryosurgical probe may also be used successfully. These procedures only give relief for 6 months to a year. Partial turbinectomy appears to give longer relief but is associated with troublesome postoperative epistaxis in about one in 80 cases.
- *Drainage of infected sinuses.* Operations on the sinuses are performed only when gross infection is present.
- *Removal of tonsils and adenoids.* Must always be a matter for careful consideration in children with a past or present history of allergy. As a rule, operation is best avoided unless infection is obvious.

Nasal polypi

Definition

A pedunculated portion of oedematous mucosa of the nose or paranasal sinuses.

Aetiology and pathology

Types

Two main types:

1. *Simple.* A simple 'mucous' polypus shows oedematous hypertrophy of the submucosa. There is a very loose fibrillar stroma, with intercellular serous (not mucinous) fluid. The surface is covered with ciliated columnar epithelium in the early stage; metaplasia to a transitional and then to a squamous type occurs in some cases. Many white cells are scattered throughout the stroma.

- *Allergic:* due to uncomplicated sensitivity to one or more allergens. The polypi are usually multiple. Eosinophils and plasma cells are found in large numbers.
- *Vasomotor:* similar to allergic, but no allergen identifiable.

- *Inflammatory:* the role of infection is unclear. Infection may be a secondary event to the stasis associated with polyp formation in polypi of non-specific origin. Allergy to bacteria or products of infection has not been proven. They are not common but may be regarded as:

  (a) 'Acute', i.e. of recent origin. This is an uncommon type, usually associated with influenza. The polypus is usually single, very soft, and slightly haemorrhagic.

  (b) 'Chronic non-specific', i.e. of long standing. These polypi are often multiple.

  (c) 'Chronic specific'. Rhinosporidiosis causes a friable bleeding polypus resembling a strawberry.
- *Mixed infective-allergic:* Probably represents secondary infection in the allergic or vasomotor type.
- *Aspirin intolerance:* the mechanism of development is not known but is not allergic. When associated with asthma the recurrence rate is particularly high.

2. *Neoplastic*
- *Benign:* The 'bleeding polypus of the septum' is a misnomer for 'fibro-angioma' or granuloma. Neurofibromas, transitional-cell tumours, and fibromas may present as polypoid tumours, as also may gliomas in infants and meningiomas in adults.
- *Malignant:* these are carcinomatous, melanotic, lymphomatous or sarcomatous, more commonly the first. They may simulate 'mucous' polypi, but are usually more solid, friable and extremely haemorrhagic.

Sites of origin

1. *Ethmoidal.* The ethmoidal cells are the commonest sites. The middle turbinate is next in frequency. Polypi from these two sites tend to grow forwards towards the anterior nares.

2. *Antral.* The antrum is less often the site of origin. There may be multiple polypi, or a single polypus may emerge from the sinus ostium and extend backwards to the posterior choana *(antrochoanal polypus).*

Age incidence

Simple ethmoidal polypi usually occur in adults but children with cystic fibrosis can have them. Antrochoanal polypi occur more commonly in children and young adults.

Clinical features

Men develop the condition approximately three times more commonly than women. Onset of symptoms is usually slow and insidious, but may be sudden and rapid after an acute infection.

Nasal obstruction is the chief symptom. Other features resulting from this obstruction include anosmia, epiphora, postnasal 'catarrh' (irritation and drip), headaches, snoring and speech defects.

Antrochoanal polypus causes marked obstruction, sometimes without any visible ethmoidal polypi.

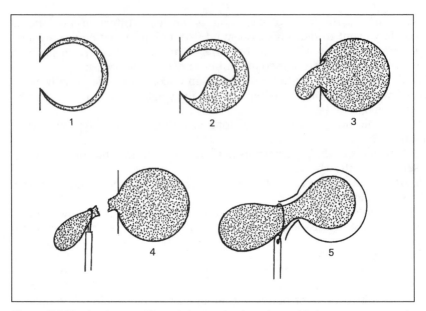

Figure 10.8 Nasal polypus. a, Normal sinus cavity; b, oedema of lining mucosa, e.g. as dome-shaped swelling on anttral floor; c, protrusion of mucosa as polypus through ostium; d, removal by cutting snare leaves mucosa in sinus. Recurrence probable; e, gentle closure of avulsion snare and then traction often will remove air-cell lining. Recurrence less likely

Sneezing and clear rhinorrhoea are common when polypi are associated with nasal hypersensitivity.

Purulent rhinorrhoea is common when infection is present and is often associated with headaches.

Expansion of the nasal bones with broadening of the nasal bridge, occurs in long-standing cases ('frog-face').

Diagnosis

A simple 'mucous' polypus can be traced up to its stalk in the middle meatal region. Gentle probing differentiates it from a turbinate. A large polypus may present at the anterior nares. *Biopsy* is essential when the polypus is unilateral and haemorrhagic. *Radiography of the sinuses* often shows widespread changes due to infection or allergy.

Treatment

Conservative

In early cases, mild symptoms may sometimes be controlled by conservative measures without resort to surgery.

1. *Antihistamine preparations* applied locally or given by mouth.
2. *Local decongestants* used as drops or sprays. 'Rebound' congestion and addiction may be promoted.

3. *Topical steroid therapy.* Beclomethasone aerosol spray 200 g t.d.s. will often shrink existing polypi and prevent recurrence of those removed surgically.

4. *Combination therapy.* This is aimed at preventing the degranulation of mast cells, the reduction of oedema and control of infection. Oral prednisolone on a reducing dose regimen is given for 15 days starting with 30 mg/day. Betnesol nasal drops are administered four times daily for a month. An antibiotic is given for a week. Finally those patients with a known allergy are given an antihistamine as well. Nasal polyposis is brought under control rapidly with this regimen. Then the patient is maintained on a steroid nasal spray with an antihistamine if appropriate.

Surgical

Required when obstructive symptoms are established.

1. *Minor procedures. Removal with the cold-wire snare* is often necessary as the first stage of treatment. This can be successfully done as an out-patient procedure, using local analgesia. It is more satisfactory with single than with multiple ethmoidal polypi. An antrochoanal polypus is rarely removed effectively by this method owing to recurrence from its antral origin.

2. *Major procedures* are indicated for recurrent multiple polypi; for gross infection; for antrochoanal polypi.

- *Ethmoidectomy* may be performed by three routes:
  (a) Intranasal, when great care must be taken to avoid damage to the orbit and its contents and to the floor of the anterior cranial fossa. Complete clearance of the polypus-bearing area is rarely attained.
  (b) Transantral, especially when the antrum is infected. It is impossible to reach the anterior ethmoidal cells by this route, especially the agger cells. It must therefore be combined with an intranasal approach.
  (c) External, is often safer and more thorough than the other two as it allows better visual access.
- *Sublabial antrostomy* is used for recurrent antrochoanal polypi.
- *Functional endoscopic surgery* is done per nares. It has the advantages of a reduced stay in hospital. The surgery may be difficult because of bleeding. It is not without considerable risk in inexperienced hands.

3. *Complications and sequelae* of operations for removal of polypi include:

- *Adhesions*
- *Anosmia*: Though often the sense of smell returns after minor or even major procedures.
- *Damage to optic nerve and other orbital contents.*
- *Meningitis*, following penetration of the floor of the anterior cranial fossa.
- *Onset of asthma* may follow surgery, often in the natural course of the disease.

Long-term management

Removal of polypi must be followed by thorough investigation and treatment of the causal factors. Persistence of the hypersensitive state may lead to recurrence of polypi and development of asthma. It is best controlled by long-continued antihistamines by mouth, and regular courses of topical steroid aerosol or drops.

Obstruction of the nasolacrimal passage

Aetiology

1. Congenital defects

- Atresia occurs rarely at some point along the line of fusion between the lateral nasal and maxillary processes when subsequent canalization along this line is incomplete.
- *Fistula* may occur in the same line. Tears discharge on to the face.

2. Trauma

- Fractures of the ascending process of the maxilla or of the lacrimal bone may sever or compress the nasolacrimal duct or sac. Stenosis or atresia results.
- *Surgical operations* on the lateral nasal wall may lead to stenosis very occasionally.

3. Infection

- Chronic dacryocystitis is the commonest cause of obstruction. Stricture or contraction of the sac is produced. Acute exacerbations are common. A *tuberculous* infection must be excluded.
- *Recurrent abscesses* frequently appear in the presence of chronic sac infection.

4. Nasal polypi

These may cause absorption of the ethmoidal bone and obstruct the sac by pressure.

5. Neoplasms

Neoplasms of the maxillary and ethmoidal sinuses may press on or invade the sac or duct, sometimes at an early stage. Rodent ulcer of the inner canthal region and subsequent scarring after irradiation may obliterate the canaliculi and sac.

6. Functional obstruction

This is inferred when the patient has epiphora but examination of the duct does not reveal any physical obstruction. It may be due to a failure of the musculature attached to the sac effectively compressing the sac and propelling the tears downwards; such as in facial palsy. There may be an abnormality of mucociliary function. This group of patients frequently do not have a successful outcome from surgery.

Clinical features

Epiphora is the cardinal symptom of obstruction. It is worse in cold weather. Pressure over the sac produces a flow of mucopurulent fluid or pus from the puncta when infection is present. The sac may be palpable if distended by retained fluid or pus; it is tender during an acute exacerbation of infection.

Diagnostic procedures

1. *Radiography* must be done routinely to exclude a causative condition in the sinuses.
2. *Syringing* of the passage is used to test its patency.
3. *Contrast radiography.* Radiopaque (iodized) oil introduced through the syringe may be useful in localizing the obstruction. This is often at the junction of the sac and duct.

Treatment

1. *Syringing and repeated passage of lacrimal probes.* Relieve cases of minor obstruction.
2. *Dacryocystorhinostomy* in which the lacrimal sac is anastomosed to the mucosa of the lateral nasal wall above the stricture. Mucosal flaps are made from the sac and from the nose via an external approach (Toti's operation).
3. *Conjunctival or mucosal grafts* may be used to reconstruct the passage when the canaliculus is destroyed or the sac is fibrotic. The graft may be carried on a fine 'Portex' tube or tantalum wire.

FACIAL PARALYSIS AND AESTHETIC SURGERY OF THE FACE

Surgery for facial paralysis

Acute traumatic facial paralysis

1. Purposeful iatrogenic

In this situation the surgeon has deliberately severed or resected the facial nerve. This may occur in tumour surgery such as malignant parotid tumours, large acoustic neuromas, or malignant tumours of the petrous temporal bone. In this situation the patient should usually have been warned beforehand and thought will have been given to the reconstruction.

Either an end-to-end anastomosis or an interposition graft will be the method of choice in most cases. In the cerebellopontine angle, the proximal stump may be inaccessible or very short making anastomosis impossible. In this situation a XII–VII anastomosis using the descendens hypoglossi is the treatment of choice. This can be performed at primary surgery or at a second operation a few days later.

2. Unexpected iatrogenic

This situation has grave medico-legal implications. It usually follows a mastoidectomy or middle ear procedure. The facial paralysis is noted in most cases immediately postoperatively. Occasionally the damaged ends of the facial nerve are identified during the surgery.

After every ear operation the facial nerve function should be checked. If normal facial movement was observed after the operation and the paralysis develops in the postoperative period then re-exploration of the ear is not immediately necessary. Any packing in the ear should be loosened or removed. Provided there are no contraindications then oral or parenteral steroids should be commenced.

If the facial paralysis is noted immediately after the operation then several hours should be allowed to go by before any decisions are made. Temporary facial paralysis due to the action of injected local anaesthetic is not uncommon and therefore time should be given to allow for such effects to wear off before alarming patients and relatives with talk of further surgery. If the paralysis does not recover then re-exploration of the ear should be arranged as soon as practically possible.

Before returning to theatre an experienced surgical colleague should be brought in and introduced to the patient and his relatives. This colleague may either perform the second operation or observe the re-exploration. If possible one member of the surgical team should have some experience in nerve grafting. At the re-exploration photographs should be taken or, better still, if the facility is available a video should be made of the findings. At this surgery it may be necessary to take a peripheral nerve for grafting purposes and consent should be taken for this.

Occasionally the decision to re-explore can be difficult. For example the patient may have had a successful stapedectomy and developed an immediate facial paralysis. Total decompression of the facial nerve in this situation would be accompanied by a grave risk to inner ear function. Here an immediate tympanotomy and inspection of the footplate region and the second genu may be justified. Another alternative is to wait about 15 days and then perform neurophysiological studies in an attempt to establish if the prognosis for recovery is poor or good. Then a frank discussion can be made with the patient.

However, as a general rule early exploration and repair is accompanied by a better prognosis.

Traumatic

Peripheral branch injuries caused by lacerations of the face should be explored and the divided ends of the nerve anastomosed.

Incomplete or delayed onset facial paralysis is usually accompanied by a good prognosis and exploration is not required.

Immediate and total facial paralysis following head trauma carries a worse prognosis. If nerve excitability remains normal at 5 days then a neuropraxia can be diagnosed and surgical exploration is not warranted. If radiological investigations demonstrate that the nerve is divided or neurophysiological studies suggest total denervation then surgical exploration is warranted provided the patient's overall condition permits. Studies have shown that the geniculate ganglion region and the labyrinthine segment are frequently injured in major trauma and consequently a middle fossa approach may be required as well as the mastoid approach.

Established facial paralysis

After time the peripheral nerve atrophies and it can be virtually impossible to find. In this case other techniques have been devised to improve facial appearance and if possible to restore some function.

Static repairs

1. *Face lift.* This removes redundant skin. On its own it is only of temporary help. It is usually combined with other procedures.
2. *Brow suspension.* This lifts the eyebrow on the paralysed side so that it is symmetrical with the good side.
3. *Fascial sling.* Fascia lata is implanted in the face between the angle of the mouth and the zygomatic arch. This lifts the corner of the mouth and gives a more symmetrical appearance to the face. It is a reliable technique which improves facial appearance a great deal, though there is no movement.

Dynamic repairs

1. *Masseter transposition.* Two slips of the masseter muscle are detached from their insertion and transferred to be implanted into the upper and lower lips. This can give good tone at rest and voluntary movement of the corner of the mouth.
2. *Temporalis transposition.* Slips of temporalis can be implanted into the brow and cheek. This helps to give some tone to this area as well as movement of the brow.
3. *Cross face anastomosis.* This technique is unreliable in many surgeons' hands. Peripheral branches of the facial nerve with some muscle are transferred across the midline and the muscle is implanted.
4. *Free muscle grafts.* First the sural nerve is taken and grafted to the buccal branch of the facial nerve on the unparalysed side and led through a tunnel in the upper lip to the paralysed side. Six months later pectoralis minor with its blood supply and nerve supply is taken and transferred to the paralysed side of the face. Then a microvascular anastomosis is made with the facial artery and vein. The medial and lateral pectoral nerves are anastomosed with the implanted sural nerve.

The eye in facial paralysis

Temporary facial paralysis

Often nothing needs to be done as the Bell's phenomenon protects the cornea. Glasses can be of a protective value in this situation. Other methods of treatment are listed below.

1. Taping the eye closed. The tape can be uncomfortable and frequently have to be renewed.
2. Botulinum toxin can be used to paralyse the levator; the lid then drops to protect the cornea for a period of about 6 weeks. It is unsuitable when the best seeing eye is on the paralysed side.
3. Subcutaneous air has been injected into the lids to force the eye closed. Once the air is absorbed the eye will open. The technique is unsuitable when the best seeing eye is on the paralysed side.
4. Tarsorraphy. This has the advantage of giving the cornea some protection and maintaining the use of the eye at the same time. However, after the operation is undone it is not uncommon to have problems with inturning of lashes causing irritation.

The eye in established facial paralysis

The aim is to facilitate eye closure. There is no problem opening the eye as levator palpebrae superiores is functioning. Ideally the technique should also reduce an ectropion of the lower lid.

1. *Gold weight* can be implanted into the upper lid.
2. *Metal spring* can be implanted into the upper lid.
3. *Silicon rods* such as O'Donaghue's rods can be implanted into both eye lids. All these techniques can be combined with a wedge resection of the lower lid for any gross ectropion. Blepharoplasty and brow suspension should also be considered to improve the overall appearance.

Aesthetic surgery of the ageing face

Women, people in the public eye and politicians are the main groups of people that are concerned enough about their image to request surgery that apparently makes them look younger. These people need to be counselled very carefully lest their expectations are greater than what is possible and to ensure that they fully understand the procedure and the risks. If necessary, the surgeon should not hesitate in obtaining an opinion from a psychiatrist. In this way litigation may be avoided.

As with all plastic surgery photographs should be taken pre- and postoperatively.

1. Face lift (rhytidectomy)

Via an extensive hair line incision that goes inferiorly round the ear, the skin of the face and neck is undermined. Redundant skin is resected and the wounds closed. In this way wrinkles are smoothed out and sagging jowls lifted. It is a major operation. Risks include, loss of temporal hair, skin necrosis, facial nerve injury.

2. Blepharoplasty

Wrinkles, 'hooding' of the upper eyelid, and sagging of the skin of the lower lid can be corrected by this technique. Serious complications are rare but blindness has occurred.

3. Collagen injections

Bovine collagen can be injected to correct lines, wrinkles, shallow acne scars and postoperative defects. A test dose should be given because of the risk of allergy. The effect is temporary, lasting from 3 to 48 months.

4. Liposuction

Unsightly pads of subcutaneous fat can be literally sucked out by this technique.

5. Chemical peel

Using a buffered solution of phenol. It is helpful in reducing small wrinkles, e.g. in the perioral region.

6. Dermabrasion

Useful in controlling small wrinkles. It is must not be done deeply as there is a risk of scarring.

Rhinoplasty

Patient selection

The surgeon and patient should have a clear idea what surgery will offer. Although surgery may help to restore patient confidence socially it will not correct psychosocial problems of interaction with the opposite sex. The surgeon should therefore beware of people (particularly young men) requesting rhinoplasty for what appear to be minor or trivial abnormalities. A psychiatric opinion may be of great value.

The surgeon should consider the face as a whole. The patient complaining of a large nose may have a normal nose that only appears large because of a small or receding chin. In this case a mentoplasty may be more appropriate than a reduction rhinoplasty.

The surgeon should beware of the patient with thin skin, as changes to the bony or cartilaginous skeleton may show through. Some patients have a tendency to produce hypertrophic scars or keloid and these patients may be unsuitable for rhinoplasty.

Nasal function must be borne in mind when planning surgery and counselling the patient. Surgery may have to be staged to obtain the best results. Photographs should be taken pre- and postoperatively.

Reduction rhinoplasty

Rhinoplasty is an art. No two operations are exactly the same though each operation consists of the same stages or components. These are hump reduction, medial and lateral osteotomies, septoplasty, infracture and tip work. The reader is advised to read a textbook devoted to the subject as it is too complex to give even the minimum of information here.

Augmentation rhinoplasty

In this situation there is a lack of tissue. This frequently presents as a saddle deformity, the result of trauma or infection. Material has to be implanted to restore the profile of the nose. This may be obtained from the patient, such as conchal or costal cartilage, rib, or iliac crest. This material is usually well tolerated though it may resorb over a period of time. Artificial material can also be used such as silastic. However, there is a marked problem of extrusion. To minimize this it is advisable that the implant is inserted with the minimum amount of surgical opening of the tissues and it should not be implanted at the same time as performing other components of rhinoplasty surgery.

Pinnaplasty

Indications

Commonly performed for protruberant ears. Children are usually being teased at school. Usually done after the age of 5 years.

Stenström technique

The new antihelix is marked with ink by passing a straight cutting needle through the skin and cartilage. A dumb-bell shape of postauricular skin is excised in most cases. An incision is made through the cartilage of the scapha and the lateral aspect of the cartilage is exposed. The cartilage here is scored either using a knife or special instrument. Thus tension is removed from the cartilage and the antihelix is formed.

Converse technique

After exposure of the postauricular aspect of the cartilage, side by side incisions are made. Non-absorbable mattress sutures are then used to fold the cartilage over, to form the antihelix.

Mustardé technique

This technique is similar to the Converse technique except that the cartilage is not incised.

Hyperkinetic conditions of facial movement

Common conditions include blepharospasm, hemifacial spasm, spastic torticollis, synkinesia following reinnervation.

Blepharospasm

A dyskinesia, commencing in middle and late life characterized by progressive attacks of spasm of the orbiculari oculi. The spasms lead to intermittent functional blindness such that driving or operating machinery becomes impossible. The worst of the spasms can be controlled by a selective neurectomy. Many patients obtain significant relief by regular botulinum toxin injections.

Hemifacial spasm

Believed to be due to irritation of the facial nerve in the cerebellopontine angle. This irritation is often due to a vascular loop of the anterior inferior cerebellar artery rubbing against the nerve. The facial nerve can be protected by sponge placed at open surgery. Many patients feel that this effective surgical treatment is too drastic for this non-life-threatening condition. Other alternative treatments include selective facial neurectomy or botulinum toxin injections.

Spastic torticollis

A progressive dystonia of the sternomastoid, trapezius, scalene and splenius capitis muscles which comes on in middle life. It presents with an intermittent turning of the head which becomes permanent. Surgical treatment consists of section of the anterior and posterior roots of the cervical nerves, however, this has given way to the regular use of botulinum toxin injections in recent years.

PART III
The mouth and pharynx

Chapter 11

Surgical anatomy

DEVELOPMENT OF THE MOUTH AND PHARYNX

The pharynx develops from the anterior end of the *primitive foregut.* Towards the end of the first fetal month the foregut ends blindly at the *buccopharyngeal membrane;* this soon ruptures and the stomatodeum (primitive mouth) becomes continuous with the pharynx.

Pharyngeal pouches and arches

(Described on p. 3.) From these are developed the following parts of the adult pharynx:

Stomatodeum, or primitive mouth, is the space which exists between the frontonasal process above and the first visceral arch below and laterally *(see* Figure 8.1, p. 169). It constitutes the beginning of the oral and nasal cavities. That portion of the mouth which originates from the stomatodeum is lined by ectoderm. The epithelium of the hard palate, sides of mouth, lips, enamel of the teeth, and parotid gland are ectodermal in origin, probably also the submandibular gland. Rathke's pouch arises from this ectoderm to form the anterior lobe of the pituitary gland. The buccopharyngeal membrane, however, breaks down so early that it is difficult to say where ectoderm and entoderm meet. It is possible that the mucous membrane of the anterior two-thirds of the tongue is ectodermal in origin, and the remainder of the epithelium of the mouth entodermal. On completion of the formation of the palate *(see* Figure 8.2, p. 171), the oral and nasal cavities become separated.

Tongue develops from the tuberculum impar *(see* Figure 1.1, p. 3), two lateral tubercules and the hypobranchial eminence. The two lateral tubercles are situated on the first arch and fuse with the tuberculum impar to form the anterior two-thirds of the tongue. The hypobranchial eminence, or copula, arises from the second visceral arch with a contribution from third arch mesoderm. It forms the posterior one-third of the tongue and unites with the other rudiments mentioned above. Between the copula and the tuberculum impar there is a median diverticulum, which is the site of origin of the thyroid gland. The *thyroglossal duct* is the connection between the diverticulum and the pharynx. This is soon obliterated and its former connection with the floor of the mouth is marked by the foramen caecum. Remnants of this tract are a potential source of cyst formation.

Mandible develops in the first visceral arch from Meckel's cartilage *(see* Figure 1.2, p. 4), arising as two parts, the one from each side of the arch meeting its fellow of the opposite side anteriorly.

Posterior pharyngeal wall is derived from the remainder of the dorsal part of the second pharyngeal pouch.

Lateral wall of the nasopharynx, in front of the orifice of the eustachian tube is formed by the entodermal aspect of the first visceral arch.

(Palatine) tonsil is said to develop round the *intratonsillar cleft,* which was formerly thought to represent the site of the second pharyngeal pouch. The cleft is often wrongly called the *supratonsillar fossa.* This latter term is correctly applied to the triangular area of mucous membrane which lies above the tonsil, in the upper angle between the anterior and posterior pillars of the fauces. It is likely that the true supratonsillar fossa represents the site of the second pharyngeal pouch.

Pharyngo-epiglottic folds arise from the third visceral arch. They are paired folds which bound the valleculae laterally.

ANATOMY OF THE MOUTH AND PHARYNX

Mouth

The mouth extends from the lips to the anterior pillar of the fauces, and consists of two parts:

1. *The vestibule.* Between the lips and cheeks, and the teeth and alveoli. Anteriorly, the vestibule opens on to the face by means of the *oral fissure;* posteriorly, it communicates on each side with the mouth proper between the ramus of the mandible and the last standing teeth. This posterior communication is of importance when the jaw has to be fixed, as it is a means by which fluids can be introduced.

2. *The mouth proper.* Being the space enclosed by the teeth and alveolus.

The mouth is lined by a mucous membrane which is adherent to the deeper structures: on the lips, cheeks and tongue to the muscles; on the hard palate and alveolar bone to the periosteum, so forming a mucoperiosteum. It consists of stratified squamous epithelium. The mucous glands of the lips and buccal mucosa open into the vestibule; so also do the parotid ducts, one on each side, through a small papilla opposite the upper second molar tooth. The mouth cavity proper is bounded anteriorly and laterally by the alveolus, teeth, and gums; posteriorly it communicates with the pharynx by means of the *oropharyngeal isthmus.* The floor is formed mainly by the anterior two-thirds of the tongue, and the submandibular and sublingual ducts open into the floor of the mouth beneath the tongue. The roof is formed by the hard and soft palates.

The gums

The gingivae or gums consist of dense fibrous tissue covered with the mucous membrane after its reflection from the vestibule. It is called mucoperiosteum where the mucous membrane is firmly attached to the alveolus and palate by this fibrous tissue, which is also firmly attached to the periosteum. The mucoperiosteum is thus attached to the alveolus of the jaw and also to the cervical margin of the roots of the teeth.

The teeth

Deciduous dentition

There are 10 teeth in each jaw: edcba/abcde
                                edcba/abcde

Eruption times: a/a   6 months   d/d   14 months
                               d/d

                  a/a   7 months   c/c   18 months
                               c/c

                  b/b   8–9 months e/e   2 years
                  b/b   e/e

Permanent dentition

There are 16 teeth in each jaw: 87654321/12345678
                                87654321/12345678

Eruption times: 1/1   6 years   4/4   10 years
                              4\4

                  1/1   7 years   53/35 11–13 years
                              53/35

                  6/6   6 years   7/7   12 years
                  6/6   7/7

                  2/2   8 years   8/8   18–25 years
                  2/2   9 years   8/8

The wisdom teeth, being the last to erupt, are not infrequently impacted.

Structure of teeth (Figure 5.1)

The teeth consist of:

1. *Crown* consisting of an outer layer of hard enamel, a central body of dentine, and a pulp chamber containing nerve, blood vessels and lymphatics.
2. *Neck* being that portion of the alveolar margin to which the alveolar mucous membrane is attached.
3. *Root* consisting of an outer layer of cementum which is a bone-like structure and to which the periodontal membrane is attached. This is a ligament suspending the tooth into the alveolus. This ligament contains blood vessels, nerves and lymphatics, and in it may also be found epithelial remains.

- *The dentine* of the root continues from the dentine of the crown.
- *The central root canal* continues from the pulp cavity and is the means by which blood vessels and nerves enter the pulp of the tooth from the jaw.

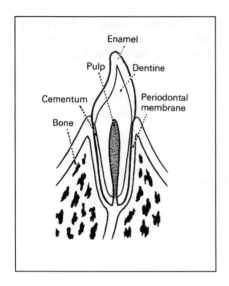

Figure 11.1 The structure of a tooth

The mandible

Two halves at birth, but ossification occurs at the symphysis during the first year of life to produce a complete single bone. The body or horizontal ramus of the mandible is traversed by the *inferior alveolar canal,* which enters the bone on the medial aspect at the *mandibular foramen* and emerges on the lateral aspect in the region of the premolar teeth at the *mental foramen.* This canal contains the *inferior alveolar nerve and vessels* which supply the teeth and soft tissues overlying the mandible; the nerve is also responsible for the sensory supply to one-half of the lip. The ascending ramus has two processes: anteriorly, the coronoid process; posteriorly, the condylar process. With eruption of the teeth the alveolar bone develops, thus increasing the depth of the jaw. At the same time growth also takes place in the condylar region to produce an elongation of the ramus. In the adult the mental foramen lies approximately half-way between the upper and lower borders of the mandible. With the loss of teeth, however, the alveolar bone resorbs and the mental foramen becomes nearer the upper border of the bone and may be exposed to the pressure of a denture.

Temporomandibular joint (Figure 11.2)

A synovial joint between the condyle of the mandible and the glenoid fossa on the under surface of the squamous part of the temporal bone. It is separated into an upper and a lower cavity by a fibrous disc which is attached to the inside of the joint capsule. The articulating surfaces of both bones and the disc are covered with a synovial membrane. The anterior margin of the disc and the capsule receive the insertion of the upper fibres of the lateral pterygoid muscles.

Muscles of mastication

The muscles chiefly engaged in producing masticatory movements are:

1. Depressors

- Mylohyoid.
- Anterior belly of digastric.

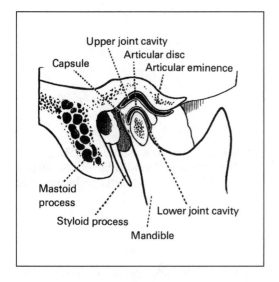

Figure 11.2 The right temporo-mandibular joint

2. Elevators

- Temporalis.
- Masseter.
- Medial pterygoid.

3. Protractors

- Lateral pterygoid.
- Medial pterygoid.
- Masseter, superficial fibres.

4. Retractors

- Temporalis, posterior fibres.
- Masseter, deep fibres.

5. Side-to-side movements

Produced by the muscles of opposite sides acting alternately.

Tongue

Consists of a mass of muscles covered with mucous membrane. They are:

Extrinsic

- Genioglossus.
- Hyoglossus.
- Styloglossus.
- Palatoglossus.

Intrinsic

- Superior and inferior longitudinal.
- Vertical and transverse.

Floor of mouth

The mylohyoid muscle is the main muscle of the floor of the mouth and is a thin sheet arising from the whole length of the mylohyoid ridge on the lingual side of the mandible and running downwards and forwards to be inserted into the hyoid bone and median raphe.

Buccinator muscle

Lies next to the mucous membrane of the cheek and forms most of its substance. It arises from the outer surface of the maxilla and mandible opposite the sockets of the molar teeth, and between these bony attachments it also arises from the pterygomandibular ligament. Anteriorly the fibres of the buccinator converge towards the angle of the mouth and blend with and form a large part of the orbicularis oris. The lower and upper fibres cross at the angle of the mouth, the lower ones entering the upper lip, the higher ones entering the lower lip. It is used to press the cheek against the teeth and prevent food escaping into the vestibule. It is covered by fascia which extends backwards to cover the constrictor muscles of the pharynx. The parotid duct pierces it on its way to the vestibule. Several small mucous glands lie on the fascia around the parotid duct, their ducts also passing through the fascia and the buccinator muscle, to open into the vestibule of the mouth. Several lymph nodes are also occasionally found on the surface of the fascia of the muscle.

Salivary glands

1. Small mucosal and submucosal glands in the buccal cavity: *labial, lingual* and *palatine.*
2. Three pairs of large glands which open by ducts into the oral cavity:

● *Parotid.* With serous cells, secreting a watery saliva. This is the largest gland and it has two lobes—superficial and deep—separated from one another by the main branches of the facial nerve. There are three surfaces:

(a) Superficial. Extending upwards to the zygomatic arch, backwards to the external auditory meatus and forwards over the masseter muscle.
(b) Anteromedial. In contact with the posterior surface of the ramus of the mandible.
(c) Posteromedial. Lying against the mastoid process, sternomastoid and posterior belly of digastric muscles.

The *parotid duct* arises from the anterior border of the gland, passes forwards over the masseter muscle and turns around its anterior border to pierce the buccinator, entering the vestibule of the mouth at the level of the second upper molar tooth.

● *Submandibular.* A 'mixed' gland with serous and mucous secretion. It has a superficial part in the digastric triangle, under cover of the body of the mandible and a deep part in the floor of the mouth, above the mylohyoid muscle. Medially the deep portion is related to the *hypoglossal* and *lingual nerves.* The *facial artery* grooves the posterior part of the gland, and emerges between it and the mandible.

The *submandibular duct* is formed in the superficial part and passes into the deep portion; then forwards, above the lingual nerve, to open in the mouth at the side of the frenulum of the tongue.

● *Sublingual.* The smallest, with mucous and mixed alveoli, in the floor of the mouth, where it produces the sublingual fold, between tongue and mandible.

Cavity of the pharynx

This is the upper part of the respiratory and digestive passages. It is about 10 cm in length in the adult.

It extends from the base of the skull (basi-occiput and basisphenoid) to the level of the sixth cervical vertebra, at the lower border of the cricoid cartilage.

The pharynx is roughly funnel-shaped, being broadest at its upper end.

Its lower end, where it becomes continuous with the oesophagus, is the narrowest part of the digestive tract.

The cavity opens in front into the nose, mouth and larynx, from above downwards, and is thus divided into three parts:

1. *Nasopharynx* opens anteriorly into the nasal fossae. It is bounded above by the base of the skull, below by the soft palate.
First cervical vertebra is separated from its posterior wall by the prevertebral fascia and the underlying longus capitis and cervicis muscles.
Lower opening of the Eustachian tube is situated in the lateral wall of the nasopharynx, about 1–1.5 cm behind the posterior end of the inferior turbinate. It is bounded above and behind by the tubal elevation *(torus tubarius)* which is formed by the tubal cartilage covered by mucous membrane.

Pharyngeal recess (fossa of Rosenmüller) lies behind the tubal elevation.

Nasopharyngeal tonsil (adenoid pad) sits at the junction of the roof and posterior wall of the nasopharynx.

Nasopharyngeal isthmus leads from the nasopharynx into the oropharynx. It is closed during swallowing by raising of the soft palate and contraction of the palatopharyngeal sphincter.

2. *Oropharynx* opens anteriorly into the mouth. It is bounded above by the soft palate, below by the upper border of the epiglottis.

Second and third cervical vertebrae lie behind it.

(Palatine) tonsils are situated in its lateral wall, between the anterior and posterior pillars of the fauces.

Anterior faucial pillar contains the palatoglossus muscle. *Posterior faucial pillar* contains the palatopharyngeus muscle.

Supratonsillar fossa is a triangular area of mucous membrane which lies above the tonsil, in the angle between the faucial pillars.

3. *Laryngopharynx (hypopharynx)* opens anteriorly into the larynx through the sloping laryngeal inlet. It is bounded above by the upper border of the epiglottis, below by the lower border of the cricoid cartilage.

Third, fourth, fifth and sixth cervical vertebrae lie behind it.

Pyriform fossae are small recesses lying on each side of the laryngeal inlet. Each is bounded by:

- *Ary-epiglottic fold,* medially.
- *Thyroid cartilage and thyrohyoid membrane,* laterally. The internal division of the superior laryngeal nerve runs beneath the mucous membrane of its floor. A dental roll wrung out of local analgesic solution and held against the floor of the pyriform fossa produces effective local analgesia for minor intralaryngeal procedures.

Valleculae are paired shallow recesses lying between the base of the tongue anteriorly and the anterior surface of the epiglottis posteriorly. They are separated by the midline glosso-epiglottic fold and are bounded laterally by the pharyngo-epiglottic folds.

Structure of the pharynx

The pharynx is a fibromuscular tube. It has four layers.

1. Mucous membrane

This is continuous with the mucous membranes of the Eustachian tubes, nasal fossae, mouth, larynx and oesophagus.

Ciliated columnar epithelium. Found in the upper half of the nasopharynx.

Stratified squamous epithelium. Lines the oro- and laryngopharynx.

Transitional epithelium. Occurs between the oro- and nasopharynx.

Subepithelial lymphoid tissue of pharynx. There are scattered collections of lymphoid tissue widely distributed beneath the pharyngeal mucosa. Collectively they form *Waldeyer's ring* (Figure 11.3). They have efferent lymph vessels but no afferent vessels. They consist of:

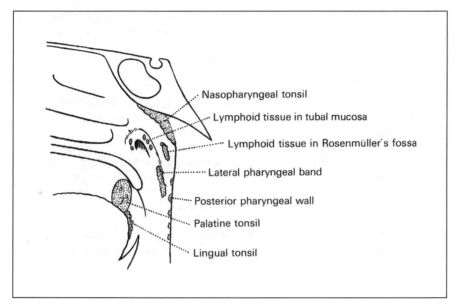

Nasopharyngeal tonsil

Lymphoid tissue in tubal mucosa

Lymphoid tissue in Rosenmüller's fossa

Lateral pharyngeal band

Posterior pharyngeal wall

Palatine tonsil

Lingual tonsil

Figure 11.3 Waldeyer's ring, lateral view

- *(Palatine) tonsils.* Lying between the anterior and posterior pillars of the fauces, on each side of the oropharynx. The *free surface* is covered by stratified, squamous epithelium. 12–15 *crypts* open on this surface and each is lined with squamous epithelium. The intratonsillar cleft *(crypta magna)* is the largest. *Mucous glands* open into the crypts. The *lymphoid tissue* is arranged in follicles, with light-staining centres where lymphocytes are actively produced. The *deep surface* is separated from the constrictor muscles of the pharynx by a connective-tissue *'capsule'*. This makes complete removal by dissection usually possible. The *'capsule'* is strengthened by two folds of mucous membrane:

(a) Semilunar fold: overlying the upper pole.
(b) Triangular fold: arising from the free border of the anterior faucial pillar and binding the tonsil to the base of the tongue.

- *Nasopharyngeal tonsil.* Lies between the roof and upper part of the posterior wall of the nasopharynx. It is a single midline structure. When enlarged it forms 'adenoids'. The *free surface* exhibits about five vertical *fissures.* The *deep surface* has no capsule. Complete enucleation by dissection is therefore not possible.
- *Lingual tonsils.* Clothe the upper surface of the base (posterior one-third) of the tongue. They are continuous with the lower ends of the palatine tonsils.
- *Tubal tonsils.* Lie in the fossae of Rosenmüller behind the lower opening of the Eustachian tube.
- *Lateral pharyngeal bands.* Descend from the tubal tonsil, behind the posterior faucial pillars.
- *Discrete nodules.* Occur in the subepithelial layer of the posterior pharyngeal wall.

Mucous glands. Also found in the subepithelial layer of *the pharynx. They are numerous in its upper part, but gradually diminish towards the laryngopharynx.*

2. Pharyngeal aponeurosis

An incomplete connective-tissue coat in the lateral and posterior walls of the pharynx between the muscular layers. Its thickness is greatest above but diminishes as it descends.

Pharyngobasilar fascia. The thickened upper part, where the muscle is deficient, i.e. above the upper border of the superior constrictor muscle. Superiorly it blends with the periosteum on the under-surface of the basi-occiput. Posteriorly it is strengthened by a strong band *(median raphe).* This is attached above to the pharyngeal tubercle of the basi-occiput and gives insertion to the constrictor muscles. Anteriorly it is attached to the posterior border of the medial pterygoid plate and the pterygomandibular ligament. The tensor and levator palati muscles, and the cartilaginous Eustachian tube, pass through it.

3. Muscular coat

Has two layers:

- External. Consists of the three constrictor muscles (Figure 11.4). Each is partly surrounded at its lower end by the upper fibres of the one below. They therefore overlap one another to some extent. All the constrictor muscles are inserted into the median raphe.

(a) Superior constrictor is a quadrilateral muscle. It arises from the pterygoid hamulus, pterygomandibular ligament, and posterior end of the mylohyoid line (on the inner surface of the mandible). There is a gap between its upper fibres and the base of the skull, closed by the *pharyngobasilar fascia.*

Palatopharyngeal sphincter is formed anteriorly by the tensor palati, posteriorly by fibres of the superior constrictor which arise from the torus tubarius.

Ridge of Passavant is produced by the pharyngeal wall when the sphincter contracts, during closure of the pharyngeal isthmus.

(b) Middle constrictor is fan-shaped. It arises from the lesser horn and upper border of the greater horn of the hyoid bone and from the lower part of the stylohyoid ligament. The upper fibres ascend, to overlap the superior constrictor. The stylopharyngeus muscle and the IXth cranial nerve pass through the interval between. The middle fibres pass horizontally backwards. The lower fibres descend, deep to the inferior constrictor. The internal branch of the superior laryngeal nerve and the laryngeal branch of the superior thyroid artery pass through the interval between them.

(c) Inferior constrictor has two parts:

Thyropharyngeus, above. This propels food downwards at the end of the second stage of the act of swallowing. It arises from the oblique line of the thyroid cartilage, from the inferior horn of the thyroid cartilage, and from a localized condensation of fibrous tissue covering the cricothyroid muscle. The upper fibres pass obliquely upwards and backwards to overlap the middle constrictor. The lower fibres pass almost horizontally backwards.

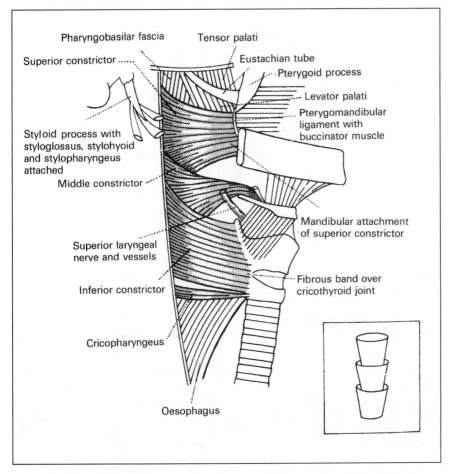

Figure 11.4 Constrictions of pharynx. (Inset: 'Flower-pot' diagram of constrictors (after Lee McGregor))

Cricopharyngeus, below. Relaxation of this sphincter allows food to pass into the oesophagus from the pharynx. It arises from the side of the cricoid cartilage. The fibres pass transversely backwards.

Killian's dehiscence (Figure 11.5). This is a potential gap between the oblique thyropharyngeus and the transverse cricopharyngeus. The mucous membrane in this situation may bulge between the two parts of the inferior constrictor when the sphincter contracts prematurely during the second stage of deglutition. A *pharyngeal pouch* is caused by this neuromuscular incoordination.

- *Internal.* This layer also has three muscles, one of which (stylopharyngeus) arises from outside the pharynx and pierces the interval between the superior and middle constrictors, to form part of the internal muscular coat.

(a) Stylopharyngeus is a long, thin muscle. It arises from the medial side of the base of the styloid process. It passes between the superior and middle constrictor muscles and spreads out beneath the mucous membrane.

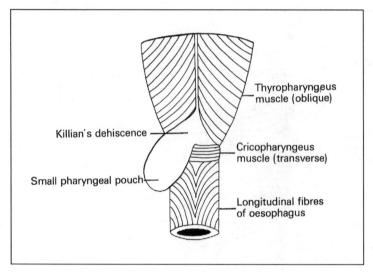

Figure 11.5 Killian's dehiscence with pharyngeal pouch (see from behind)

(b) Salpingopharyngeus arises from the lower part of the cartilage of the eustachian tube. It passes downwards and blends with the palatopharyngeus.

(c) Palatopharyngeus forms an internal longitudinal muscle coat for the pharynx. It arises from the posterior border of the hard palate and the palatine aponeurosis. It passes laterally and downwards in the palatopharyngeal arch (posterior faucial pillar) to join the salpingopharyngeus and sends a small slip to the posterior surface of the tonsil (tonsillopharyngeus muscle). These internal muscles are all inserted into the posterior border of the thyroid cartilage and into the median raphe. They elevate the larynx during swallowing.

4. Buccopharyngeal fascia

This is thin. It covers the outer surface of the constrictors and extends forwards over the prevertebral fascia. Laterally it is attached to the styloid process and its muscles, and to the carotid sheath. Superiorly, above the upper border of the superior constrictor, it is firmly united with the pharyngobasilar fascia. Here the fasciae form a single layer.

Relations of the pharynx

Posteriorly the pharynx is separated from the bodies of the cervical vertebrae by the longus capitis and cervicis muscles and the prevertebral fascia covering them. *Anteriorly* it opens into the nasal fossae, mouth and larynx, from above downwards. The wall is therefore incomplete. It is attached on each side, from above downwards, to:

1. *Medial pterygoid plate.*
2. *Pterygomandibular ligament.*

3. *Tongue.*
4. *Hyoid bone.*
5. *Thyroid and cricoid cartilages.*

Laterally the pharynx is related to:

1. Styloid process and its muscles.
2. Carotid sheath and its contents.

Parapharyngeal space

This potential space lies outside the pharynx and is of great importance surgically (Figures 11.6, 11. 7). It is triangular in cross-section, The space and its contents may become infected from surrounding structures. It extends from the base of the skull above to the superior mediastinum below.

Anteromedial wall is formed by the buccopharyngeal fascia.

Posteromedial wall consists of the transverse processes of the cervical vertebrae, covered by the prevertebral muscles and fascia.

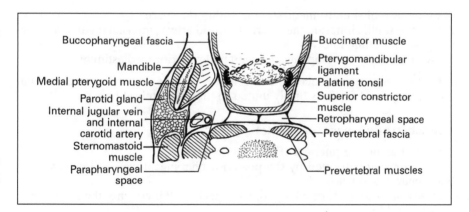

Figure 11.6 Fascial compartments of neck at level of C2

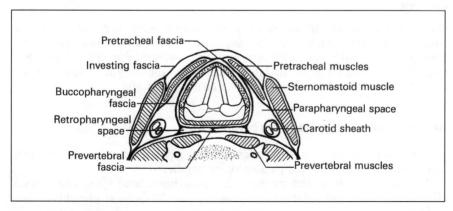

Figure 11.7 Fascial compartments of neck at level of C5

Lateral wall is formed:

In its *upper part* by the ascending ramus of the mandible (clothed internally by the medial pterygoid muscle) in front; by the parotid gland behind.

In its *lower part* by the sternomastoid muscle, the 'ribbon' or 'strap' muscles of the neck and the intervening deep fascia.

Contents

Include:

1. Great vessels of the neck.
2. Ascending palatine and ascending pharyngeal arteries.
3. Deep cervical lymph nodes.
4. The last four cranial nerves and the cervical sympathetic trunk.

Spread of infection

Infection usually enters the space from infection of the tonsils or teeth (particularly the third lower molar). It may spread:

1. From base of skull to mediastinum, within the space.
2. Into the skull, alongside the internal carotid artery, internal jugular vein, or the posterior cranial nerves.
3. Down to the paraoesophageal region and superior mediastinum.

It does not spread across the midline, as the median raphe of the buccopharyngeal fascia is firmly united to the prevertebral fascia.

Retropharyngeal space (of Gilette)

This lies behind the pharynx (Figures 11.6, 11.7).

Anterior wall is formed by the posterior pharyngeal wall and its covering buccopharyngeal fascia.

Posterior wall is formed by the cervical vertebrae and their covering muscles and fascia.

Contents

Included are the *retropharyngeal lymph nodes;* these are usually paired lateral nodes. The nodes of the two sides are separated from one another by a tough median partition which connects the prevertebral with the buccopharyngeal fascia and so lie in the lateral spaces of Gilette. They usually disappear spontaneously during the third or fourth year of life.

Relations of (palatine) tonsil (Figure 11.8)

Anteriorly the tonsil is partly covered by the palatoglossal arch (anterior faucial pillar) containing the palatoglossus muscle.

Posteriorly it is bounded by the palatopharyngeal arch (posterior faucial pillar) containing the palatopharyngeus muscle. *Medially* it presents a free surface.

Laterally it is related from within outwards to:

1. Capsule.

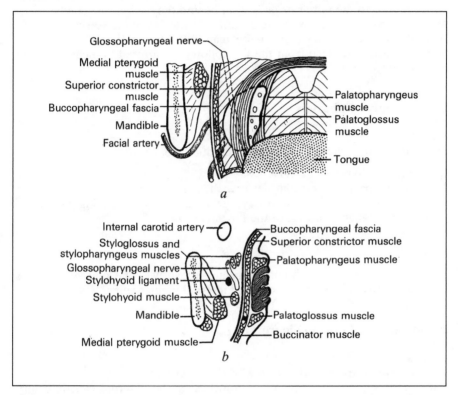

Figure 11.8 a, Schematic view of relations of the tonsil; b, horizontal section through right tonsil (seen from above)

2. Superior constrictor muscle. The IXth cranial nerve and the facial artery lie outside this muscle.
3. Buccopharyngeal fascia.
4. Medial pterygoid muscle.
5. Inner surface of angle of mandible.

Blood supply of mouth and tongue

Arteries

1. Inferior dental artery. Supplies the mandible and mandibular teeth.
2. Lingual artery. Supplies the tongue and floor of mouth.
3. Maxillary artery. Supplies the palate and upper jaw.

Veins

The veins from the tongue unite to form the *lingual vein* which joins either the common facial or internal jugular vein. The veins corresponding to the branches of the maxillary artery open into the *pterygoid plexus* and the blood passes thence to the *posterior facial vein* behind the neck of the condyle. The plexus is also connected with the cavernous sinus by an emissary vein. Similarly, the venous drainage from the mandible also ends in the pterygoid plexus. Venous drainage from the lips follows the arterial branches to enter the *anterior facial vein*.

Blood supply of pharynx

Arteries
These are all branches of the external carotid artery.

1. Ascending pharyngeal artery.
2. Ascending palatine and tonsillar branches of the facial artery.
3. Branches of the internal maxillary artery, chiefly the ascending palatine.
4. Dorsales linguae branches of the lingual artery.

Veins

These form a plexus which communicates above with the pterygoid plexus and drains into the common facial and internal jugular veins.

Blood supply of tonsil (Figure 11.9)

Arteries.
The chief one is the *tonsillar branch of the facial artery.*
   It is also supplied by the other branches of the external carotid artery enumerated above.

Veins

The most important is the paratonsillar vein. It emerges from the lateral surface of the tonsil and runs down its lateral surface outside the capsule. It then pierces the superior constrictor muscle and ends in the pharyngeal plexus. It is a troublesome site of bleeding in tonsillectomy.

Nerve supply of mouth

1. Mandibular branch of Vth cranial nerve. Supplies:
● Muscles of mastication.
● Mandibular teeth.
● Anterior two-thirds of tongue.
2. Maxillary branch of Vth cranial nerve. Supplies:
● Palate.
● Upper teeth.

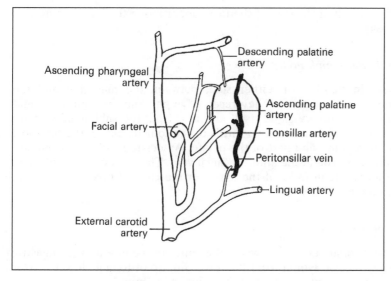

Figure 11.9 Blood supply of the right tonsil

3. Auriculotemporal nerve. Supplies:
● Temporomandibular joint.
4. VIIth cranial nerve. Supplies:
● Buccinator muscle.
5. XIth cranial nerve. Supplies:
● Palatoglossus muscle.
6. XIIth cranial nerve. Supplies:
● The other muscles of the tongue.

Nerve supply of pharynx

Derived chiefly from the *pharyngeal plexus.* This is formed by branches of the IXth and Xth cranial nerves, together with autonomic fibres. The principal *motor* element is the *cranial part of the XIth* (accessory) cranial nerve, which is distributed through the pharyngeal branches of the vagus. It supplies all the muscles of the pharynx except the stylopharyngeus (IXth) and tensor palati (Vth). The main *sensory* nerves are the IXth and Xth cranial nerves. The *nasopharynx* is supplied largely by the Vth cranial nerve. The *tonsil* is supplied partly by the IXth and partly by the Vth cranial nerve.

Lymphatic drainage of mouth and tongue

This is to the following nodes:

1. Parotid lymph nodes
These are several small nodes related to the parotid salivary gland. They

drain the upper half of the side of the face; upper molar teeth and gums; and part of the ear.

2. Submandibular lymph nodes

Three to six in number on either side, between the mandible and the submandibular salivary gland. They receive lymph from the superficial and deep parts of the salivary gland itself and also from the sublingual salivary gland; floor of mouth; anterior two-thirds of the tongue, except the tip; most of the teeth and gums; and part of the palate. Associated with this group are a few facial nodes around the anterior facial vein. The most constant of them lies on the mandible in front of the masseter muscle and takes some of the lymph from the lower lip.

3. Submental lymph nodes

Three or four small nodes between the anterior bellies of the digastric muscles. They receive lymph from the lower lip; tip of tongue; lower incisor teeth and gums; and anterior part of the floor of the mouth.

The efferent vessels from these nodes eventually pass into the cervical chain.

Lymphatic drainage of pharynx

The vessels pass to the deep cervical nodes, either directly or indirectly.

Retropharyngeal nodes

Situated between the buccopharyngeal and prevertebral fasciae. These nodes are said to atrophy in childhood. Efferent vessels pass to the upper deep cervical nodes.

'Tonsillar' node

This is the jugulodigastric node. It is a member of the upper deep cervical group and is situated around the internal jugular vein, where it is crossed by the posterior belly of the digastric muscle.

Nasopharyngeal tonsil

Drains into the upper deep cervical nodes, either directly or indirectly through the retropharyngeal nodes.

(Palatine) tonsil

Also sends efferent vessels to the upper deep cervical group. Most of them end in the jugulodigastric node.

Epiglottis

Served by the infrahyoid lymph nodes.

Remainder of pharynx

Drains to the deep cervical nodes, either directly or indirectly through the retropharyngeal and paratracheal nodes.

PHYSICAL EXAMINATION OF THE MOUTH AND PHARYNX

Mouth

Should be examined with a good light, tongue depressor, mirror, and probe. *Inspection.* Should include:

1. Buccal mucosa and lips.
2. Palate and its movement.
3. Tongue, floor of mouth and their movement.
4. All surfaces of the teeth and gums.
5. Movements of mouth on opening and closure.
6. Occlusion of teeth.

Palpation

Where fractures are suspected, palpation must be made for lack of continuity of bony outline. The cheeks and floor of the mouth must be examined by bimanual palpation for swellings. One or two fingers are used intra-orally to fix the swelling so that extra-oral palpation may define its outline from surrounding structures. This is important in palpating the submental and submandibular lymph nodes and the salivary glands. The jaws should be palpated to ascertain if there is expansion of bone or swelling attached to bone. The temporomandibular joint must be palpated for tenderness or 'clicking'.

Percussion of teeth

Tenderness indicates surrounding pathology in the maxilla. If a fracture is present there is a 'cracked' note, the normal note being a clear sharp 'click'.

Nasopharynx

The methods of examining the nasopharynx have been described with examination of the nose (p. 185).

Oropharynx

Examined through the open mouth. A *tongue depressor* is held in one hand, to allow instrumentation with the other.

Inspection

After examining the buccal cavity the following areas should be inspected thoroughly and methodically:

1. *Anterior faucial pillars.* For colour changes, ulceration or scarring.
2. *Tonsils.* For size, mobility and the presence of pus, debris and concretions.
3. *Tonsillolingual sulcus.* Between the tonsil and base of the tongue. This is an important site for primary malignant growths which may be easily overlooked.
4. *Lateral pharyngeal bands.* For enlargement.
5. *Posterior pharyngeal wall.* For swelling or ulceration.

Movements of the palate

Are noted on phonation or retching.

Palpation

Digital examination of the above areas for induration is indicated whenever malignancy is suspected.

Laryngopharynx (hypopharynx)

Examined by:

Indirect laryngoscopy

With a laryngeal mirror at rest and during phonation.

Fibrescopic laryngoscopy

Should always be available as in almost all cases it gives a view of diagnostic quality under topical anaesthesia. Often this will resolve a difficult case without resort to general anaesthetic.

Direct laryngoscopy

With a laryngoscope under general anaesthesia, preferably with fibreoptic illumination with operating microscope. Inspection of the following areas must be undertaken in all cases:

1. *Base of tongue.*
2. *Posterior wall of laryngopharynx.*
3. *Lateral wall of laryngopharynx.*

4. *Valleculae.*
5. *Laryngeal inlet.*
6. *Pyriform fossae.*
7. *Postcricoid region.* Only the uppermost portion of this region can be seen by the indirect method.

The neck

No examination of the pharynx is complete without a systematic examination of the cervical lymph nodes, and a visual and manual search for swellings of branchiogenic or thyroid gland origin. Normal 'laryngeal crepitus' must be noted. Remember to auscultate any masses as the finding of a bruit can give a clue to diagnosis.

RADIOGRAPHIC EXAMINATION OF THE TEETH, JAWS AND PHARYNX

Teeth, jaws and salivary glands

Apart from the standard views used in radiography of the sinuses, the following are also of value:

1. *30° Lateral.* For ascending ramus of mandible and head of condyle. (Tube tilted 30° to horizontal.)
2. *Rotated 30° lateral.* For coronoid process and body of mandible. (As above, with slight rotation of face towards plate.)
3. *Postero-anterior.* For ramus and condyle.

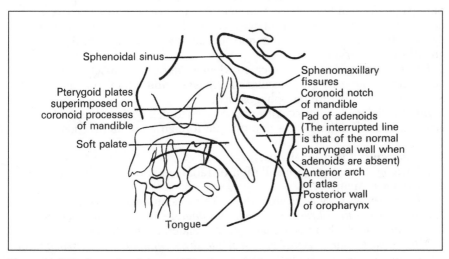

Figure 11.10 Radiography of the nasopharynx

4. *Rotated postero-anterior.* For lower incisor region.

5. *Plain films of temporomandibular joints.* Should be taken in the open and closed positions of the mouth, and tomographs when indicated.

6. *Opaque media.* May be introduced for sialograms and occasionally for cysts. Conventional films may be taken or CT.

7. *Dental films.* Which show the whole tooth and surrounding structures. They are also necessary for buried roots, cysts and impacted teeth. (With small film held inside mouth.)

8. *Bite-wing X-rays.* For interstitial caries. (With film mounted on bite-wing held between teeth.)

9. *Occlusal films.* Occasionally, for calculi in the submandibular ducts, fractures, foreign bodies or misplaced teeth. The film is held between the teeth.

10. *Orthopantomography.* Provides an invaluable 'panoramic' perspective of the upper and lower jaws and dentition.

Nasopharynx

May be examined radiologically in three ways:

1. *Lateral soft-tissue view.* Taken in attempted nasal inspiration this shows reduction of the nasopharyngeal airway.

2. *Submentovertical (basal) skull view.* Shows the degree of bony destruction in malignant tumours of the nasopharynx.

3. *Tomography and CT.* May demonstrate more accurately the extent of a tumour in this region.

4. *MR scan* is particularly useful in demonstrating soft-tissue lesions.

Oropharynx and laryngopharynx (Figure 11.10)

These areas are examined by:

1. *Plain films.* Anteroposterior or lateral views may show the presence of radiopaque foreign bodies. Reduction of the air spaces in the pharynx is seen in growths of the posterior pharyngeal wall; there is an increase in the distance between the air column and the shadow of the vertebral column in growths of the laryngopharynx.

2. *Barium swallow.* Always indicated when a tumour is suspected. It will also demonstrate strictures, 'vallecular dysphagia', and other organic lesions. Strongly advised before oesophagoscopy.

3. *Barium bolus.* A bolus of cotton-wool soaked in a barium solution may be arrested by, and adhere to, a non-opaque foreign body and so demonstrate its position.

4. *Tomography.* Occasionally useful.

5. *Laryngography.* By the instillation of radiopaque oil into the pharyngeal and laryngeal cavities.

6. *CT scan* shows very accurately the soft tissues and mass lesions.

7. *Isotope scanning, ultrasonography,* and *angiography* may all contribute to the diagnosis of neck masses anatomically related to the throat.

8. *MRI is particularly useful in soft tissue differentiation between neoplastic lesions and any associated inflammatory response.*

ANATOMICAL PRINCIPLES OF PHARYNGEAL SURGERY

Nasopharynx

Removal of adenoids

1. *By curettage.* The adenoids are shaved off the roof and posterior wall of the nasopharynx by a downwards sweep with the curette.
2. *By adenotome.* A type of guillotine that is rarely used now a days.

Transpalatal exposure of nasopharynx

The nasopharynx may be exposed through a transverse incision which separates the soft from the hard palate and is closed after inspection and biopsy. A median incision carried forwards from the transverse one allows removal of portions of the hard palate and vomer, so that treatment may be carried out, e.g. intracavitary irradiation. This opening may be left open for subsequent observation.

Oropharynx

Removal of tonsils

1. By dissection

This is now the most widely practised method. The tonsil is drawn towards the midline and an incision made through the mucous membrane, between the free edge of the anterior faucial pillar and its mucosal attachment to the tonsil, to expose the capsule. The upper 'pole' is mobilized and the tonsil then separated from the fossa by blunt dissection, from above downwards. The tonsil, thus freed, is attached to the base of the tongue (lingual tonsil) by a pedicle, which is severed with a snare.

2. By guillotine

The lower 'pole' and free surface of the tonsil are engaged in the fenestra of the guillotine. Digital pressure on the anterior faucial pillar pushes the whole tonsil through this 'ring' and the blunt blade is closed. This passes between the tonsil and the surrounding muscles. The tonsil is then avulsed from its remaining connections.

Opening of quinsy

A peritonsillar abscess may be opened and drained by:

1. Incision at site of election

This site is at the intersection of a *horizontal line* across the base of the uvula and *a vertical line* from the attachment of the anterior faucial pillar to the base of the tongue.

2. Opening through the intratonsillar cleft

With sinus forceps.

3. Abscess-tonsillectomy

Immediate tonsil dissection. This is advocated by some surgeons but is not without hazard.

Laryngopharynx

Lateral pharyngotomy

An incision is made in a skin crease or along the anterior border of the sternomastoid muscle. The great vessels of the neck are retracted laterally, the larynx and trachea medially. This separates the visceral compartment of the neck from the carotid sheath. Operations for the removal of tumours, pouches, strictures and (rarely) foreign bodies, or for the drainage of infected material in the parapharyngeal and retropharyngeal spaces employ this line of cleavage. The pharynx is opened longitudinally by detaching the middle constrictor from the thyroid ala. A posterior portion of the thyroid ala and/or the greater cornu of the hyoid may be removed to improve access. Epiglottopexy or arytenoid surgery is thus made possible.

Lateral pharyngectomy

In malignant neoplasms of the laryngopharynx it is possible in rare instances to remove the affected portion of the pharynx alone, leaving the larynx intact. After exposure of the pharynx as in lateral pharyngotomy, parts of the lateral and posterior walls may be excised, for limited growths of this region.

Pharyngolaryngectomy

Consists of removal of the larynx, together with a part or the whole of the laryngopharynx. Removal of the larynx is carried out as in total laryngectomy with the following modifications:

1. *If the growth is limited* and favourably situated, laryngectomy can be combined with removal of the affected portion of the pharynx, so leaving a strip of mucosa joining the oesophagus to the oropharynx.
2. *If the growth is advanced* or not favourably situated a complete segment of pharynx and upper oesophagus must be removed with the larynx.

Restoration of the pharyngeal lumen. May be effected by:

1. Secondary closure of a pharyngeal stoma. A large pharyngostome made from the I-shaped flap used for the incision may be closed later by one of several types of secondary plastic procedures.
2. Immediate replacement:

- Transference of a section of abdominal viscus (usually colon or stomach). The viscus, pedicled on its own vascular supply, may be brought up antesternally, or through the anterior or posterior mediastinum. In growths involving the upper oesophagus as well as the laryngopharynx, the stomach may be drawn up through the posterior mediastinum (by a 'pull-up' operation) after intra-abdominal mobilization, pyloroplasty, and total oesophagectomy.
- Free colon or small bowel graft, with anastomosis of its blood vessels to others in the neck.
- Utilizing the disease-free portions of the larynx and trachea.
- Pedicled vascularized myocutaneous flaps (e.g. deltopectoral).

Chapter 12

Physiology of the mouth, pharynx and salivary glands

FUNCTIONS OF THE SUBEPITHELIAL LYMPHOID TISSUE

From changes in the pharyngeal lymphoid tissue under known conditions, and of the general functions of lymphoid tissue, it is thought that the function is a protective one. The main collections are situated at the junction of the upper respiratory and upper digestive tracts.

Changes in Waldeyer's ring with age

The lymphoid tissue of Waldeyer's ring is present but small at birth. Its size increases progressively until puberty. Thereafter it diminishes until about the age of 20 years and, from this time onwards, maintains its adult size. These remarks apply only to healthy lymphoid tissue.

Protective functions of the subepithelial lymphoid tissue

1. Formation of lymphocytes

Lymphocytes are formed throughout the lymphatic system. While the lymph nodes are the most active site of formation, the tonsils also play a part.

2. Formation of antibodies

It is almost certain that the pharyngeal lymphoid tissue is concerned with the local formation of antibodies.

3. Acquisition of immunity

The various 'tonsils' of the pharynx may help in acquiring immunity to organisms entering the mouth and nose, but their exact role in this respect is still uncertain. It is postulated that they monitor continuously the different varieties of microorganisms in food and air, and a steady stream of 'samples' trickles through the lymphoid tissues, resulting in the routine production of antibodies to these organisms. Hypertrophy of this tissue occurs in normal children at the same time as immunity is being acquired to numerous infectious diseases.

4. Localization of infection

The pharyngeal lymphoid tissues may help to localize infections entering the body through the mouth and nose. They are ideally situated to act as 'filters' to the upper respiratory passages. Proetz demonstrated that the major aggregations of lymphoid tissue coincide with the impingement areas of the inspiratory air currents.

SALIVATION

Formation of saliva

Saliva is a secretion of the three main pairs of salivary glands and the numerous small buccal glands. Salivation is reflexly activated.

Afferent impulses

Arise from stimulation of the lingual mucosa, via the Vth and IXth cranial nerves; and of the buccal mucosa, via the Vth cranial nerve. They also arise from stimulation by irritants acting on the sensory vagal endings in the stomach, and from stimulation of the nerves of special sensation, such as the sight, taste or smell of food.

Efferent impulses

Are conveyed by fibres of the autonomic nervous system. The salivary glands are supplied by:

1. *The parasympathetic nervous system*
- From the superior salivary nucleus: secretomotor fibres run in the chorda tympani branch of the VIIth cranial nerve and finally join the lingual branch of the Vth cranial nerve; thence they pass through the submandibular ganglion, to supply the submandibular and sublingual glands.
- *From the inferior salivary nucleus:* secretomotor fibres run to the otic ganglion, from which the postganglionic fibres pass to the parotid gland via the auriculotemporal nerve.
2. *The sympathetic nervous system.*

Amount and rate of secretion

Vary enormously in different individuals but average about 0.5–1 litre in 24 h. Parasympathetic stimulation causes profuse secretion of a watery saliva low in organic content. Sympathetic stimulation causes release of small amounts of saliva rich in organic material.

Composition of saliva

Saliva has certain bactericidal and coagulating properties. The average pH is about 68. It consists of:

1. *Water. 99.42%.*
2. *Salts. 0.22%.* The salts are mainly those of calcium phosphate and carbonate.
3. *Organic content. 0.22%. Mucin* is secreted by the buccal, sublingual and submandibular glands, the parotid being serous.
4. *Enzymes. 0.14%.* These include *ptyalin,* which initiates the first stage of digestion by catalysing the hydrolysis of starches, in several stages, to maltase.

Xerostomia

Dryness of the mouth, may be caused by:

1. Lesions of the salivary glands.
2. Lesions which interrupt the central pathways of the secretory nerves.
3. Psychological disturbances.
4. Mouth-breathing due to nasal obstruction.
5. Drugs.
6. Certain general conditions, such as Paterson–Brown–Kelly (Plummer–Vinson) syndrome, uraemia, diabetes insipidus, chronic interstitial nephritis and Sjögren's syndrome, associated with rheumatoid arthritis.

Ptyalism

An increased flow of saliva, may be brought about by:

1. The action of certain drugs.
2. Morning sickness of pregnancy.
3. Certain types of mental disorder.
4. Inflammation, foreign body, or tumour of the mouth, pharynx or oesophagus.

Treatment

The drooling associated with such conditions as cerebral palsy can be managed by rerouting the submandibular gland ducts into the oropharynx.

Assessment of salivary gland function

May be made by:

1. Radioactive scan (technetium-99m injected intravenously) shows uptake in normal glandular tissue, and prompt, symmetrical emptying of the glands if their ducts are unobstructed and parasympathetic nerve supply intact.

2. Labial gland biopsy can be useful (e.g. in Sjögren's syndrome).
3. Submandibular duct cannulation and measurement of the relative amounts of saliva secreted from the two sides in response to stimulation by sucking lemon. In a comparable way parotid secretions may be collected and measured by the Carlsson-Crittenden plastic cup fitted over the papilla.

DEGLUTITION

Food is carried to the stomach after mastication by an orderly sequence of coordinated movements of the muscles of the mouth, pharynx and oesophagus.

Stages of deglutition

The act of swallowing is usually divided into three stages. There is, however, no pause between the stages and once the first stage has been initiated the whole act inevitably follows.

1. Oral stage

Voluntary. Closure of the mouth is associated with cessation of respiration and slight raising of the larynx. Sudden elevation of the tongue follows. Contraction of the mylohyoid muscles presses the tongue against the palate and pushes it backwards. This throws the previously masticated bolus backwards through the anterior faucial pillars, into the oropharynx. The palatoglossi contract, to close the faucial isthmus and prevent any food from returning towards the mouth.

2. Pharyngeal stage

Reflex. During the second stage food is carried through the oropharynx, past the laryngeal inlet. The oropharynx is common to the digestive and respiratory systems and is shut off from the nasal cavities by raising of the soft palate and contraction of the nasopharyngeal sphincter. At the same time the posterior faucial pillars are approximated. The larynx rises further and the laryngeal inlet closes. There is closure of all three tiers of the laryngeal sphincter and respiration ceases automatically. The epiglottis diverts the food stream into the lateral pharyngeal gutters on each side of the upstanding laryngeal inlet, and sometimes falls backwards over the inlet. Contraction of the constrictor muscles pushes food through the relaxed cricopharyngeal sphincter.

3. Oesophageal stage

Also reflex. Food is carried down the oesophagus by peristalsis. Gravity assists in the erect position.

Nervous mechanism of deglutition

Swallowing is a reflex act, apart from the initiation of the first stage.

Afferent fibres

Run in the second division of the Vth cranial nerve, in the IXth and in the pharyngeal branches of the Xth.

Centre

Situated in the medulla, close to the vagus nucleus.

Efferent fibres

Pass mainly in the Xth and XIth cranial nerves to the muscles of the pharynx; also in the XIIth cranial nerves. Impulses are mediated through these nerves to the muscles of the tongue, pharynx, larynx and oesophagus.

Closure of larynx

Effected through impulses carried in the superior and inferior (recurrent) laryngeal nerves.

Inhibition of respiration

Accompanies every act of swallowing. The deglutition centre is situated close to the respiratory centres, and they are interconnected. In some animals this is effected reflexly through the IXth cranial nerve.

RESPIRATION, SPEECH AND TASTE

Respiration

All parts of the pharynx form part of the upper respiratory tract, between the nasal cavities and the larynx.

Speech

Vocal resonance

The pharynx, mouth and nose act as resonating cavities which modify the basic laryngeal sounds. Certain overtones (harmonics) are picked out or exaggerated by modifications in the size and shape of these cavities. The vowel sounds of speech are produced in this way.

Articulation

The pharynx, soft palate, tongue and lips, i.e. the whole vocal tract above the larynx, all play a part in the articulation of the various sounds which make up speech.

The two basic classes of speech sounds are: *vowels,* in which the vocal tract is relatively open above the larynx; and *consonants,* in which it is constricted or completely obstructed for some time. Within these classes, much of the differentiation is based on the movements of the tongue.

Consonants are determined in large measure by the point within the supraglottic vocal tract at which constriction or closure is made.

In *bilabial* sounds, the lips are brought together; *labiodental* sounds are produced by approximating the upper teeth and lower lip; in *alveolar* sounds, the edge of the tongue is brought into contact with the upper alveolar ridge; in *palatal* sounds, the front of the tongue is carried up under the hard palate; and in *velar* sound, the back of the tongue is brought up under the soft palate.

Consonants are also determined in part by the *mode* of articulation. *Plosive* consonants are those in which the vocal tract is completely obstructed for a short time; if instead of complete closure the articulatory movement merely narrows the vocal tract at some point, a *fricative* results; *affricatives* require a combination of plosive and fricative movements.

Finally, consonants may be *voiceless* or *voiced.*

Production of normal speech requires the stringing together of all these types of movement, in a great variety of sequences, each movement running smoothly into the next.

Examination of speech

1. *Content.* The vocabulary range should be noted. The ability to form sentences of increasing grammatical complexity. The ability to name objects.
2. *Diction.* Fluency of the voice should be noted. The presence of mispronounciation of specific vowels or consonants intermittently or continuously in the flow of speech is looked for.
3. *Quality.* The volume, pitch and frequency range should be noted. The presence of hypo- or hypernasality should be observed as should hoarseness of the voice. The entire upper respiratory tract should be examined by endoscopy if necessary.

Special investigations include stroboscopy, phonetogram and voice recording.

Taste

Taste buds

These are the end-organs of taste. They are found mainly on the tongue but also occur on the hard palate, anterior faucial pillars, tonsils, posterior wall of the pharynx, epiglottis and inner surface of the cheek.

Taste cells

Thin fusiform cells contained in the buds (Figure 12.1). The peripheral end of the cell projects as a delicate process through the orifice of the taste bud, so that it is in contact with the fluids in the mouth.

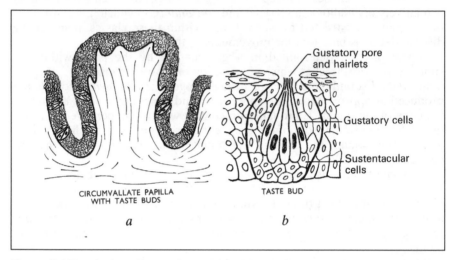

Figure 12.1 Taste buds. a, Circumvallate papilla with taste buds; b, taste bud

Mechanism of taste

To stimulate the taste cells, a sapid substance must be in solution. There are four primitive tastes:

1. *Sweet.*
2. *Salt.*
3. *Sour.*
4. *Bitter.*

The tip and sides of the tongue are most sensitive to sweet, salt and sour respectively.

The back of the tongue is most sensitive to bitter.

The taste of any particular substance is related to its chemical composition. Flavours depend largely upon the sense of smell.

The distinctive character of many ingested substances depends not only on stimulation of the nerves of taste, but also on stimulation of the endings of tactile sensation. Acids, for example, have an astringent character as well as a sour taste in weak solutions.

Nerves of taste

1. *IXth cranial nerve* from the posterior one-third of the tongue (bitter).
2. *Lingual branch of Vth and chorda tympani* branch of VIIth cranial nerves from the anterior two-thirds of the tongue (sweet, sour and salt).
3. *Xth cranial nerve* from epiglottis (not known).

Examination of taste

With the tongue extended, test solutions can be placed on the anterior two-thirds. Electrogustometry gives a quantifiable reading of taste threshold but no information concerning quality.

Chapter 13

Diseases of the mouth and pharynx

CONGENITAL ANOMALIES OF THE MOUTH AND PHARYNX

Fordyce spots

These are small, elevated yellowish spots found on the lips and buccal mucosa. They are due to sebaceous glands in the oral mucosa and are apparent in adult life. Present in about 60% of the population. More common in males.

Congenital anomalies of the teeth

Anomalies in size, shape and number of the teeth are not uncommon.

Total anodontia

Rare. Sometimes associated with an ectodermal dysplasia and is due to lack of development of the dental lamina.

Partial anodontia

Far more common.

Supernumerary teeth

Additional teeth due to an accessory bud being given off from the dental lamina. They are not uncommon and may take the form of a normal tooth, or may be conical or tuberculated. Supernumerary teeth may prevent the eruption of normal teeth or produce irregularity.

Malocclusion of the teeth

Lies in the province of the orthodontic specialist but may be due to local causes, e.g. premature loss of deciduous teeth, supernumerary teeth, or absence of one or more teeth; or to general causes, in which there is a disparity in size between the teeth and jaws, or malrelationship between the two jaws. If teeth are to be placed in their correct position and relationship it is necessary for the tongue, mouth and lips to function normally. Where mouth breathing has become a habit due to nasal obstruction it must be remembered that the habit may well persist after the obstruction has been removed and an orthodontic opinion is advisable.

Congenital malformations of the tongue

1. Bifid tongue

A rare condition, probably due to failure of the lateral tubercules of the mandibular arch to coalesce during development.

2. Macroglossia

Also a rare condition. It may occur in cretinism, mongolism and acromegaly. Macroglossia may also be caused by a lymphangioma. When teeth are present their indentations can be seen on the side of the tongue and eventually this will cause proclination of the teeth. Treatment is surgical, when a wedge-shaped portion of the tongue should be removed.

3. Microglossia or aglossia

Smallness or complete absence of the tongue, extremely rare.

4. Ankyloglossia (tongue tie)

Produced by a short lingual frenum which is attached to the tip of the tongue. If it produces difficulty in speech, the tongue should be freed by surgical division of the tie.

5. Median rhomboid 'glossitis'

Consists of a smooth oval patch on the dorsum of the tongue, anterior to the vallate papillae. It is thought to be due to persistence of the tuberculum impar on the surface of the tongue.

6. Furrowed tongue

A congenital fissuring of the tongue. Particles of food debris may sometimes collect and stagnate in these fissures, producing irritation. In such cases regular cleansing of the tongue should be prescribed. It is associated with Melkersson's syndrome of furrowed tongue, swelling of the lips and recurrent facial palsy.

7. Lingual thyroid

May appear at the back of the tongue as a purplish-red swelling. Excision for obstruction may produce hypothyroidism, reimplantation in the sternomastoid muscle worth considering. Severe bleeding especially in pregnancy may occur, when early tracheostomy with a cuffed tube is advised.

8. Accessory thyroid tissue

May be found along the line of the original thyroglossal tract. Fragments of this tract may also give rise to cysts. Where accessory thyroid tissue occurs, the thyroid gland itself may never have developed in its normal position. Before the removal of any accessory thyroid tissue is contemplated, it must be determined whether the gland itself is present and functioning normally.

9. Thyroglossal cysts

May appear anywhere between the suprasternal notch and the foramen caecum on the tongue. They occur in the midline. Treatment is by surgical excision, which includes the middle third of the hyoid bone (Sistrunk's operation).

Perforation of anterior faucial pillars

Bilateral and symmetrical in some cases.

Bifid uvula

Relatively common. It is regarded as a very minor degree of cleft palate.

Stenosis of the pharynx

May involve the nasopharyngeal isthmus. If the degree of stenosis is marked it may interfere with speech, smell, swallowing, and even respiration.

Web or stricture of the pharynx

A rare affection of the postcricoid region of the laryngopharynx, Dysphagia may be produced and can be relieved by the passage of bougies.

Branchial cysts and fistulae.

See p. 376.

INJURIES OF THE PHARYNX

Lacerations

May result from accidental trauma by foreign bodies entering the mouth. It is rarely necessary to suture these, but antibiotics should be given to prevent secondary infection. Tonsillectomy may lead rarely to a hole in one of the faucial pillars.

Penetrating wounds

The pharynx may be involved in stab wounds of the neck or may be entered by high-velocity missiles. Such injuries are almost invariably fatal owing to associated damage to vital structures.

Foreign bodies

Less common in the pharynx than in the oesophagus. Smooth rounded objects are usually held up at, or just below, the cricopharyngeal sphincter. These are considered with oesophageal foreign bodies.

Sharp and irregular foreign bodies may be arrested in the tonsils, fauces, base of tongue, valleculae or pyriform fossae. Small fishbones and toothbrush bristles are the commonest and are usually impacted in the tonsil. They can be removed perorally by forceps, but direct endoscopy under general anaesthesia is preferable for foreign bodies in the pyriform fossae or valleculae.

Caustic burns

Usually self-inflicted. The oral and pharyngeal mucosae are involved by the resultant strictures. In non-fatal cases they involve mainly the oesophagus.

INFLAMMATIONS OF THE ORAL AND PHARYNGEAL MUCOUS MEMBRANES (STOMATITIS AND PHARYNGITIS)

Stomatitis

Inflammatory lesions of the oral mucosa are produced by a variety of causes which may be local or systemic.

Recurrent ulcerative ('aphthous') stomatitis

Aetiology

A common condition of unknown cause. Viral, psychogenic, vitamin deficiency, hormonal and autoimmune factors have been suggested.

Clinical features

Small vesicles: the earliest sign and may occur on any portion of the buccopharyngeal mucosa.

Ulceration: soon occurs, leaving an ulcer which varies in size from that of a pin-head to one of 2–3 cm. The ulcers have a sloughing base with a marked ring of hyperaemia where bacterial attack occurs.

Pain: may be extreme, and may last for days or weeks.

Recurrence: a characteristic feature of the ulcers, tending to appear in a fresh site as another disappears.

Treatment

1. *Attention to oral hygiene*, topical chlorhexidine effective.
2. *Hydrocortisone.* As Corlan pellets, locally, may be very helpful.
3. *Topical application* of local anaesthetic preparations gives temporary relief. Aspirin has an immediate local analgesic effect.

Behçet's syndrome

Definition

A clinical entity comprising both oropharyngeal and genital ulceration, with iritis and hypopyon.

Aetiology

Not yet established. The condition occurs more commonly in males.

Pathology

Non-specific inflammatory changes, with perivascular infiltration.

Clinical features

Painful ulcers: appear in crops in the mouth, pharynx and anogenital region. They are punched out, with a sloughing base, and are usually surrounded by a red areola. They heal within days or a few weeks but recurrence is usual.

Neurological manifestations: may appear after a delay of 2–5 years and may resemble acute encephalitis or acute lesions of the brainstem and pyramidal tracts.

Blindness: may result from ocular lesions.

Treatment

Non-specific.
Steroids: e.g. 20 mg prednisolone daily, have produced relief.

Traumatic stomatitis

Quite common, and incorrect use of the toothbrush is the most frequent cause. The epithelium becomes abraded, producing shallow ulcers on the gums; or a bristle may become detached and caught in the gums causing a small abscess. Dentures produce acute ulceration if they are ill-fitting or if the patient is sensitive to the material used. If left uncorrected the ulceration becomes chronic, producing varying degrees of hyperplasia. Jagged and rough teeth produce acute ulceration similar to that caused by the ill-fitting denture, the lesions being extremely painful, with a sloughing base and a marked hyperaemia around a ragged outline.

1. Thermal, chemical and physical injuries

Hot foods or drinks will produce burns of the oral mucosa, as also will chemical injuries similar to those found in the pharynx. Heavy tobacco smoking may produce hyperkeratosis and/or ulceration of the oral mucosa. These results are due partly to generated heat and partly to the chemical composition of the fumes.

2. Actinic cheilitis

Certain people react severely to exposure to the sun's rays, and the lips may become severely inflamed.

3. Radiation stomatitis

Radiation may produce an inflammatory reaction in the oral mucosa similar to that seen in the skin. Initially there is simply a hyperaemia but later irradiation may produce changes in the blood supply to the jaws. Extraction of teeth after radiation may produce necrosis of the jaws (osteoradionecrosis).

4. Angular cheilitis (perlèche)

This is a symptom rather than a disease. It is characterized by ulceration and *cracking at the angle of the mouth.*
Aetiology: ill-fitting dentures are probably the commonest cause. Candida, saccharomycetes, and streptococci may be found in the lesion, probably as secondary invaders. It may also occur in the avitaminoses, notably in that due to riboflavin deficiency and in chronic anaemic states.
Treatment: the cause must be removed. If candida are present nystatin ointment is used.

Stomatitis due to metals and drugs

Metals

1. *Mercury and bismuth:* stomatitis may occur when these metals are used medicinally, or in workers using these metals. The gums become red and swollen and the periodontal membrane becomes involved. A *black or purplish line* appears around the gingival margin. This is due to the fact that the soluble salts circulating in the bloodstream come into contact with hydrogen sulphide (formed during decomposition of debris around the teeth), and the insoluble sulphide of the metal is deposited. If untreated the condition is progressive, and sloughing and necrosis of the jaws may occur. The salivary glands may also be involved.

2. *Lead:* the lesions are similar to those produced by mercury and bismuth, but lead is not used in drugs. They occur in lead metal workers and painters.
3. *Gold:* used in the treatment of certain arthritic conditions and it may produce a gingivitis.

Drugs

l. *Epanutin:* used in the treatment of epilepsy. It may produce a *hyperplasia of the gums* due to an increase in fibrous tissue. This may be considerable, almost covering the teeth in some cases. There is no direct inflammatory reaction except from secondary causes. Drug should be stopped; gingivectomy may be necessary.
2. *Antibiotics:* may produce a stomatitis and glossitis, especially when administered locally.
3. *Antidepressants:* may also produce oral symptoms, with dry mouth.
4. *Bromides, iodides and salicylates:* may sometimes produce inflammatory lesions in the oral mucosa.

Allergic stomatitis

Lipstick: a cause of cheilitis of the lips.
   Dental materials: particularly the acrylic resins used in denture materials, may rarely produce an allergic condition of the mouth.

Stomatitis associated with virus diseases

Occurs in the following forms:

1. Catarrhal stomatitis

Acute catarrhal inflammation usually arises in conjunction with coryza, pharyngeal infection or the exanthemata. The mouth usually shows signs of inflammation similar to those in the oropharynx. Lack of oral hygiene is always a contributory factor.

2. Measles

The eruption appears in the oral cavity about 3 days before the skin is affected. The lesions are known as *Koplik's spots* and appear as whitish specks surrounded by an erythematous area, usually on the labial and buccal mucosa.

3. Herpes simplex

In this condition, small vesicles appear, with shallow painful ulcers. The margins of the ulcer are very hyperaemic and although they may appear in any part of the oral mucosa the commonest site is round the palatal gingival margin. Acyclovir is effective by mouth.

4. Hand-foot-and-mouth disease

Oral ulceration with a vesicular eruption on the extremities due to Coxsackie A virus. It is highly contagious with an incubation period between 3 and 10 days.

Acute infective stomatitis

1. Acute coccal (pyogenic) stomatitis

Usually an acute gingivitis superimposed upon a chronic inflammatory condition already present in the gums. It is more commonly seen in young adults, when the gingival margin is acutely inflamed and painful, and slight ulceration may occur. Strict attention to *oral hygiene* is essential, and *systemic* antibiotics are required in severe cases.

Modern dental practice is now orientated to the prevention of gingival disease by plaque control, and prevention of dental caries. Fluoridation, good oral hygiene and regular dental check ups are the mainstay in the control of this problem.

2. Acute ulcerative (Vincent's) stomatitis

Aetiology: it is now thought that a virus may be the actual exciting cause, the Vincent's organisms being secondary invaders. However, these organisms are always present in the fully developed clinical condition.

Clinical features: the inflammation originates in and spreads around the gum margins and is most likely to occur in patients with bad oral hygiene. Ulcers are found and foetor is present.

Treatment: in severe cases, systemic antibiotics. Daily treatment by a dental surgeon initially is essential, all calculus being removed from the teeth and the area cleaned as much as possible without undue trauma. After the acute phase has passed, strict attention to the teeth and gums must continue, otherwise the infection will recur.

Stomatitis associated with tooth eruption

Pericoronitis is an infection of the soft tissues surrounding the crown of an erupting or partially erupted tooth. Any tooth may be involved but most commonly the impacted partially erupted lower wisdom is involved. The acute phase can be most serious.

Clinical features

1. Pain: often severe.
2. Swelling: over and around the tooth which can lead rapidly to cellulitis of the cheek and submandibular tissues.
3. Trismus: frequently present in some degree.
4. Pyrexia: may be severe. Sequelae: oedema of the larynx, and septicaemia.

Treatment

1. Systemic antibiotics.
2. Hot saline mouth washes.
3. The soft tissues over the tooth (gum flaps) may be cauterized by applying a little acetic acid or liquid phenol beneath the flaps.
4. Not infrequently the opposing upper wisdom tooth has erupted and traumatizes the gum flap. This upper tooth should be removed as soon as possible.
5. If submandibular tissues are involved and pus present extra-oral drainage is needed. Drainage may also be necessary intra-orally.
6. When acute phase under control impacted tooth should be removed.

Chronic specific infective stomatitis

Tuberculosis of the oral cavity

A primary lesion in the mouth is extremely rare. However, tuberculosis may be seen in the miliary form, or as a single painful ulcer on the tip of the tongue.

Syphilis

May be present in the mouth in any of its stages.

1. *Chancre:* may be seen on the tongue and lips, in the primary stage.
2. *'Mucous patches':* occur occasionally on the oral mucosa in the secondary stage ('snail-track' ulcers).
3. *Gumma:* may appear on the palate, usually in the midline, or on the tongue, in the tertiary stage.

Fungous infections of the mouth

Candida (thrush)

The commonest and is usually due to *Candida albicans.* Lesions may occur on the oral mucosa and tongue. It is especially likely in infants, in patients receiving broad spectrum antibiotics, and in immunodeficiency states. Treatment is to remove the plaques and apply nystatin ointment or gentian violet three times daily.

Actinomycosis, blastomycosis and histoplasmosis

Occur in the mouth, but are extremely rare.

Gangrenous stomatitis (cancrum oris)

A rare disease, the cause of which is obscure. It is frequently fatal.

Predisposing causes

1. Severe malnutrition.
2. The micro-organisms found in Vincent's stomatitis.

Clinical features

1. *Ulceration* usually commences in the buccal mucosa and spreads very rapidly.
2. *Gangrene* supervenes, with destruction of areas of the cheeks.

Treatment

Five per cent solution of sodium bicarbonate should be used locally to clean the area.
   Systemic antibiotics.
   Reconstructive surgery if the condition is arrested.

Lichen planus

An inflammatory disease of the skin and mucous membranes. The aetiology is unknown. On the skin it appears as pinkish patches which are irritable. Lesions on the skin and oral mucosa may appear separately or together.

Clinical features

The condition may be symptomless.

1. *Glistening white papules* appear in the mouth. They form varied patterns which may be plaque-like or arranged in lines, giving a lace-like appearance.
2. *Hyperkeratosis* may be present in varying degrees.
3. *Pain* though rare, may be severe, if the lesions erode and ulcerate.

Differential diagnosis

This condition must always be differentiated from hyperkeratosis, carcinoma-in-situ and carcinoma. A biopsy is generally necessary.

Treatment

Reassurance is required in symptomless cases.
   Local application of steroids with antifungals (in orabase) is helpful.
   Oral hygiene is necessary if ulcers occur.

Prognosis

Spontaneous remissions occur occasionally.

Pemphigus

A rare and severe condition and may occur in acute or chronic form. The onset is usually between the ages of 35 and 50. Several types have been described but the most common is pemphigus vulgaris. The aetiology is unknown but it is thought to be an 'autoimmune' disease. It is characterized by the formation of large bullae which rupture easily leaving a denuded area which tends to increase in size by progressive detachment of the epidermis.

Clinical features

1. Oral lesions are frequently the first to appear as severe ulceration, the bullae having ruptured.
2. The erosions are shallow and large with tags of mucosa at the margins. Occasionally bullae or collapsed bullae may be seen.
3. The mucosa splits easily when a gentle labial force is applied.
4. Oral lesions extremely painful.

Differential diagnosis

From pemphigoid, ulcerative lichen planus, recurrent major aphthae.

Treatment

Hospitalization for large doses of steroids. Prior to the advent of steroids this was a fatal condition.

Pemphigoid (benign mucous membrane pemphigoid; ocular pemphigus)

Presents with subepithelial bullae on the mucosa and conjunctiva and skin lesions are sometimes present. It most commonly occurs after the age of 55. Unlike pemphigus this is not a fatal condition. The aetiology is unknown.

Clinical features

The oral lesions are similar to those described under pemphigus, and although not as serious a condition, blindness may result and the oral lesions cause great discomfort.

Differential diagnosis

As for pemphigus.

Treatment

Topical steroids and possibly systemic steroids.

Hyperkeratosis

Occurs in the form of *white patches*. There are several types some of which are harmless. Leucoplakia, the most important, is often precancerous.

Aetiology

Hyperkeratosis is usually associated with local irritation, as from heavy smoking, strong alcohol, or spiced foods. *Endocrine changes* may also play a part. Syphilis is not now considered to be a cause of this disease.

Pathology

Hyperkeratosis should be regarded as a *precancerous* condition. *Biopsy* is necessary to differentiate it from lichen planus or carcinoma.

Clinical features

1. *No symptoms* may be present in the early stages.
2. *Whitish plaques* appear. Several plaques may coalesce and the condition may be seen as a whitish band in the cheeks, along the line of the occlusal surfaces of the teeth where biting of the cheeks has been the cause. In heavy smokers the lesions are commoner on the dorsum of the tongue and the palate. The normal mucosa may disappear completely when the keratotic lesion is very marked.
3. *Pain* follows, when the plaques crack and ulcerate.

Treatment

1. Removal of any recognizable cause.
2. Regular observation for carcinomatous change.
3. Removal of the lesion, in some cases.

Acquired immune deficiency syndrome (AIDS)

First recognized in 1981, infection with the human immunodeficiency virus (HIV) has spread quickly. Aphthous ulceration which persists, thrush, gingivitis, angular cheilitis and scaly red dermatitis in a young male suggest immunosuppression and are known as AIDS-related complex (ARC). Kaposi's sarcoma or a life-threatening infection like pneumocystosis caused by *Pneumocystis carinii* make the diagnosis certain. It is best to consider saliva and blood to be infected from such patients.

The incubation period from infection to development of AIDS is variable and can extend to many years. AIDS is fatal. AZT has been shown to prolong the onset of the syndrome after infection.

Chronic oral sepsis

Many types of organism may be found in a normal healthy mouth as in the normal nasal cavities, sinuses and pharynx. In chronic gingival conditions and periodontal disease, some of these organisms are enormously increased in numbers.

Chronic gingivitis

Aetiology

Local causes

1. *Neglected oral hygiene:* Food debris clings around the teeth and deposits of salivary calculus are hastened and increased. Bacteria multiply in these areas and produce irritation and gingivitis.

2. *Irregular teeth, poor occlusion, partial dentures and tooth roots:* make cleaning of the teeth difficult and lead to poor oral hygiene.

3. *Mouth breathing:* A frequent cause of hyperplastic gingivitis and is usually confined in the early stages to the gum margins around the maxillary teeth. The habit of breathing through the mouth may continue even after the nasal obstruction has been removed.

Systemic causes. During pregnancy, gingivitis may result from a disturbance in the endocrine secretions.

Clinical features

If left untreated, chronic gingivitis proceeds to periodontal disease. Bacteria and their toxins may be conveyed to any other part of the body by:

1. *Extension along the alimentary tract and its ducts* due to chronic gingivitis and periodontal disease. Organisms and their products may be swallowed or inhaled. Dental caries does not in itself cause any considerable increase in the bacterial content of a clean mouth.

    Sequelae include:

- Cheilitis.
- Tonsillitis, pharyngitis and otitis media.
- Infection of salivary glands.
- Pulmonary infections.

2. *Transmission into systemic circulation* from the site of infection. Periapical infections, periodontal disease and chronic gingivitis may all become foci of infection, and the products from such foci may enter the body by the bloodstream or lymphatics. Chronic oral sepsis may be responsible for *subacute bacterial endocarditis.*

Treatment of chronic oral sepsis

1. Scaling and polishing of the teeth.
2. Removal of infected teeth or roots.
3. Instruction to the patient on how to maintain oral hygiene.

Nasopharyngitis

Acute nasopharyngitis

Usually accompanies acute inflammation of the subepithelial lymphoid tissue. Infection may be:

1. *Viral* especially by influenza, para-influenza, rhinovirus, and adenovirus.
2. *Bacterial* especially by streptococci, pneumococci and *Haemophilus influenzae.*

    Diphtheritic infection is rarely seen nowadays.

    A *dry, hot sensation* in the nasopharynx is often the first symptom of an acute upper respiratory infection, as in the common cold. *Localized simple acute nasopharyngitis* does occur occasionally. Clinical features include:

1. *Localized pain or discomfort,* exaggerated by swallowing.
2. *Pyrexia*
3. *Cervical adenitis.* Treatment is expectant. Paracetamol may be required in children.

Chronic nasopharyngitis

Simple

Aetiology. Chronic nasopharyngitis is usually associated with an inflammation of the nose or oropharynx. It is seen most commonly in early adult life.

Aggravating factors are nasal obstruction; exposure to dust and fumes; excessive alcohol and tobacco; and overuse of astringent nasal medications. Remnants of adenoid tissue, or persistence of the median recess, predispose to the condition. Rarely foetid pus draining from a chronic otitis media may cause it.

Clinical features
1. Postnasal irritation is the main symptom.
2. *Inspiratory snorting* results from the irritation, which becomes further aggravated by the snorting. Hence a vicious circle is established.
3. *Congestion of the mucosa* may be accompanied by viscid mucopus and the membrane may look granular.
4. *Chronic abscesses* with adenoid remnants or in Thornwaldt's disease, rarely (*see* p. 375).

Differential diagnosis
1. Malignant neoplasm is the most important condition to exclude.
2. *Enlarged posterior ends of the inferior turbinates.*
3. *Antrochoanal polypus* can be seen on posterior rhinoscopy.
4. *Specific infective conditions around the eustachian orifice.* Rarely.
5. *Psychoneurosis:* commonly causes the same symptoms.

Treatment
1. *Attention to any predisposing cause:* in the nose, sinuses or pharynx. Adenoids must be removed. Any marked nasal obstruction must be corrected.
2. *Conservative measures:* aim at maintaining a high level of general health and excluding any aggravating factors. A *warm alkaline nasal douche* will dislodge any viscid mucus.

Atrophic

This is a special form of chronic nasopharyngitis usually seen in conjunction with atrophic rhinitis and pharyngitis. Syphilis must be excluded.

Excessive dryness and crusting are associated with wide nasal airways, but nasopharyngeal symptoms are usually less pronounced than in simple nasopharyngitis. Treatment is similar to that for atrophic rhinitis.

Inflammations of the oropharynx and laryngopharynx

Acute non-specific pharyngitis

Aetiology

The inflammation is usually caused by both viruses and bacteria, the former often primarily.

1. *Viruses.* Especially adenovirus and rhinovirus, particularly in children.
2. *Bacterial.* Especially the haemolytic streptococcus, less commonly the non-haemolytic streptococcus, pneumococcus, or *Haemophilus influenzae.*
   It is more common in cold, damp weather and more likely to attack persons with lowered resistance.
   It may occur in epidemic form in schools, wards or camps.
   It is a common and important prodromal manifestation of measles, scarlet fever, glandular fever and influenza and also rarely of typhoid, smallpox and secondary syphilis.
   It may be caused by local trauma from operations; swallowing of hot fluids or corrosives; or from abrasion by foreign bodies.

Clinical features

There are varying degrees of acute non-specific pharyngitis:

1. Mild (simple) in which the following features are present:

- *Sore throat* especially on swallowing.
- *Earache* sometimes.
- *Enlargement and tenderness of the cervical lymph nodes.*
- Low pyrexia.
- Marked injection of the mucosa sometimes with oedema of the soft palate and mouth. Small, shallow ulcers are sometimes seen.
- *Complications are rare* but acute rheumatism and nephritis must be watched for.

2. Severe (septic) in which all the symptoms are more severe.

- *High pyrexia,* up to 38.9– 40.5°C (102°–105°F).
- *Rigor* may initiate the attack.
- *Relatively slow pulse.*
- Oedema of soft palate and uvula.
- Mucopurulent exudate. A soft, non-adherent membrane may be present, imitating diphtheria. This may be extensive and involve the mouth.
- *Circumoral pallor and flushed face* are common. In streptococcal cases the rash of 'scarlet fever' may appear.
- *Complications are common* especially in children. They include otitis media and *oedema of the 'glottis'.* The soft tissues of the submandibular region may be involved, leading to a firm brawny swelling *(Ludwig's angina).* Septicaemia, pleurisy, pericarditis, nephritis and meningitis were relatively common before the antibiotic era.

Differential diagnosis

Distinction between viral and bacterial types may be difficult. The incubation of viral infections is 34 days, while streptococcal is 2 days. Children under 5 years are more prone to viral than streptococcal infections. Association with conjunctivitis suggests an adenovirus, and with diarrhoea an enterovirus. Glandular fever and Vincent's angina must be considered in some cases. Leucocytosis is much more marked in bacterial infections.

Diphtheria must be excluded by swabs. The high pyrexia with relatively low pulse rate and the lack of foetor oris, favour a diagnosis of acute septic pharyngitis.

Prodromal manifestations of the exanthemata must be remembered.

Blood dyscrasias can be excluded by a full blood count.

Treatment

In many patients, resolution occurs within 3–7 days on simple conservative therapy of isolation, rest, fluids, aspirin or one of its derivatives.

Systemic antibiotics are necessary in more severe cases. Penicillin should be started in full dosage while the bacteriological results of a swab are awaited. In young children, where viral infections are commoner, antibiotics are of questionable value. Adverse reactions to treatment, such as a drug rash or glossitis, must be watched for.

Intubation or tracheostomy may be required if oedema spreads to the laryngeal inlet.

External incisions must be made if the infection spreads to the fascial spaces in the soft tissues of the submandibular region and neck. These are rarely necessary nowadays.

Acute membranous -pharyngitis (Vincent's angina)

Definition

An acute ulcerative lesion, usually involving one or both tonsils and spreading to the fauces, soft palate and gums.

Aetiology

The infection is characterized by a Gram-negative fusiform bacillus and a spirillum *(Spirochaeta denticola)* often with a secondary anaerobic streptococcus. It is now thought that a virus may be the primary cause. Predisposing factors are carious teeth and pyorrhoea, poor diet and overcrowding. It was common in troops during World War I ('trench mouth').

Clinical features

The onset is sudden.
1. *Pain* is marked.
2. *Foetor oris.*
3. High fever at first.
4. *Cervical adenitis.*
5. *Grey, membranous slough* soon separates, with considerable loss of tissue.

The base of the deep ulcers bleeds easily when the membranous slough is removed; the slough re-forms.

The acute symptoms usually subside in 4–7 days, but the ulcer persists for several weeks, with characteristic foetor.

Differential diagnosis

From diphtheria; acute suppurative pharyngitis of streptococcal origin; membranous mononucleosis (glandular fever); tertiary syphilis; malignant growths; agranulocytic angina; acute lymphatic leukaemia and acquired immune deficiency syndrome.

Treatment

Consists of:
1. *Systemic antibiotics* particularly metronidazole.
2. *Antiseptic mouthwashes and paints* to gums and fauces.

Acute diphtheritic pharyngitis

Definition

A severe infection due to the *Corynebacterium diphtheriae.*

Incidence

The incidence of faucial diphtheria has fallen markedly in the last quarter of a century. The severity and type have also changed in most cases. Children were particularly affected, especially those between 2 and 5 years old.

Clinical features

1. *Sore throat* is the first local symptom.
2. *Enlargement and tenderness of cervical glands* are moderate.
3. *Pyrexia.* The temperature is rarely above 38.3°C (101°F), but the pulse rate is usually raised out of proportion.
4. *Toxaemia* is marked.
5. *Vomiting and prostration* occur.
6. *Proteinuria* is common.
7. *Patches of false membrane* are present on the tonsils, faucial pillars, soft palate, and occasionally on the posterior pharyngeal wall. It is usually grey in colour. It is firmly attached and, when detached, leaves a bleeding surface on which it tends to re-form. It often has a strong foetor. In atypical cases no false membrane is present and the picture resembles a simple streptococcal infection.
8. *Nasal discharge.* Serosanguineous or purulent rhinorrhoea may occur, from nasal involvement.

Treatment

1. *Antitoxin* must be given immediately, without waiting for the bacteriological

results of a swab, when the disease is suspected; 20 000–100 000 units are injected.

2. *Systemic penicillin* helps to control the primary and any secondary infection.

Fungous infections of the pharynx

Candida (thrush)

This is the commonest. *White patches* appear on the fauces, palate, gums, tongue and buccal mucosa. These are caused by the *Candida albicans* fungus. *Very little discomfort* is present. It occurs chiefly in debilitated patients.

 Treatment. Nystatin or amphotericin suspension may be painted on the affected parts. Also useful are gentian violet 1% or dilute hydrogen peroxide.

Other fungi

Rarely seen. They include:

1. *Actinomycosis.* With deep ulcers containing 'sulphur granules'.
2. *Blastomycosis.* With shallow granulating ulcers.

Herpetic lesions of the pharynx

Simplex

A common condition which may be associated with herpes on the lips or face, together with:

1. *Mild pyrexia and toxaemia.* Initially.
2. *Small vesicles.* Present in the mouth and oropharynx, and sometimes on the epiglottis and arytenoid processes. Their sites follow no particular nerve distribution.
3. *Shallow painful ulcers.* Formed when the vesicles burst. The surrounding area is reddened.

Treatment
- Simple antiseptic mouthwashes are usually efficient.
- *2% gentian violet paint* can be used.
- *Acyclovir* is effective if given in the very earliest stage.

Zoster

A rare condition except in the immunosuppressed or debilitated patient.
1. *Vesicles* occur in the distribution of the IXth and Xth cranial nerves which may be paralysed. They are found unilaterally in the pharynx; on the palate; and in the region of the laryngeal inlet. The pharyngeal condition may be associated with geniculate herpes. Cranial nerves affected by zoster often suffer permanent loss of function.
2. *Pain* may be complained of both in the pharynx and in the ear.

Treatment is the same as in the simplex type. Acyclovir used early may be effective.

Chronic non-specific pharyngitis

This is a common condition, especially in patients who have had their tonsils removed. When the tonsils are present, they are usually involved in the chronic inflammatory process.

Aetiology

There are many causative and contributory factors:

1. Recurrent attacks of acute pharyngitis.
2. Nasal obstruction and infections.
3. Excess of alcohol and tobacco.
4. Prolonged exposure to dry and dusty atmospheres.
5. Infected gums and teeth.
6. Pharyngeal 'neuroses', leading to excessive hawking.
7. Faulty or excessive use of the voice.

Clinical types

1. *'Catarrhal'*. In which there is either a dusky red congestion of the mucosa or a pale mauvish oedema. The uvula may appear enlarged or elongated.
2. *Hypertrophic*. Small nodules of lymphoid tissue are scattered over the pharyngeal wall, giving a granular appearance. The lateral pharyngeal bands may be very prominent.
3. *Follicular*. Usually accompanied by a similar infection in the tonsils, when they are present. Small yellowish cysts are seen, commonly in the valleculae, which often escape notice.
4. *Atrophic*. This is usually coexistent with atrophic rhinitis. The pharyngeal mucosa is dry and glazed, with some viscid mucus on the surface.

Symptoms

1. *Irritation in the throat.*
2. *Constant hawking.*
3. *Tiring of the voice* occurs readily.
4. *Snoring.*

Treatment

1. *Cause must be eradicated.* Disease in the nose, sinuses, mouth or tonsils must be eliminated. Hawking must be checked, as it aggravates the condition.
2. *Speech therapy* may be useful.
3. *Reassurance.* The exclusion of cancer helps many psychologically. Strong astringent or antibiotic lozenges are contraindicated.
4. *Cautery to the lymphoid patches* is sometimes advocated.

Chronic pharyngo-oesophagitis *(Paterson–Brown–Kelly disease; Plummer–Vinson syndrome; Chronic hypopharyngitis)*

Definition

A chronic atrophic type of inflammation of the mucous membrane, involving the cricopharyngeal region of the laryngopharynx and the upper part of the oesophagus.

Aetiology

Iron deficiency is probably the basic cause. Approximately half the patients have a pyridoxine deficiency with evidence of abnormal tryptophan metabolism. Gastrectomy increases the risk of developing an upper oesophageal web eightfold. It occurs almost exclusively in women, usually over 40 years of age.

Pathology

A chronic superficial pharyngo-oesophagitis occurs, with subepithelial inflammation. These changes gradually lead to an atrophic mucosa and a subepithelial fibrosis which may be responsible for the web formation which is sometimes found at the pharyngo-oesophageal junction. At an early stage there is some spasm of the cricopharyngeal sphincter but true stenosis occurs later. A hypochromic, microcytic anaemia is present and often severe. Achlorhydria is usually present. Occasionally the condition complicates pernicious anaemia. Between one-third and two-thirds of postcricoid carcinoma patients have had preceding Paterson–Brown–Kelly syndrome.

Clinical features

1. *Increasing dysphagia* occurs, first for solids, later for fluids also. There is often a long history of a 'small swallow' or inability to swallow a normal-sized bolus of food. There may also be a complaint of a 'lump in the throat'.
2. *Pallor* due to the anaemia.
3. *Fissures at the angles of the mouth* result from the angular stomatitis. They are similar to those seen in avitaminosis.
4. *Koilonychia.* Spoon-shaped nails, are common.
5. *Loss of weight.*
6. Dryness of the tongue is caused by a superficial glossitis ('bald tongue').

Differential diagnosis

All other causes of dysphagia. Barium swallow and endoscopy with biopsy should always be done. Full blood count, serum iron, and B_{12} levels are required.

Postcricoid neoplasm is the most important condition to exclude, especially as it not uncommonly follows a chronic pharyngo-oesophagitis.

Functional dysphagia ('globus hystericus') can produce somewhat similar local symptoms.

Treatment

1. *Iron and vitamins* must be given in large doses, viz. ferrous sulphate or gluconate and vitamin B preparations.
2. *Non-irritating soft foods* are desirable.
3. *Repeated endoscopic dilatation* is indicated if the condition is marked and resistant to medical treatment. Any granular area must be removed for biopsy, to exclude carcinoma.

Prognosis

Must be guarded. The disease can improve rapidly with massive doses of iron and vitamins but some cases tend to relapse and must therefore be kept under regular observation.

Tuberculosis of the pharynx

1. Acute miliary tuberculosis

An uncommon complication of pulmonary tuberculosis, usually of an advanced degree.

Clinical features
Painful ulcers, tending to coalesce, with marked salivation, and emaciation.

2. Chronic tuberculous ulceration

Single ulcers occur, especially on the tonsil. Pain may be severe.

3. Lupus vulgaris of the pharynx

Uncommon now. Usually associated with lupus of the face or nose, and is secondary to the latter. Occasionally it is seen with lupus of the larynx. It is most common in young women.

Clinical features
The condition is painless, causing very little inconvenience, but it is slowly progressive. Discrete yellowish-pink nodules arise on the fauces, uvula and palate. These ulcerate and coalesce, forming a pale granular area. Scarring occurs in some parts, simultaneously with nodulation and ulceration in others. The uvula tends to shrink and the soft palate is stiff. There is no adenitis.

Differential diagnosis
From tertiary syphilitic ulceration, leprosy and lymphoma.

Treatment of tuberculosis
Rifampicin, ethambutol, INAH, streptomycin, and PAS are used in combinations chosen to minimize side effects and emergence of drug-resistant bacilli.
   Oral hygiene is essential, as also is attention to any coexistent nasal condition.

Syphilis of the pharynx

Primary syphilis

A chancre is rare in the pharynx but when present is usually on the tonsil as a *unilateral hard, red swelling. Ulceration* takes place within a few days. *Pain is slight. Adenitis is considerable.*

The *Treponema pallidum* is identified in a smear and must be distinguished from other spirochaetes which are often found in buccal and pharyngeal ulcers.

Differential diagnosis is chiefly from quinsy, tuberculosis, lymphoma, sarcoma, agranulocytosis, Vincent's angina and diphtheria.

Secondary syphilis

Clinical features
1. *'Mucus patches',* preceded by erythema, are a relatively common manifestation of the secondary stage.

The lesions may have a greyish translucent surface, often described as a 'snail-track' in appearance, and are surrounded by a narrow zone of injection. They spread on to the tonsil, fauces, tongue, and buccal mucosa.
2. *Cervical and epitrochlear adenitis* are usually present.
3. *Skin rashes* are also found.

Tertiary syphilis

1. *Superficial ulceration* may occur in the early phases of this stage. The ulcers are *serpiginous* in shape, with a dark red areola and occur most commonly on the soft palate and uvula.
2. *Localized gumma* found on the posterior pharyngeal wall, palate, tonsils or vallecula.

A firm red swelling is seen first.

Ulceration follows, with rapid destruction of tissue, often on the posterior surface of the soft palate.

Perforations result from destruction of tissue. When the palate is affected, voice changes occur and there is regurgitation of fluids through the nose. Abundant sticky mucopus adds to the patient's discomfort.
3. *Diffuse infiltration* of gummatous material may lead to confusing bands of thickened tissue on the pharyngeal walls or to swelling of the tonsil.
4. *Scarring* is a common sequel to ulceration and perforation It may be so marked that adhesions are formed between the palate and the posterior pharyngeal wall.
5. *Absence of pain, pyrexia or adenitis* is characteristic of all the above manifestations of the tertiary stage.

Differential diagnosis

Chiefly from lupus vulgaris, malignant disease, scleroma, actinomycosis, Wegener's granulomatosis and a subacute type of Vincent's infection.

Treatment

Systemic penicillin is of prime importance. Local treatment consists of mouth-washes and deodorants, e.g. alkaline solutions and hydrogen peroxide.

Scleroma of the pharynx

This rare chronic induration of the pharynx, probably due to the Frisch bacillus, is met with mainly in inhabitants of Central and Eastern Europe, but also occurs in Central and South America. The nose, nasopharynx and larynx are commonly involved.

Clinical features

A painless, hard, almost cartilaginous induration replaces the pharyngeal wall. This usually spreads down from the nasopharynx, which may become almost closed off by the bulky tissue and by cicatrization. There is no ulceration. General health suffers little.

Differential diagnosis

From lupus, tuberculosis, syphilis, lymphoma, leprosy, and malignant disease.

Treatment

1. *Systemic antibiotics.* Streptomycin and the tetracyclines have given good results, and are often used together with systemic steroids.
2. *Surgery.* Obstructive tissue may be removed surgically from the nasopharynx.

Leprosy of the pharynx

Very rare in UK. Pharyngeal involvement usually follows nasal disease. The tongue, mouth and larynx are also involved and skin lesions are present. *Leprous nodules* become *ulcerated* and then healing occurs, leaving *pale stellate scars* on the pharynx and palate. The uvula becomes granular and ulcerated and may be destroyed. *Perforation* of the *palate* may occur. The leprous tissue is *painless.*

Treatment

Long-term chemotherapy with rifampicin, clofazimine, and dapsone.

Sarcoidosis of the pharynx

A rare chronic granulomatous condition, which occasionally involves the palate though it is more common in the nose, larynx and skin of the face. The lungs are usually affected. *Painless nodules* appear. They are white, brown or bluish, with an injected areola. The patient remains well and spontaneous resolution of the disease is recorded. Evidence of sarcoidosis may be found in the lungs, phalanges, eyes, central nervous system and reticulo-endothelial system. The Kveim test may be positive.

Diagnosis

By biopsy.

Treatment

Empirical. Includes systemic steroids and vitamin D.

Wegener's granulomatosis

Due to a periarteritis, and associated with lung and kidney changes. It is a rare form of *painless progressive ulceration,* similar to that seen in the nose. It appears to start more often on the anterior faucial pillars and later destroys tonsil tissue. The antipolymorpholeucocytic antibody test is frequently positive. Treatment does not always prevent a fatal outcome, though steroids and high dose cyclophosphamide have cured some patients. Oral azathioprine or cyclophosphamide can be used for maintenance therapy.

INFLAMMATIONS OF THE PHARYNGEAL LYMPHOID TISSUE

Adenoids

Definition

A hypertrophy of the nasopharyngeal tonsil sufficient to produce symptoms, most commonly between the ages of 3 and 7 years.

Pathological types

1. *Simple inflammatory.* Usually at the time of physiological enlargement.
2. *Tuberculosis.* Rare.
   In either form there may be some variation in the actual localization of the hypertrophy. It may take the form of a generalized enlargement with many fleshy folds; a firm midline pyramid; or lateral masses around the eustachian cushions. Atrophy usually begins after 10 years of age, and is complete before the age of 20.

Clinical features

Symptoms and signs may be due to simple enlargement, to inflammation, or to both. It is the size of the mass relative to that of the nasopharyngeal space that is of importance, not its absolute size. Certain children show a marked tendency to generalized lymphoid hyperplasia in which the adenoids take a part.

Symptoms and signs due to hypertrophy

1. *Nasal obstruction* leads to mouth-breathing; difficulty in eating, especially in infants; noisy breathing and eating; drooling; snoring; and toneless voice. Later the true 'adenoid facies' may develop, with pinched nostrils and prominent incisors. There may also be a lack of development of the thorax, with flat chest and round shoulders. The open mouth leads to spongy gums and excessive thirst.

2. *Eustachian obstruction* leads to *deafness* from diminished air entry into the tympanum and subsequent retraction of the drumheads. Deafness without otorrhoea, commencing insidiously after the age of 3, must suggest obstruction from adenoids. It can become quite severe and will tend to persist for long periods if not relieved. Obstruction by adenoids predisposes to salpingitis and to the presence of fluid in the middle ear (secretory otitis media). Intermittent earache is common.

Symptoms and signs due to inflammation

1. *Nasal discharge, postnasal drip and cough* are the commonest. The appearance of an egg-white plug of mucus, seen behind the uvula on gagging, is almost diagnostic. An acute infection occurs occasionally, when there is pyrexia and mucopus covers the surface of the adenoids.

2. *Otitis media* is the most serious effect. It may present as recurrent acute attacks, or in a chronic form, often non-suppurative.

3. *Rhinitis and sinusitis* may occur and fail to resolve.

4. *Cervical adenitis* involves the upper deep cervical glands and those in the posterior triangles.

Generalized disturbances

Mental dullness and apathy may be marked and are due to poor breathing, bad posture, or deafness. Nocturnal enuresis, habit tics and night terrors may occasionally be aggravated by adenoids.

Diagnosis

Very large adenoids may rarely be visible through the open mouth. Inspection with a postnasal mirror can often be made in quite young children (i.e. over the age of 3). Narrowing of the nasopharyngeal air space may be seen in the lateral soft-tissue view on an X-ray film.

Differential diagnosis

Many children have their adenoids wrongly blamed for:

1. *Other causes of nasal obstruction* including vasomotor rhinitis; foreign bodies; hypertrophied posterior ends of inferior turbinates; deflected nasal septum; collapsed alae nasi; congenital choanal atresia; sinusitis; antrochoanal polypus; rarely syphilitic 'snuffles' and septal haematoma or abscess.
2. *Orthodontic abnormalities.* High-arched palates, wedge-shaped faces, narrow upper jaws, and crowded teeth predispose to mouth breathing in children and are usually familial. Adenoids may coexist but are not necessarily causative.
3. *Thornwaldt's disease* in which there is a cystic persistence of the median furrow of the nasopharyngeal tonsil.

Treatment

1. Conservative

When symptoms are not marked.
   Non-irritant decongestant nasal drops may give relief. Sinusitis and nasal allergy must be treated. Fresh air, sensible diet, breathing and postural exercises, and tuition in nose-blowing are all important. 'Politzerization' may be useful if there is persistent deafness.

2. Surgical

Adenoidectomy is indicated when the symptoms are marked. Nasal obstruction, deafness, chronic otorrhoea, recurrent otitis media, and sinusitis are the chief indications. In secretory otitis myringotomy and possibly insertion of ventilation tube ('grommet') will be done together with adenoidectomy. Removal of adenoids at the same time as antral lavage is usually more effective in maxillary sinusitis than either of these manoeuvres alone. The tonsils should be only removed if there is a specific indication and not as a routine.

Acute tonsillitis

Aetiology

Infection is often caused by the haemolytic streptococcus, but a great variety of other organisms may be responsible. In many cases a virus infection may be primary. It may occur in epidemic form, especially in schools and camps.

Pathological types

1. *Acute parenchymatous* where the whole tonsil is infected, causing marked generalized swelling. The surface appears reddened and oedematous, with the orifices of the crypts even more injected but not exuding frank pus.
2. *Acute follicular* in which the crypts are filled with infected fibrin, and the mouths of the crypts contain pus, leading to the characteristic spotted appearance. Occasionally these follicular exudates coalesce, giving the appearance of a whitish-yellow false membrane.

These types are not always clearly distinct but tend to merge. In both the cervical lymph nodes are enlarged and tender, the jugulodigastric ('tonsillar') node especially.

Clinical features

1. *Sore throat.*
2. *Pain on swallowing.*
3. *Pyrexia* tends to be very high in children.
4. *Malaise.*
5. *Constipation.*
6. *Earache* is relatively common.

The pulse rate is not raised above 120. The tongue is furred and the breath foetid. The skin is often flushed.

Other complaints include headache, thickened speech from impedance of palatal movements and slight difficulty in opening the mouth.

In severe cases a rigor may occur and the patient may show signs of marked toxaemia, with thirst and oliguria. A slight rash may occur.

Pyrexia and malaise are often the presenting features in children, and especially in infants, when there may be no complaint referable to the throat itself. Pneumonia or appendicitis may be simulated.

Acute tonsillitis occurs in scarlet fever, in which there is very marked injection of the whole pharynx. The tongue has a 'strawberry' appearance and the whole skin is hot and soon develops a punctate erythema.

Complications and sequelae

These are uncommon since the introduction of antibiotics. The most important are:

1. *Peritonsillar abscess.*
2. *Parapharyngeal and retropharyngeal abscesses.*
3. *Oedema of the larynx.*
4. *Acute rheumatism.* Often after a latent period of about 6 weeks. The joints are attacked by antibodies produced against the streptococci.
5. *Acute nephritis.*
6. *Acute infection of the middle ear cleft.*
7. *Septicaemia.*
8. *Chronic tonsillitis.*

Differential diagnosis

Must be made from the many conditions causing an acute pharyngitis. The most important are:

1. *Scarlet fever.*
2. *Diphtheria,* especially from the attenuated form seen in inoculated persons.
3. *Vincent's infection.*
4. *Agranulocytosis.*
5. *Glandular fever (infectious mononucleosis).*

Treatment

1. *Bed rest, soft diet, and ample fluid intake.*
2. *Soluble aspirin.* Effective in mild cases.
3. *Systemic antibiotics.* Given immediately if the infection is severe.

Chronic tonsillitis

Chronic parenchymatous tonsillitis

Usually follows acute or subacute attacks of tonsillitis, and is more common in children between the ages of 4 and 15 years. It may follow any of the exanthemata. There is a chronic inflammatory hypertrophy, usually associated with enlargement of the nasopharyngeal tonsil.

Clinical features

1. *Persistent or recurrent sore throats.*
2. *Persistent cervical adenitis.*
3. *Marked tonsillar enlargement.* Enlarged upper poles may render swallowing difficult and obstruct the eustachian orifices. As time passes the tonsils may shrink due to fibrosis.
4. *Injected anterior faucial pillars.*
5. *Irritating cough.*

Differential diagnosis

Mainly from physiological enlargement, especially in childhood. Sinusitis must be excluded.

Treatment

May be conservative at first, with attention to general health and diet. Lozenges and throat paints are of little use.

Tonsillectomy is advisable if the symptoms persist. Size alone is not an indication unless breathing and feeding are seriously embarrassed.

Chronic follicular tonsillitis

Follows repeated attacks of acute follicular tonsillitis and is seen most commonly in adults.

Clinical features

1. *Chronic irritation or repeated sore throats.* Often with whitish-yellow plugs in the crypts.
2. *Cervical adenitis.* Sometimes.
3. *Cough* is common.
4. *Bad taste and halitosis.*

Differential diagnosis

Mainly from keratosis pharyngis, in which the horny outgrowths are adherent. Small follicular cysts in fibrous tonsils may be mistaken for malignant disease.

Treatment

May be conservative at first. Debris can be expressed with a spatula. Cysts can be incised under local analgesia and the contents expressed or aspirated. Diathermy and other forms of local destruction are deprecated.

Tonsillectomy is indicated if symptoms persist.

Chronic enlargement of the lingual tonsil

May occur in children but more often in adults, especially as a delayed result of tonsillectomy. In the former it may follow whooping-cough. It leads to persistent irritation and cough.

Treatment

Astringent lozenges and paints may suffice. Rarely, in persistent cases in adults, laser or cryosurgical reduction may be warranted.

Tonsilloliths

These arise as a result of chronic infection through calcification of the contents of follicular cysts. One or more of these concretions may be present. They may vary greatly in size. They may lie deep in the tonsil tissue and simulate carcinoma or elongated styloid process on palpation.

Treatment

Consists of simple removal of the concretion or calculus under local analgesia. Tonsillectomy is indicated if this proves ineffective or impossible.

Intra-tonsillar abscess

An abscess is rarely large enough to produce marked local symptoms and is then usually the result of infection around a tonsillolith. Its clinical features vary between those of a chronic follicular tonsillitis and those of a peritonsillar abscess.

Asymptomatic tuberculous infection of the tonsil

Rare now. There are no special characteristics in the tonsils themselves but they may appear more pale and bulky than usual. Large painless cervical lymph nodes are common and typical. Proof of the tuberculous nature of the infection is found only on microscopy. The adenoids are often similarly infected.

Treatment

It is usually wise to perform tonsillectomy in children with tuberculous cervical adenitis. Operation is best done in the quiescent period, after appropriate chemotherapy.

PERITONSILLAR ABSCESS; PARAPHARYNGEAL ABSCESS; RETROPHARYNGEAL ABSCESS

Peritonsillar abscess (quinsy)

Definition

An abscess between the tonsil 'capsule' and the adjacent lateral pharyngeal wall (superior constrictor muscle).

Aetiology

Peritonsillar infection follows an attack of tonsillitis, which is often relatively mild. The size of the tonsils has no bearing on the condition, which may also occur in persons with a post-tonsillectomy 'remnant'. In the great majority the abscess is unilateral and lies above the tonsil near the soft palate. There is first a cellulitis, later frank pus.

Clinical features

1. *Severe pain in the throat.*
2. *Pyrexia. Up to 40°C (104°F).*
3. *Malaise.*
4. *Headache.*
5. *Rigors* may occur.
6. *Trismus* is common, making examination difficult.
7. *Earache.*
8. *Intense salivation and dribbling.*
9. *Thickened speech.*
10. *Foetor oris.*
11. *Cervical adenitis* is marked, with tenderness.
12. *Marked hyperaemia and oedema* of the tonsillar and palatal regions. The uvula is oedematous and pushed to the unaffected side. The tonsil itself may be almost or completely obscured. The reddened mucosa may be covered with festoons of mucopus. Without treatment the abscess usually bursts spontaneously at the end of a week, discharging through a sinus in the fauces, soft palate or tonsil. Aphagia followed by stridor is an indication for urgent drainage.

Complications

Rare with modern therapy. Parapharyngeal abscess is the commonest. Haemorrhages, oedema of the larynx and septicaemia have occurred.

Differential diagnosis

From neoplasms of the tonsil, parapharyngeal abscess, and retropharyngeal abscess.

Treatment

1. *Conservative.* In the early stages of cellulitis, conservative treatment may cure the infection.
   Systemic antibiotics in large intravenous doses. If there is no response to in 48 hours the antibiotics may be changed in the light of bacteriological findings.
   If soluble aspirin fails to control the pain intramuscular opiates are advised.
   Rest in bed, and ample fluids, if necessary by nasogastric tube or intravenously.
2. *Surgical.* When considerable swelling is present, drainage is advisable.
   Incision of the abscess is the standard and accepted treatment. Topical anaesthesia is used and the patient sits upright. Efficient suction should be available. Even if pus has not formed, some relief of pain may follow and resolution may take place quickly. Tonsillectomy is advisable not less than 1 month after the attack has subsided.
   'Abscess-tonsillectomy' is practised by some surgeons, with reports of surprising ease of operation. This technique is appropriate for a child with a quinsy (rare). Systemic antibiotics must be given as a cover. A very experienced anaesthetist is required.

Parapharyngeal abscess

Definition

A suppurative infection of the parapharyngeal space.

Aetiology

Infection spreads from the tonsils, the tonsillar fossa, a penetrating foreign body or from a lower wisdom tooth and its surrounding gums and bone. The abscess may occur at any age, but is more frequent in adolescents and adults.

Clinical features

1. *Painful throat is usual.*
2. *Trismus* is sometimes marked.
3. *Pyrexia* is usually between 38.3 and 38.9°C (101° and 102°F) and the patient feels ill.

4. *Swelling of the* neck may be considerable and is very tender.
5. *Pharyngeal wall and tonsil are pushed medially.* At first there is marked phlegmon, later localized pus.

Complications

These include:

1. Acute oedema of the larynx.
2. Thrombophlebitis of the internal jugular vein, with septicaemia and pyaemia.
3. Direct spread of infection:
- To the fascial planes and 'spaces' of the neck, causing a localized swelling behind the sternomastoid muscle.
- To the mediastinum *(mediastinitis)*.

Differential diagnosis

From peritonsillar abscess, retropharyngeal abscess, tumours and aneurysms.

Treatment

1. *Systemic antibiotics.*
2. Incision of the abscess is performed if fluctuation exists. This may be done through the pharynx or through the neck, depending on the point of maximum swelling but preferably by the latter route. Inhalation of blood and pus must be prevented by efficient suction when the former route is used. Tracheostomy may rarely be necessary.

Retropharyngeal abscess

Definition

The abscess lies in the potential space between the buccopharyngeal and prevertebral fasciae.
    There are two distinct types:

(a) Acute retropharyngeal abscess

Tends to be limited to one side of the midline by the central adherence of the fascia, in the laterally placed space of Gilette.

Aetiology

The acute abscess is caused by suppuration in the retropharyngeal lymph nodes, which become infected from the nasopharynx or oropharynx. Penetration of the pharyngeal wall by a sharp foreign body (e.g. bone) or a neoplasm must be excluded.

Rarely, infection tracks from an acute suppurative otitis media or mastoiditis, either along the tissues around the eustachian tube or by formation of an abscess below the petrous bone.

The commonest organism is *Streptococcus pneumoniae.*

Clinical features

May be misleading, as the patient is often a suckling infant. At least one-half of the patients are under one year of age. This is due to the tendency of the lymph nodes to atrophy in childhood. Boys are said to be more commonly affected than girls.

1. *Difficulty in breathing and suckling* are the prominent features. They are caused by obstruction to the opening of the high and obliquely placed infant's larynx.
2. *Croupy cough* is common. The cry may resemble a 'squawk'.
3. *Nasal obstruction* may be present, when the abscess is highly placed.
4. *Stiffness of the neck or torticollis.*
5. *Pyrexia and toxaemia.*
6. *Lateral swelling of the posterior pharyngeal wall* is seen on inspection through the mouth. The whole pharynx is congested. Palpation is useful, though fluctuation is not always present.
7. *Oedema of the larynx* may develop quickly.
8. *Spontaneous rupture of the abscess* may occur occasionally, and can cause sudden death from aspiration.

Treatment

1. *Incision of the abscess* is made vertically through the open mouth into the swelling. No anaesthetic is used in infants, who must be placed in the prone position, with the head low. Suction should be available.
2. *Systemic antibiotics.*
3. *Tracheostomy* may become necessary when laryngeal obstruction threatens or supervenes.

(b) Chronic retropharyngeal abscess

Aetiology

The chronic abscess is caused by a tuberculous infection. There are two types:

1. Tuberculous caries of the cervical vertebrae, when the abscess lies centrally behind the prevertebral fascia.
2. Tuberculous infection of the retropharyngeal lymph nodes, due to spread of infection from the deep cervical nodes. This abscess lies laterally in the space of Gilette.

Clinical features

A chronic abscess is seen in older children. It also occurs in adolescents and adults. Local symptoms and signs are slow in onset and may be minimal or absent.

1. *Dysphagia* is slight.
2. *Sore throat and cough* may be complained of.
3. *'Cold' abscess* is present on the posterior pharyngeal wall. It is in the midline in cases of spinal caries.
4. *Enlarged painless lymph nodes* are present in the deep cervical group in patients without caries.

Diagnosis

Radiography reveals vertebral disease or calcification in tuberculous lymph nodes. Chronic infection in a branchial cyst must be excluded.

Treatment

Incision of the abscess is made through the neck, never through the mouth. The approach is made in front of the sternomastoid muscle, in the plane between the carotid sheath and the visceral compartment of the neck. If the abscess is highly situated it is better approached from behind the carotid sheath, through an incision behind the sternomastoid.

Any spinal caries is treated appropriately. Large cervical nodes may need to be dissected at a later quiescent stage.

System antibiotics: Rifampicin, ethambutol, INAH, PAS, as appropriate.

ADENOIDECTOMY AND TONSILLECTOMY

Adenoidectomy

Indications

These have been discussed in the section on adenoids (p. 234).

Technique

This has been described briefly under the anatomical principles of pharyngeal surgery (p. 310).

Complications and sequelae

1. Haemorrhage

Is the main one. It is usually primary or reactionary in type, occurring any time up to 24 hours after operation. Secondary haemorrhage from the adenoid bed is less common.

Prevention

● No operation should be done on patients with blood dyscrasias, jaundice, or acute infection.

- Haemorrhage is less likely to occur if the following conditions are observed:
  (a) Curettes are sharp.
  (b) No 'tags' are left behind.
  (c) The operation is unhurried. A dry field should be obtained before the patient is allowed to leave the operating table.
- Known cases of haemophilia and similar disorders should be operated on only with appropriate cover in a Regional Haemophilia Centre.

Treatment

- *Postnasal* pack must be inserted without delay in serious cases of bleeding, after any clots or 'tags' have been removed.
  A general anaesthetic is preferred.
  An inflatable rubber tampon can be introduced through the nose without anaesthesia.
- *Blood transfusion,* when indicated, should not be delayed.

2. Acute otitis media

3. Recurrence

Unfortunately not an uncommon sequel. It may be due to incomplete removal or to an inherent tendency for regrowth of lymphoid tissue in certain children, especially the very young. Further removal may be indicated.

4. Chronic nasopharyngitis

May result from the formation of areas of postoperative fibrosis after excessive removal of mucosa. Simulates Thornwaldt's disease.

5. Granular pharyngitis

Along with enlarged lateral pharyngeal bands are sometimes seen as a late sequel to adenoidectomy.

6. Other complications

Include trauma to the uvula, soft palate, and eustachian cushions; retropharyngeal abscess; cervical cellulitis; sinusitis; and septicaemia. Injury to the internal carotid artery has been reported.

Tonsillectomy

Indications

There are still considerable differences of opinion, but the last decade or two have witnessed a general change to a more conservative attitude.

Local indications

1. *An attack of peritonsillar abscess (quinsy).*
2. *Repeated attacks of acute tonsillitis,* severe enough to cause invalidity. Each case must be judged on its own merits.
3. *Chronic tonsillitis,* when other treatment gives no relief.
4. *Gross obstruction to breathing and swallowing,* where conservative measures have failed.
5. As a preliminary stage to operations for cleft palate, sometimes.
6. For avulsion of the glossopharyngeal nerve and/or removal of the styloid process for neuralgia, by the pharyngeal route.
7. As a precautionary and diagnostic measure for any tonsil suspected of malignancy, where simple biopsy is insufficient.

Contraindications

1. *Allergic rhinitis and asthma.* Unless there is convincing evidence of true tonsillar infection.
2. *Bleeding tendency.* Any suspicion of a bleeding tendency in the patient or family calls for full investigation and correction. Haemophiliacs and other cases of bleeding disorders should only have surgery in recognized Haemophilia Centres. Even if all tests are negative, vitamins K and C may have some preventive value when the history is suggestive. Cryosurgical reduction should be considered in such cases.
3. *Epidemics.* Tonsillectomy (and adenoidectomy) being operations of election should not be performed during an epidemic of any infectious disease. This applies particularly to epidemics of poliomyelitis, in which there is some evidence that the bulbar type of infection is more likely to occur than the spinal type during the postoperative period.

Technique

This has been described briefly under the anatomical principles of pharyngeal surgery (p. 262).

Complications

1. Haemorrhage

1. Reactionary
Occurs within the first few hours after return from the operating theatre.
Causes. The bleeding results from:

- Failure to ligate all bleeding vessels.
- Oozing from the vessels after relaxation of the stretched faucial tissues, on removal of the mouth gag.
- Failure of a vessel to contract and retract after crushing or cutting.
- Rise of blood pressure, during recovery from the anaesthetic. Coughing and straining dislodge an insecure thrombus.
- Slipping of a ligature.

Contributory factors:
- Active or recent acute infection.
- Fibrosis of the tonsil capsule.
- Hurried operations.
- Use of sharp instruments, whereby the vessels are cut across and not torn across.
- Anoxia, from failure to maintain adequate airway.

Nature of the bleeding
Veins are less capable of retraction than arteries, especially if there is much fibrosis in the fossa. A large clot in the fossa tends to keep the torn vessel open, and oozing occurs beneath the clot. Copious fresh blood may appear in the mouth, or a large clot may be seen in the fossa, with fresh blood oozing around it. There is a danger of blood or clot entering the larynx so that the patient should be kept in the correct prone or lateral position.

Other features
The pulse rate rises steadily and must be carefully watched every 15 min. The patient becomes more exsanguinated and shocked. The amount of blood loss may be deceptive, especially in children. Vomiting and collapse may be caused by the presence of swallowed blood in the stomach. In rare cases, submucosal bleeding may extend down to the larynx or into the soft palate, necessitating tracheostomy or laryngotomy.

Prevention
Measures are adopted to exclude causative factors wherever possible.

Treatment
If the patient has not recovered from the anaesthetic the lateral or prone position must be ensured and an adequate airway maintained. Opiates must not be given if restlessness is due to blood loss.
- Removal of clot from the fossae must be attempted as a first-aid measure and a swab held firmly against the fossa for several minutes. It can be soaked in hydrogen peroxide solution. This is often impossible in children and is not dependable.
- Ligature of bleeding vessels should be performed under general anaesthesia *without delay* and, in any event, when signs of blood loss are evident. Delay leads to tragedy.
- Blood transfusion: necessary in severe cases. It must precede ligature if the blood volume is dangerously depleted. (In small children the normal blood volume approximates 80 ml/kg body-weight.)
- Clotting disorders, if suspected, should be urgently tested for, and suitable factor concentrate or fresh blood must be given if appropriate. In some cases intravenous injection of aminocaproic acid is effective.
- Bronchial aspiration through a bronchoscope:
- Iron may be prescribed in the convalescent period.
- Ligature of external carotid artery should rarely be required.

Secondary
Usually occurs between the 3rd and 10th postoperative days. Less commonly it may occur even later.

Cause
Infection in the tonsillar fossa causes secondary haemorrhage, after separation of the slough.

Nature of the bleeding
Bleeding is usually slight, rarely copious. The initial bleeding usually presents as a slight tinge in the saliva; later a frank ooze occurs.

Other features
Postoperative pyrexia usually persists and acts as a warning. The tongue is furred and foetor oris is marked.

Treatment
Secondary haemorrhage usually stops spontaneously.
- Systemic antibiotics should be given whenever postoperative pyrexia persists.
- Rest in bed and minimal sedation will control the bleeding in most cases. The sitting-up position aids haemostasis in the throat and is preferred unless hypotensive shock is present.
- Suture of faucial pillars: is necessary when the bleeding is severe. Oedema or granulations make ligation of the bleeding difficult.
- Blood transfusion may be indicated.

2. Otitis media

Must be distinguished from referred otalgia, which is a very common sequel to tonsillectomy. Deafness will suggest a middle ear infection, but the ears must always be examined when there is a complaint of pain, and routinely at discharge from hospital.

3. Oedema of the soft palate leading to nasal speech.

4. Cervical lymphadenitis

5. Parapharyngeal abscess

6. Septicaemia

7. Pneumonia or lung abscess

May result from inhalation of blood, a deciduous tooth, or infected tissues. The danger is greater when premedication is excessive. They have become rare since the advent of systemic antibiotics and improvements in anaesthesia.

8. Flare-up of distant infections

Tonsillectomy occasionally leads to recrudescences of infections in the joints, kidneys, conjunctivae, or skin. Rheumatic conditions are most commonly affected. Penicillin cover for the operation in such cases usually prevents these occurrences.

9. Dental injuries

Loosened or extracted permanent teeth may sometimes be re-implanted if a dental surgeon is called in immediately.

10. Rare complications

Include burns of the mouth and lips from hot instruments, atrophy or paresis of the uvula, emphysema of the neck, dislocation of the cervical vertebrae or lower jaw, and prolapse of the intervertebral discs.

TUMOURS AND CYSTS OF THE MOUTH, SALIVARY GLANDS AND PHARYNX

Pathology of oral and pharyngeal tumours

Besides primary tumours, the mouth and pharynx may be invaded by tumours originating in the nose, larynx, oesophagus, and other related structures in the neck, such as the thyroid gland.

Benign tumours

Benign epithelial tumours

Papilloma occurs commonly as a discrete pedunculated tumour in the mouth, fauces, palate and tonsils; rarely as a large area of papillomatosis.

'*Mixed' salivary tumour* is always potentially malignant.

Adenoma occurs rarely in the mouth, the most common site being in the palate. It should be removed completely.

Benign connective-tissue tumours

Benign tumours may arise from any of the connective tissues in the pharynx.

Fibroma is not uncommon in the mouth. May be found in any site but most frequently on the buccal mucosa. It is painless unless ulcerated by the teeth, and may be pedunculated or sessile. Fibromas also occur in the pharynx. They should be excised completely.

Lipoma may be found in the floor of the mouth, lips, tongue and pharynx.

Myxoma is an extremely rare tumour in the mouth and pharynx.

Muscle tumours are rare in the mouth and pharynx.

Haemangiomatous formations

- *Scattered telangiectases*
- *Cavernous type*
- *Cirsoid type*

These are not true neoplasms, but rather vascular malformations.

Neurilemmoma is rare in the mouth and pharynx. It usually arises from the sheath of the vagus nerve.

Chordomas are derived from the notochord, which resembles cartilage microscopically. The cells of the notochord, however, are larger and vacuolated and have small nuclei (physaliphorous cell). Chordomas are locally invasive but rarely metastasize.

Teratomas are derived from embryonic tissues not normally present in the pharynx. They may be benign or malignant.

Melanomas are potentially malignant.

Malignant tumours

Not infrequent.

Malignant epithelial tumours

Squamous-cell carcinoma is by far the commonest. It varies in type from highly keratinized to anaplastic.

Polygonal-cell carcinoma (lympho-epithelioma) is next in order of frequency, and occurs more commonly in the proximal than in the distal parts of the pharynx.

Usually considered to be an anaplastic carcinoma occurring in epithelium which is in close association with lymphoid tissue. Consists of an epithelial syncytium with lymphoid cells in the interstices. More common in younger patients and is highly malignant and radiosensitive.

Adenocarcinoma. Tumours of the seromucinous glands of the pharyngeal mucosa mimic one another histologically because of the excessive mucin and mucoid degeneration that separates surviving tumour cells.

Adenoid cystic carcinoma. Once called cylindroma because of its histological form, arises in small salivary glands. Slow growing but definitely malignant, spreads by invading perineural space and following cranial nerves. Metastasizes to lung after some years.

Malignant connective-tissue tumours

Lymphoma. Both the Hodgkin's and non-Hodgkin's malignant lymphomas may be encountered. They are often successfully treated by radiotherapy and cytotoxic drugs.

Solitary plasmacytoma has a tendency to recur; multiple myelomatosis may follow. Excision and radiotherapy are indicated.

Tumours of the mouth and tongue

Benign tumours

All of the benign tumours mentioned in the preceding section on pathology may occur in the mouth. Treatment is by surgical excision.

Pleomorphic adenoma usually occurs in minor salivary glands of the hard palate. They are well circumscribed and treated by excision. A flap repair may be necessary in large defects.

Premalignant lesions

A white patch in the mouth is called leucoplakia. Approximately 3% of white patches will undergo malignant change in 5 years. Biopsy is essential. Dysplasia indicated by nuclear hyperchromatism, nuclear pleomorphism, mitosis and deep cell keratinization, is associated with a higher risk of developing malignancy. Erythroplasia (red patches in the mouth) has a higher risk of undergoing malignant change than leucoplakia.

Oral cavity carcinoma

Carcinoma is the commonest malignant tumour of the oral cavity. Mesothelial malignancies are rare.

Aetiology of oral cavity carcinoma

Smokers are six times more likely to get this condition than non-smokers. Reverse smokers develop hard palate carcinoma. It is more common in pipe than cigarette smokers.

Chewing of tobacco and betel nut (common in India) is a predisposing factor. High alcohol intake, particularly in smokers dramatically increases the likelihood of developing malignancy. Cirrhotics are more likely to develop an oral cavity carcinoma.

The incidence is less than one in 20 000 and decreasing over the recent years.

TNM classification for oral carcinoma

Primary tumour
Tis   Carcinoma in situ
T0   No evidence of primary tumour.
T1   Tumour 2 cm or less in its greatest dimension.
T2   Tumour greater than 2 cm but less than 4 cm in its greatest dimension.
T3   Tumour more than 4 cm in its greatest dimension.
T4   Tumour with extension to bone, muscle, skin, etc.
TX   The minimum requirements to assess the tumour cannot be met.
N   Regional lymph nodes
N0   No evidence of regional lymph node involvement.
N1   Evidence of involvement of movable homolateral regional lymph nodes.
N2   Evidence of involvement of movable contralateral or bilateral regional lymph nodes.
N3   Evidence of involvement of fixed regional lymph nodes.
NX   The minimum requirement to assess the regional lymph nodes cannot be met.

Carcinoma of anterior two-thirds of tongue

Clinical features.

1. *A small warty growth:* may occur.
2. *Ulceration:* may appear in an area of hyperkeratosis, usually on the side of the tongue. The base of the ulcer is indurated and sloughing and there is an everted edge. The tumour is usually considerably larger than the ulcer. It extends on to the floor of the mouth and gingiva as it grows making the exact site of origin uncertain.
3. *Pain:* common.
4. *Foetor:* often a marked feature.
5. *The tongue is fixed:* in advanced cases it deviates to the side of the lesion when protruded.
6. *Lymph node metastases:* Common and often bilateral. If the lesion is at the tip of the tongue, the submental nodes are involved first.

Diagnosis

Any doubtful lesion should be subjected to biopsy, and if it is ulcerated *cytological examination* can be useful.

Carcinoma of buccal mucosa and floor of mouth

Presents similar clinical features. Usually occurs in patients in their fifties and sixties. May occur primarily in any part of the mouth, especially in the region of the opening of the submandibular ducts. The oral mucosa may also be affected by spread from the tongue or alveolus. In floor of mouth cases, fixation of the tumours usually indicates that the mandible has been invaded. Most cases present at the T3 and T4 stage.

Carcinoma of the alveolar ridge

Eighty per cent affect the lower ridge 80% present at least T2 stage. It invades the mandible and once it has entered the inferior alveolar canal will grow along the nerve to the skull base. Such spread is not clinically obvious.

Carcinoma of the retromolar trigone

These tumours appear to be more aggressive than most oral cavity sites with early metastasis in over 50% of cases to the regional nodes.

Treatment of oral cavity carcinoma

Radiation
T1 and T2 lesions do equally well with surgery or radiotherapy. 65 Grays are delivered in fractions over 4–5 weeks. Radioactive needles can be given to lesions of the lateral border or tip of the tongue. Palpable neck nodes should be controlled by block dissection.

T3 and T4 lesions do badly when treated with radiation alone. Postoperative radiation may reduce recurrence.

Surgery

The standard procedure is a partial or total glossectomy with resection of adjacent mandible and floor of mouth. Reconstruction is effected by using one of the following:

1. Regional random flaps, e.g. nasolabial flaps, lateral or median cervical flaps.
2. Distant axial flaps, e.g. temporal flap or deltopectoral flap.
3. Pectoralis major myocutaneous flap. The primary blood supply is from the pectoral branch of the acromiothoracic artery.
4. Free vascular forearm flap based on the radial artery and two forearm veins.

The mandible can be repaired by pedicled bone grafts, free bone grafts or metal plate (usually temporary).

Neck nodes

Unilateral nodes are best dealt with by a radical neck dissection. Bilateral nodes or fixed nodes carry such a poor prognosis that palliative treatment will be all that is appropriate in many cases. Irradiation to both sides of the neck is possible as is bilateral neck dissection with preservation of one jugular vein.

Carcinoma of the lip

Aetiology

More common in males. Sun exposure and tobacco smoking predispose. More common in outdoor workers and in Caucasians living in hot climates such as Australia and the southern states of the USA.

UICC classification

T   Primary tumour
Tis   Carcinoma in situ.
T0   No evidence of primary tumour.
T1   Tumour limited to the lip: 2 cm or less in its greatest dimension.
T2   Tumour limited to the lip: more than 2 cm but not more than 4 cm in its greatest dimension.
T3   Tumour limited to the lip: more than 4 cm in its greatest dimension.
T4   Tumour extending beyond the lip to neighbouring structures such as skin, bone, tongue etc.
TX   The minimum requirements to assess the primary tumour cannot be met.

Treatment

Has a more favourable prognosis than other oral lesions. Surgery is preferred to radiotherapy. Most cases present early and can be reconstructed after resection with an Abbé flap.

Tumours of the nasopharynx

Juvenile nasopharyngeal angiofibroma

The commonest of the rare benign tumours of the nasopharynx.

Pathology

A firm tumour, consisting of fibrous tissue with varying degrees of vascularity. The blood channels may or may not have a muscle coat. Originates from the periosteum of one or other side of the roof of the nasopharynx.
Extensions occur:

1. *Into the nose:* To bend the lateral nasal wall into the antral cavity, and the septum into the opposite nasal cavity.
2. *Into the pterygoid fossa:* To wind round the outside of the maxilla and later to lie under the cheek.
3. *Into the ethmoidal region:* To push the inner wall of the orbit outwards, and to enter the orbit through the sphenomaxillary (inferior orbital) fissure.

Incidence

Patients usually present between the ages of 18 and 20 years, but the tumour may occur at any time between 8 and 50. There is a predilection for males, but females are not exempt.

Clinical features

1. *Progressive nasal obstruction.*
2. *Recurrent severe epistaxes.*
3. *'Nasal' speech (rhinolalia clausa).*
4. *Conductive deafness* occurs from pressure on the eustachian tube, usually of one side.
5. *A smooth, lobulated, rubbery tumour* is found in the nasopharynx. It is reddish or grey in colour.
6. *Late features due to extension.* Include:
● *Broadening of the nasal bridge* ('frog-face' deformity).
● *Unilateral prominence of the cheek.*
● *Displacement of the globe of the eye.*

Radiography

The tumour may be shown in the nasopharynx, with a small area of attachment sometimes discernible. It may show displacement of the lateral nasal wall into the antrum, and of the septum to the opposite side. There may also be widening of the space between the outer wall of the maxilla and the mandible, in the anteroposterior projection. Angiography demonstrates the size and vascular supply of the tumour and offers the radiologist the opportunity to embolize the feeding vessels.

Differential diagnosis

From an antrochonal polypus undergoing fibrosis. Biopsy may be helpful but precautions must be taken to treat the excessive bleeding which may result.

Treatment

Conservative treatment. Not justifiable, as it is doubtful whether spontaneous regression ever occurs.

Irradiation. May decrease the vascularity of the tumour but does not cure it. It is therefore reserved for preoperative treatment.

Cryosurgery. Has also been used to decrease vascularity, but results have been disappointing.

Surgery. The tumour may be approached by two routes: *(a) Transpalatal approach. (b) Combined lateral rhinotomy and per-oral approach.* Haemorrhage is the main danger of operation, but it can be minimized by separating the tumour from the base of the skull in a plane between the bone and periosteum. Staged reduction of the tumour by electrocoagulation or cryoprobe has been used. Hypotensive anaesthesia is invaluable.

Other benign tumours

Give rise to nasal obstruction. Nasal discharge and epistaxis are variable features. Diagnosis depends upon biopsy. Salivary gland tumours, chordomas, and teratomas are liable to malignant change; they should therefore be extirpated by surgical removal and/or electrocoagulation.

Squamous-cell carcinoma

The commonest tumour of the nasopharynx, is especially common in the Chinese peoples. HLA-A2, HLA-8Sin2 and HLA-A8 are usually found in the affected Chinese. High titres of Epstein-Barr virus are usually found in association with the disease. The exact aetiological role of the virus is unknown. Varying degrees of differentiation occur. The fossa of Rosenmüller is a common site.

Clinical types

1. *Proliferative.* Sometimes polypoid, giving rise to signs of obstruction in the nasopharynx.
2. *Ulcerative.* When epistaxis may be a prominent feature.
3. *Infiltrative and non-ulcerative.* In which neuro-ophthalmological signs result.

Clinical features

1. *Metastases in the lymph nodes of the neck.* Often the presenting sign. They may be unilateral or bilateral. The retropharyngeal nodes are said to be involved sometimes. The primary lesion may remain submucosal and invisible for many months after the nodes have appeared. It has been suggested

that such primary tumours may arise from the submerged portion of the lining of the primitive pharynx.

2. *Symptoms of local invasion (Trotter's triad)*

● Conductive deafness: due to infiltration of the eustachian tube. This may proceed to secretory otitis media.

● *Elevation and immobility of the homolateral soft palate:* due to direct infiltration.

● *Pain in the side of the head:* due to involvement of the Vth cranial nerve, from infiltration via the foramen lacerum. Pain may also be felt in the ear, upper or lower jaws, and the tongue.

3. *Other symptoms of invasion*

● *Internal strabismus:* caused by involvement of the VIth cranial nerve.

● Exophthalmos: from orbital invasion via the sphenoidal (superior orbital) fissure. This leads to paralysis of the IInd, IIIrd and IVth cranial nerves.

● *Jugular foramen syndrome:* shown by pareses of the IXth, Xth and XIth cranial nerves.

4. *Nasal obstruction.* In the proliferative type of tumour.

5. *Epistaxis.* In the ulcerative type.

Diagnosis

The postnasal mirror, the flexible fibrescope and the finger should be used in all cases of suspected nasopharyngeal neoplasm.

Radiography, including tomography and CT scan, may show a lesion in the base of the skull, even when the above clinical examinations are negative.

Biopsy is essential. In cases of doubt the transpalatal removal of a 'melon slice' of mucosa and submucosa from the region of fossa of Rosenmüller is justified, when symptoms suggest an infiltrative tumour, even in the absence of an obvious tumour mass in that situation.

UICC classification

Tis Carcinoma in situ.
T0   No evidence of primary tumour.
T1   Tumour confined to one site (including tumour identified from positive biopsy).
T2   Tumour involving two sites.
T3   Tumour extension to nasal cavity and/or oropharynx.
T4   Tumour with extension to base of skull and/or involving cranial nerves.
TX   The minimum requirements to assess the primary tumour cannot be met.

Regional lymph nodes are classified the same as for carcinoma of the oral cavity.

The sites in the nasopharynx are:

1. Posterosuperior wall: extending from the junction of the hard and soft palates to the skull base.

2. Lateral wall: including the fossa of Rosenmüller.

3. Inferior wall: consists of the superior surface of the soft palate.

Treatment

Radiotherapy. The method of choice, because surgical removal of the primary growth is rarely possible; metastases are often present when the patient is first seen; and the tumours are usually anaplastic and highly radiosensitive. Treatment must include the whole lymphatic field.

A central palatal fenestration allows inspection and the destruction of any residual growth by diathermy. A permanent palatal obturator can be worn without great inconvenience.

Other malignant tumours

The lymphomas are usually seen in younger patients. They are usually highly radiosensitive; external irradiation to the primary focus and lymphatic fields is therefore the method of choice, whether or not lymph node involvement is evident, and cytotoxic drugs form a part of the management.

Tumours of the oropharynx

Benign tumours

1. Papilloma

The common pedunculated and fimbriated papilloma of the tonsil, fauces and palate may be single or multiple. It has a fibrovascular core. It may be large enough to make its presence felt but is usually small and can be snipped off.

2. Adenoma

Rare. The salivary gland tumour is the commonest 'adenoma' and should always be regarded as potentially malignant.

3. Benign connective-tissue tumours

Rare. They include lipoma and fibroma, which may be pedunculated or submucosal.

4. Neurilemmoma

May appear in the lateral part of the pharynx, behind the tonsil, as an encapsulated tumour arising from the sheath of the vagus or other cranial nerves. A homolateral Horner's syndrome may be associated with the tumour. It shells out easily but may leave a palsy.

5. Haemangiomatous formations

Occur in the palate, tonsils, and posterior and lateral walls of the oropharynx.

Treatment
May be required for haemorrhage or obstructive symptoms. The choice lies between:
● *Diathermy coagulation:* with ligature of the external carotid artery if necessary.
● *Cryotherapy or laser excision.*

Malignant tumours

1. Squamous-cell carcinoma

Aetiology
Occurs most commonly in a keratinized form in elderly males; a less differentiated type is sometimes seen in younger patients. Tobacco and alcohol are believed to be important factors in aetiology. Dental sepsis and syphilis are still important factors in the Third World but not routinely in the western countries.

Site

The commonest site of origin is the tonsillo-lingual sulcus, but the tumour may also arise from the tonsil itself; from the palate or uvula; and from the lower part of the posterior wall of the oropharynx. An intraepithelial form of carcinoma (carcinoma-in-situ, or Bowen's disease) may precede the clinically obvious malignant change by a long period, especially on the palate. There may be local infiltration into the tongue, hard and soft palates, alveolus and mandible. Lymphatic metastases appear in the upper deep cervical nodes.

UICC classification
Primary tumour
Tis   Carcinoma in situ
T0   No evidence of primary tumour
T1   Tumour 2 cm or less in its greatest dimension.
T2   Tumour greater than 2 cm but not more than 4 cm in its greatest dimension.
T3   Tumour more than 4 cm in its greater dimension.
T4   Tumour with extension to bone, muscle, antrum, neck etc.
TX   The minimum requirements to assess the primary tumour cannot be met.

Nodal classification
Same as for oral cavity.

Clinical features
● *Early*
  (a) A persistent sore throat, often mild in character.
  (b) Slight difficulty in swallowing is sometimes the first symptom, occasionally with referred ear pain.
● *Late*
  (a) Pain in the ear.
  (b) Enlarged cervical nodes.
  (c) Salivation.

(d) Haemorrhage from the mouth. The tumour is usually ulcerated and infiltration into the tongue causes it to be partly immobilized and pulled towards the side of the lesion when it is protruded.

Diagnosis
Some cases have been mistaken for a quinsy, especially when trismus is present. Biopsy is essential. Tuberculous and syphilitic infections must be excluded.

Treatment
- External irradiation: to the tumour and to the entire lymphatic field. Midline growths of the soft palate require irradiation to both sides of the neck.
- *Monoblock removal:* wide removal of the tumour and cervical nodes en bloc. A portion of the mandible, tongue, cheek, tonsil and palate is included as required in the excision (commando operation). A free flap repair gives the best results cosmetically.
- *Cytotoxic drugs:* at present best regarded as possibly offering temporary palliation and relief from pain.
- *Symptomatic treatment.* Many patients have such a poor prognosis e.g. those with distant metastases, fixed bilateral nodes, anaplastic tumour, advanced debilitation with age that active surgical or radiotherapy turns their last few weeks into a misery. In these patients, pain relief and supportive nursing care ideally in the home gives the best option.

Prognosis
In favourable cases of oropharyngeal squamous-cell carcinoma (i.e. without lymph-node involvement) about 30% may be expected to survive a 5-year period.

2. Lymphoepithelioma

Now known to be a highly anaplastic squamous-cell carcinoma. Not uncommon, especially in younger patients, and usually affects the tonsil, base of tongue and vallecula. Often a bulky, non-ulcerating tumour, but ulceration may occur later. Metastasizes readily. Digital palpation of the posterior third of the tongue will often reveal a suspected growth, endoscopy always. Biopsy of a tumour in this position is important. A lingual thyroid can always be recognized by a radio-isotope scan.

Treatment
By *radiotherapy* to the growth; must include bilateral lymphatic areas, from the clavicles to the base of the skull. Extremely radiosensitive.

3. Adenocarcinoma

Most of these are salivary gland tumours usually adenoid cystic carcinomas. They occur in the palatal and faucial regions as swellings and constitute about 3% of oropharyngeal tumours. A swelling at the fauces may occasionally be an extension from a tumour within the parotid gland. In this case an external approach may be required. Radiotherapy is required when there is infiltration into surrounding areas.

4. Lymphoma

Most cases are non-Hodgkins lymphoma B-cell type. The aetiology of most cases is unknown. In the high grade B-cell lymphoma, lymphoblastic type known as Burkitt's lymphoma there is a high Epstein-Barr virus titre with evidence of chronic immunosuppression due to malaria. T-cell lymphoma is associated with HTLV-I infection especially in Japan and the Caribbean.

Classification
Kiel classification of non-Hodgkins lymphoma (Lennert, 1978).
Low grade malignant lymphomas.

i. lymphocytic lymphoma (B cell, T cell, mycosis fungoides, hairy cell leukaemia)
ii. immunocytoma
iii. plasmacytoma
iv. centrocytic lymphoma
v. centroblastic/centrocytic lymphoma.

High grade malignant lymphomas.

i.centroblastic lymphoma
ii. lymphoblastic lymphoma (B or T)
iii. immunoblastic lymphoma

The commonest types of lymphoma in the oropharynx are centroblastic/centrocytic and centroblastic.

Once a diagnosis of non-Hodgkins lymphoma has been made the disease needs to be staged.

Staging of non-Hodgkin's lymphoma
I Involvement of a single lymph node region or of a single extralymphatic organ (IE).
II Involvement of two or more lymph node regions on the same side of the diaphragm; or localized involvement of an extralymphatic organ or site of one or more lymph node regions on the same side of the diaphragm (IIE).
III Involvement of lymph node regions on both sides of the diaphragm which may also be accompanied by local involvement of extralymphatic organs or site (IIIE) by involvement of the spleen (IIIS), or both (IIIE(S))
IV Diffuse or disseminated involvement of one or more extralymphatic organ tissues with or without associated lymph node enlargement. The reason for classifying the patient as stage IV is identified further by specifying the site.

Staging is facilitated by bone marrow aspiration and biopsy, chest radiography, skeletal survey, bipedal lymphography, liver biopsy and CT scan. Staging laparotomy has no place to play in non-Hodgkin's lymphoma.

Treatment
Radiotherapy is used to control localized disease. Disseminated lymphoma is managed by combination chemotherapy. Combinations of vincristine, cyclophosphamide and prednisolone (COP) and COP with doxorubicin (CHOP) are widely used.

Tumours of the hypopharynx (laryngopharynx)

Benign tumours

Rare but pedunculated fibromas and angiofibromas have been seen to originate from the aryepiglottic fold and pyriform fossa. They may grow quite large and can sometimes lodge in the laryngeal inlet and may undergo torsion of the pedicle. Some can be removed by *endoscopic division of the pedicle.*

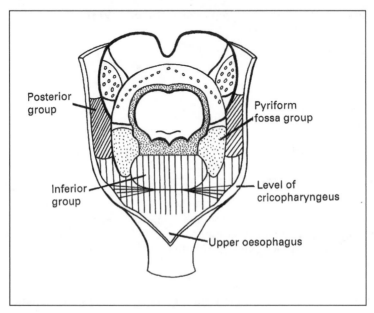

Figure 13.1

Malignant tumours

Squamous-cell carcinoma (Figure 13.1)

The commonest neoplasm and all grades of differentiation are seen. Any other type of neoplasm is of extreme rarity in this situation. Prognosis is bad with any treatment. Not more than 40% can be expected to survive 5 years.

UICC classification of hypopharyngeal carcinoma
Tis   Carcinoma in situ.
T0   No evidence of primary tumour.
T1   Tumour confined to one site.
T2   Tumour with extension to adjacent site or region without fixation of hemilarynx.
T3   Tumour with extension to adjacent site or region with fixation of hemilarynx.
T4   Tumour with extension to bone, cartilage or soft tissues.
TX   The minimum requirements to assess the primary tumour cannot be met.

Regional nodes are classified the same as for carcinoma of the oral cavity. They are best named according to their position.

1. *Pyriform fossa*

Clinical features

The largest group, commoner in men than women. At first there may be no more than a *'catch in the throat'. Pain on swallowing* occurs later and radiates to the ear. *Increasing dysphagia* follows. *A hard mass high in the neck is usually direct extension of tumour rather than a nodal metastasis and* is often the first sign. *Hoarseness* indicates infiltration or oedema of the larynx or paralysis of the recurrent laryngeal nerve.

Diagnosis

A pool of mucus in the pyriform fossa may be seen on indirect laryngoscopy. Tomography and a barium swallow often indicate the size of the tumour. *Endoscopy* is always necessary for biopsy and to assess the extent of the disease.

Treatment

- *Surgical removal* by pharyngolaryngectomy, together with the homolateral cervical nodes as a monoblock dissection is the usual practice. This may be:

  (a) Multistaged procedure using skin or myocutaneous flaps for reconstruction, or

  (b) Single-stage operation in which the immediate reconstruction is made by: (i) utilizing the retained disease-free contralateral side of pharynx, larynx, and trachea. The latter is joined to the oesophagus. (ii) A portion of an abdominal viscus (colon or stomach) replacing the pharynx as a graft pedicled on its own artery and vein and brought to the neck antesternally or through the anterior or posterior mediastinum. This is absolutely indicated when the oesophagus is involved to an extent that renders skin flaps impracticable. It is combined with total oesophagectomy. (iii) As a free graft of colon, revascularized by anastomosing the inferior mesenteric artery to the external carotid and the inferior mesenteric vein to the common facial vein.

- *Radiotherapy* is used by some as the method of choice. Radiotherapy is also employed as a palliative measure in inoperable cases or may be divided into preoperative and postoperative courses to 'sandwich' the operation. Block dissection of the neck is necessary when the primary growth, but not the nodes, is brought under control by irradiation.

- *Cytotoxic drugs* may be helpful as adjuncts to either surgery or radiotherapy. It should be recognized that some patients are untreatable.

2. *Posterior and lateral pharyngeal wall*

Clinical features

Commoner in men than women. Dysphagia is the presenting symptom. Spitting up blood may be the first sign when the tumour is traumatized by food. The midline position of the posterior tumours makes bilateral lymph node metastases frequent. Endoscopy and radiography are essential; lateral views show the thickness of the tumour and extensions upwards and downwards in the retropharyngeal tissues.

Treatment

Most are treated by external irradiation especially as many of these growths tend to be anaplastic. One or two courses of combination chemotherapy may be given a few days before radiotherapy is begun. In a few cases small growths can be removed surgically, through a lateral pharyngotomy. Operations involving varying degrees of supraglottic laryngectomy have been revived recently. These are often accompanied by 'block dissection' as lymph node involvement is so common.

3. *Postcricoid carcinoma*

Situated between the upper border of the cricoid cartilage above and the oesophageal opening below. This group is second in incidence and 90% occur in females. The anterior (cricoid) wall of the postcricoid space is more often attacked than the posterior (vertebral) wall. Lateral extensions form an annular growth, while downward extensions invade the oesophagus. There is frequently a submucosal lymphatic spread in all directions, particularly downwards, giving a mammillated appearance to the pharyngeal and oesophageal mucosae.

Clinical features

Dysphagia is the predominant symptom. The patient, sometimes as young as 30, may give a long history of moderate dysphagia due to a chronic pharyngo-oesophagitis. This is may be associated with a hypochromic, microcytic anaemia, and other manifestations of the Paterson–Brown Kelly syndrome.

   Lymph-node metastases are often bilateral and may be in the mediastinum.

Diagnosis

Endoscopy and radiography are required to assess the extent of the tumour and especially to define its lower border. Lateral views of the soft parts may show an increase in the distance between the vertebral column behind and the larynx and trachea in front. Barium swallow should be done always.

Treatment

● Surgery is preferred by many but the prospect of cure is poor with any form of treatment. Many hold that radiotherapy deserves initial trial in most if not all cases.

(a) Lateral pharyngectomy. Rarely it is possible to remove the growth, with preservation of the larynx. The pharynx is reconstructed with a skin flap from the neck which makes a gutter behind the larynx. This gutter is closed and buried at a later stage.

(b) Pharyngolaryngectomy and pharyngo-oesophago-laryngectomy. These have been briefly described under the Anatomical principles of pharyngeal surgery (p. 310). One-stage operations utilizing the disease-free anterior half of the larynx and trachea or by the use of grafts of abdominal viscera, either pedicled or revascularized, are alternatives to the multi-stage procedures.

   Postoperative care after these operations is important and consists of: systemic antibiotics to prevent local and pulmonary infections; suction for clearance of the tracheal stoma; short-term intravenous feeding, with saline and dextrose; long-term tube feeding, by intermittent or continuous drip, with a diet of 2000 calories per day, containing protein, fat, carbohydrate, vitamins and water. These feeds can be made by liquidizing natural foods in a high-speed mixer, or by using proprietary preparations such as Complan; replacement of thyroid and parathyroid hormones, when necessary, by:

   Thyroxine 0.1 mg daily and calcium lactate 3 g t.d.s. A.T. 10 (dihydrotachysterol) 3 ml t.d.s. or with calciferol 1–5 mg daily. Alcohol is a useful addition to the diet, and electrolyte and fluid balance must be maintained.

Complications include chest and gut infections, as well as poor healing leading to fistulae in the neck. Prolonged hospitalization and poor quality of life may defeat the purpose of the operation.
● *Palliative radiotherapy:* Indicated when:
(a) Lymph-node metastases are bilateral or inoperable.
(b) The patient is unfit for major operative procedures.
● *Cytotoxic drugs* can have a palliative role in combination with radiotherapy.
4. *Carcinoma of the cervical oesophagus*
 Can invade the pharynx. In such cases obstructive symptoms may be slight, despite the presence of a large ulcer, until it has caused a stricture in the gullet. Diagnosis and treatment is the same as for postcricoid carcinoma.

Tumours of the salivary glands

As a rough guide the site and nature of salivary gland tumours may be summarized by the following three statements.
● 90% of salivary tumours involve the parotid.
● 90% of parotid tumours are benign.
● 90% of minor salivary gland tumours are malignant.

Pleomorphic adenoma

A benign epithelial tumour with a mucopolysaccharide stroma. It has a pseudocapsule which is incomplete such that protruberances of tumour extend beyond the apparent capsule. They must be excised with as large a margin as is possible to reduce the high recurrence rate. Most occur in the parotid gland. The longer the tumour is in place the higher the chance of malignant change.
   Treatment is by surgical excision of the gland. In cases where the tumour has ruptured during removal or there is suspected tumour remnant radiation may be given in order to reduce the risk of a recurrence. Recurrence after formal parotidectomy is a difficult situation to deal with as the facial nerve is at great risk in revision surgery.

Adenolymphoma (Warthin's tumour)

Benign. Almost exclusively seen in middle-aged and elderly men. Nearly always occurs in the tail of the parotid. It is susceptible to inflammation associated with upper respiratory tract infection. The history may include one of pain and fluctuating swelling.
   Treatment is by surgical excision. Unlike pleomorphic adenoma recurrence is unusual.

Oncocytoma

Rare benign eosinophilic tumour that demonstrates some pleomorphism. Can occur in the lacrimal and submandibular glands but usually in the superficial parotid. It can undergo malignant change. Treatment is by excision.

Mucoepidermoid

Malignant often low grade. Predominantly affects the parotid and minor salivary glands. Consists of epidermoid and mucus producing cells. May contain large 'lakes' of mucus. Low grade tumours are best dealt by a local resection whereas high grade tumours require a radical resection with radiotherapy.

Acinic cell tumour

Very slow growing malignant tumour. Usually seen in the parotid gland. Distant metastases or local recurrence can appear many years after control of the primary site. Regional nodes are rarely involved at presentation. Treatment is by wide excision of the gland. Usually the main branches of the facial nerve can be preserved in cases involving the parotid. Adjunctive radiotherapy should be considered.

Adenoid cystic carcinoma

Commonest salivary gland malignancy. Parotid tumours are rarely of this type. It commonly occurs in the minor glands and the submandibular. It grows slowly spreading along the perineural pathways and bony canals. Twenty-one per cent of patients will survive 20 years with this condition. Distant metastases occur late.

Treatment is by radical excision and radiotherapy.

Adenocarcinoma

Accounts for about 3% of parotid neoplasms and about 11% of neoplasms of the minor glands. Most cases present as a painless lump. The commonest indication of malignancy is fixation to surrounding tissues. Facial palsy only present in about 5% of cases. One in five have involvement of regional nodes at presentation.

Recurrence is usually local but distant metastases do occur. Initial treatment is radical local excision followed by radiotherapy.

Cysts of the mouth and pharynx

Simple retention cysts

1. Mucous retention cysts

May occur on the lips and buccal mucosa as smooth roundish swellings containing fluid and are usually bluish or yellow in colour. They may also occur in any part of the pharyngeal mucosa, most commonly in the vallecula. They are usually asymptomatic.

Treatment is by total removal of cysts in the lips and by *uncapping* with forceps when symptoms are caused by a pharyngeal cyst.

2. Ranula

Ranula is a retention cyst in the floor of the mouth arising from the submandibular or sublingual ducts, or from mucous glands in the floor of the mouth. The cyst may develop to a large size, penetrating the deep structures of the floor of the mouth. It occurs on one side of the midline of the tongue which may be pushed up.

Treatment is best effected in most cases by marsupialization.

Complete excision is often difficult owing to the ramifications of the cyst; if it arises from the ducts of the sublingual gland, the gland may have to be removed.

3. Cysts of (palatine) tonsillar crypts

Commonly seen in the tonsil after inflammation as yellow cysts, often multiple.

Treatment is by *slitting* to release the contents in which concretions may be present. *Tonsillectomy* is advisable if recurrent or multiple cysts are causing symptoms.

4. Cysts of nasopharyngeal tonsil

Result from adhesions between the vertical folds subsequent upon incomplete adenoidectomy or inflammation. The enclosed submucosal glands and goblet cells produce a mucous cyst. Rupture and intermittent leakage may result.

Thornwaldt's disease is an abscess resulting from secondary infection.

Treatment is by *incision and curettage*.

Midline cysts of developmental origin

1. Cysts of median nasopharyngeal sinus

This entodermal sinus is of doubtful significance. It is thought to have remnants of notochord adherent to it when it persists and these are held responsible for the cystic formations. The cystic or suppurative condition resembles that of a cyst of the nasopharyngeal tonsil.

2. Other midline cysts of nasopharynx

Cysts developing from the remnants of Rathke's pouch and Sessel's pouch are of extreme rarity.

Branchial cysts, fistulae and sinuses

General considerations

A cyst, a sinus in the pharynx (internal) or neck (external), or even a complete fistula running between the pharyngeal mucosa and the skin of the neck, can result from abnormal development of the primitive entodermal pharyngeal pouches.

The *embryonic cervical sinus* is perceived by embryologists to be an external depression at the site of the third and fourth pharyngeal arches which later becomes obliterated. Incomplete obliteration leads to the formation of a sinus or fistula in front of the anterior border of the sternomastoid muscle.

Abnormal development of the *first entodermal pouch* involves malformation of the middle ear cleft. The unobliterated first ectodermal groove presents as a sinus in the neck above the hyoid tracking towards the external auditory canal (collaural fistula). This is quite a separate entity from the preauricular sinus and cyst.

Complete branchial fistula

Results from the persistence of the *second pouch* together with a persistent embryonic cervical sinus, the membrane between the pouch and the sinus being perforated in such a case.

The internal opening is usually in the upper half of the posterior faucial pillar. The supratonsillar fossa and the tonsil itself are other sites. Dye gently syringed up a branchial fistula with a lacrimal cannula spills into the pharynx revealing the internal opening. Radiographic contrast medium introduced in the same way shows the track beautifully on a plain neck film (sinogram). This track passes between the internal and external carotid arteries, superficial to the hypoglossal and glossopharyngeal nerves but deep to the posterior belly of digastric muscle. There is little doubt of its embryological origins.

Branchial cysts

May occur in any part of the track taken by a complete fistula, but a branchial cyst often lacks a fibrous attachment passing inwards between the internal and external carotid arteries suggesting that it is not always a branchial arch developmental abnormality but may be due to epithelial tissue within a lymph node.

Clinical features

A branchial cyst usually lies deep to the anterior border of the sternomastoid muscle. Because the tumour in the neck is usually painless and because fluctuation is difficult to elicit, it is frequently mistaken for tuberculous adenitis. The swelling may show variations in size, increasing in the presence of infection and decreasing as this subsides.

Very rarely squamous-cell carcinoma may develop as a primary tumour in a branchial cyst because squamous epithelium may turn malignant wherever it is found.

Treatment

The cyst or the fistulous track must be *dissected out* in its entirety. Staining the lumen with blue dye before skin incision makes dissection easier. Simple evacuation of the mucoid or cheesy contents of a cyst leads to recurrent intermittent discharge through the operative incision.

Pharyngocele

This is a diverticulum, usually bilateral, opening from the pyriform fossa. It is held to be a occupational risk of trumpet players and glass blowers. It can be distended by the patient blowing with the mouth and nose closed.

Treatment. Excision is necessary if large, or if swallowed fluids collect in it.

MISCELLANEOUS CONDITIONS OF THE MOUTH AND PHARYNX

Fracture of mandible

Aetiology

This injury is usually caused by a blow, but indirect fractures are not uncommon and pathological fracture through a cyst or an unerupted tooth may also occur.

Clinical features

1. *Difficulty in moving the mandible.*
2. *Swelling and bruising.* Over the site of the blow.
3. *Pain.*
4. *Derangement of occlusion.*
5. *Lack of continuity.* In the bony outline.
6. *Rupture.* Of the oral mucous membrane.
7. *Abnormal mobility.* Of the lower jaw.
8. *Tenderness.* Over the site of the fracture.
9. *Anaesthesia or paraesthesia.* Over the distribution of the mental nerve, occasionally.
10. *Bleeding from the ear.* When the tympanic plate is involved.

Diagnosis

Depends on:

1. *Displacement.* Apart from that occurring in the direction of the force causing the fracture, the displacement will also depend upon the direction of the fracture line and the direction of muscular traction, e.g. a fracture at the angle of the mandible, with an unfavourable fracture line, will result in an upward and forward displacement of the ascending ramus by the temporalis and masseter muscles. It will also tend to be pulled medially by the pterygoids.

A bilateral fracture of the mandible may also result in a downward and backward displacement of the symphysis by the digastric muscle. This results in the tongue falling backwards as its attachment from the genioglossus muscle becomes ineffective. Tracheostomy may be required.

2. *Radiography.* The interpretation of radiographs of the facial bones is very difficult owing to the superimposition of other structures; several views are therefore necessary. The most helpful are:

- *Postero-anterior.* Which should show the condyle and coronoid process, and the outline of the lower border of the mandible.
- *Right and left 30°rotated mandibular lateral.* Which shows the ascending ramus, angle, condyle and body of the mandible to the canine region.
- *Occlusal.* Sometimes useful.
- *Orthopantomography.* Shows the whole body of the mandible and both condyles on one film.

Treatment

Entails fixation of the mandible to the maxilla for a period of 3–6 weeks according to the type of fracture. This is necessary in order that the occlusion of the mandible and maxilla be as near perfect as possible for the normal restoration of function.

Generally a tooth in the line of fracture should be removed.

Methods of immobilization. Include:

1. Barrel bandage.
2. Interdental wiring.
3. Cast-metal cap splint.
4. Pins.
5. Circumferential and alveolar wiring, using the patient's dentures or Gunning splints.
6. Plating very useful in certain cases. Does not need intermaxillary fixation.

Choice of method will vary according to position and type of fracture. Generally speaking, the barrel bandage is a first-aid method and if interdental wiring or the patient's own dentures can be used, the help of a technician is not required; this may be an important consideration. Occasionally it is necessary, to carry out an open reduction to secure the bone ends with stainless-steel wire, either in the alveolus or in the lower border, e.g. where the posterior fragment is edentulous or displaced. A condylar fracture is treated by fixation for 3 weeks.

Postoperative treatment

1. *Feeding.* Fluid diet is necessary and the intake should amount to 3 litres per day. Vitamins and roughage in the form of bran are required and the calorific intake should be at least 2000 calories per day. The food should be varied and it is better to feed the patient frequently with small quantities.
2. *Oral hygiene.* Frequent and thorough cleansing of the mouth is essential. Hot salt mouthwashes are helpful.

Dislocation of the jaws

Forward dislocation

This is the commoner injury and may be caused by a blow on the chin when the mouth is open; extraction of teeth; or the use of a gag during tonsillectomy. It may also be caused by yawning.

1. *In bilateral dislocation.* The mandible is protruded and the front teeth are gagged in the open position.
2. *In unilateral dislocation.* The symphysis is deviated to the side opposite to the injury, in the open position.

Treatment

By reduction, as soon as possible. The surgeon's thumbs exert downward steady pressure on the lower molar teeth. Severe muscle spasm preventing reduction usually relaxes after intramuscular diazepam. Fixation may be necessary in some cases.

Backward dislocation

Rare and there is usually an associated fracture of the neck of the condyle.

Temporomandibular joint dysfunction

Costen first drew attention to dysfunction of the temporomandibular joint as a cause of earache. Clicking noises in the joint however do not always signify an underlying pathological condition.

Clinical features

This condition is much more common in young women, and the complaint may be of:

1. *Clicking of the jaw* on movement, with or without pain.
2. *Pain in the ear or side of face* with or without clicking. The pain in the ear is a referred otalgia, that in the face due to spasm of the associated muscles.
3. *Loss of mobility or stiffness* due to muscle spasm, and especially noticeable on waking. The onset of symptoms may be associated with a blow, yawning or instrumentation of the mouth. There may be a history of recurring subluxation. The main cause is *malocclusion,* but symptoms may be related to grinding the teeth during sleep (bruxism).

Radiography

Is usually negative, unless osteoarthritic changes have occurred.

Treatment

1. *Relaxation exercises and soft diet are helpful to begin with.*
2. *Bite plate temporary* in the first instance, to restore the occlusion, and in some cases when bruxism occurs, to be worn at night only.
3. *Correction of occlusion, by orthodontic techniques.*
4. *Hydrocortisone injection* may be of use in cases of sudden onset, but treatment of the cause must also follow.
5. *Surgery. Condylotomy* may become necessary in cases that do not respond to treatment or where there is established arthritis of the joint.

Geographical tongue

Aetiology

Unknown.

Clinical features

Red patches. Surrounded by yellowing elevated borders, are seen on the dorsum of the tongue, usually in the shape of a circle. Several patches may develop and coalesce. The characteristic feature of this condition is that its configuration changes from time to time. In the red patches the filiform papillae have disappeared but at the borders they become prolific. The condition may start in childhood and proceed throughout life, or it may remit spontaneously.

Treatment

Reassurance only is necessary.

Hairy tongue

Aetiology

Not completely understood, but this condition has followed the local application of antibiotics and antiseptics, especially oxidizing agents.

Pathology

Hairy tongue is caused by an overgrowth of the filiform papillae, up to half an inch long. These become brown or black, possibly due to chromogenic bacteria, tobacco smoking or medicaments.

Clinical features and treatment.

Blackish hairy appearance of dorsum. The elongated papillae may cause the tongue to stick and irritate the throat. The filaments should be scraped away and the patient made to brush the tongue twice a day with a weak solution of bicarbonate of soda or hydrogen peroxide.

Pharyngeal pouch (*diverticulum*)

Definition

A herniation of the pharyngeal mucosa through Killian's dehiscence.

Aetiology

A pouch probably results from neuromuscular incoordination causing failure of relaxation of the cricopharyngeal sphincter during the act of swallowing. There may be a congenital weakness of the muscle wall.

Pathology

The pouch is composed of mucosa and fibrous tissue only. As it enlarges the pouch sags downwards behind the oesophagus and may reach the mediastinum. The opening of the pouch becomes more and more a direct continuation of the pharynx and the oesophageal opening becomes concealed in front of the mouth of the pouch. As more food enters the pouch pressure is exerted on the oesophagus from behind to cause oesophageal obstruction which may become complete.

Clinical features

1. *Usually seen in the elderly.*
2. *Dysphagia* is of long standing.
3. *Regurgitation of undigested food.*
4. *Swelling in the neck* may be present. It is nearly always on the left side. It may gurgle and empty on external pressure.
5. *Cough* is caused by aspiration of fluid which eventually results in fatal pneumonia.
6. *Emaciation* may result from oesophageal obstruction and aspiration. Carcinoma may rarely occur in a pouch. Small pouches are commonly asymptomatic.

Diagnosis

Radiography with a *barium swallow* shows a characteristic retort-shaped swelling which may extend downwards into the mediastinum.

Treatment

1. Conservative

No treatment is necessary for very small symptomless pouches. Endoscopic dilatation of the cricopharyngeus muscle can be of palliative value.

2. Surgical

By a *one-stage excision* of the pouch, through an incision in a skin crease or along the anterior border of the sternomastoid muscle. The neck of the pouch is exposed and the pouch pulled up.It is easier to find if it has been packed with gauze. After division of the neck the opening is closed and buried under a second line of sutures.

The circular muscle fibres of the cricopharyngeal sphincter should be cut by a vertical incision carried down to the mucosa, to prevent recurrence (cricopharyngeal myotomy). The operating microscope facilitates this. Systemic antibiotics are essential. Drainage and tube-feeding are not always required.

- *Inversion of the sac.* After the sac is dissected out it is inverted and the pharyngeal musculature is repaired. The cricopharyngeus is divided.
- *Endoscopic division of the party-wall* between the lumen of the pharynx and that of the oesophagus may be performed by diathermy (Dohlman's operation). The cricopharyngeus is included in this partition. Specially designed forceps make this a rapid and safe procedure in practised hands.
- *Oesophagodiverticular anastomosis* has been used successfully in very large pouches in the superior mediastinum.

Oral and pharyngeal manifestations of blood diseases

Hypochromic microcytic anaemia

Occurs in association with chronic pharyngo-oesophagitis (Paterson–Brown–Kelly syndrome). A similar association has been observed with macrocytic anaemia.

Pernicious anaemia

Due to atrophic gastritis. The intrinsic factor is not present in the gastric juices and this leads to the non-absorption of vitamin B_{12}, the extrinsic factor. The haemopoietic principle is therefore not formed and not stored in the liver. The red-cell count and percentage of haemoglobin are low. Macrocytosis is characteristic.

Clinical features

1. *Extreme pallor* of lips and oral mucosa.
2. *Smoothness, redness and soreness* of tongue (Hunter's glossitis). This may be the first sign of pernicious anaemia and it may also be associated with chronic pharyngo-oesophagitis.
3. *Angular cheilitis.*

Treatment

By repeated injections of vitamin B_{12}.

Polycythaemia

Characterized by an increase in the total red-cell count. The cause is unknown.

Clinical features

1. *Bluish-red discoloration* of the oral mucosa.
2. *Glossitis and cheilitis* may be present.

Infectious mononucleosis (glandular fever)

Aetiology and pathology

Caused by the Epstein-Barr virus which leads to a considerable increase in total white cells (up to 18 000 × 10^6/l). There is a relatively great increase in number of large mononuclear cells (from 40 to 90%).

Clinical features

There is no characteristic appearance in the pharynx which often shows little abnormality, although petechiae may appear on the palate in the early stages.
Local
1. *Enlargement of cervical lymph nodes:* bilateral and usually all groups.
2. *Sore throat:* not always present.
3. *Injection of the buccopharyngeal mucosa:* as in simple pharyngitis.
4. *Pseudomembrane:* secondary infection can result in the formation of a pseudomembrane in the mouth or pharynx (anginose type). The adenopathy may be characteristically out of all proportion to the pharyngeal changes (glandular type). Spleen palpable in 50% of cases.
General
1. *Enlargement of all lymph nodes and spleen.*
2. *Pyrexia.* Up to 37.8°C (100°F).
3. *Headache.*
4. *Malaise.*
5. *Rash.* Sometimes rubella-like and late.
Rare complications
1. Jaundice.
2. Meningitis or encephalitis.
3. Splenic rupture.

Diagnosis

Confirmed by the white-cell count and by the *Paul-Bunnell test* in which sheep's red cells are agglutinated by the patient's serum. The test may be negative up to 5 days from onset. The throat condition must be differentiated from diphtheria and Vincent's infection and leukaemia.

Prognosis

The acute condition lasts about 2–3 weeks but is often followed by a long convalescence, sometimes for 6 months or more, and relapse may even occur thereafter.

Treatment

No specific treatment. Antiseptic mouthwashes may be given and systemic antibiotics when secondary infection is present. Swollen tonsils sometimes obstruct respiration, tonsillectomy is preferable to tracheostomy should steroids fail to reduce the swelling.

Acquired immune deficiency syndrome (AIDS)

Aetiology

1. Forty per cent of AIDS patients present with otolaryngological symptoms some of which are in the mouth. The agent responsible for AIDS is the human T cell lymphotrophic virus type III (HLTV III or HIV) which is transmitted by sexual contact or through blood products.

Clinical features

1. *Karposi's sarcoma.* Raised or flat red patches which may ulcerate on mucous membrane. Histological examination shows sarcomatous change. Thirty per cent of AIDS patients have Karposi's sarcoma and 25% present with it.
2. *Hairy leucoplakia.* White patches on the tongue which regress and recur. Histology shows leucoplakia with marked keratinization.
3. *Candidiasis.* Appearance in a young male must be viewed with suspicion unless there are obvious predisposing factors.
4. *Non-specific pharyngitis, tonsillitis or rhinitis* may also be the presenting symptoms of immune deficiency.
5. Persistent *cervical lymphadenopathy.* May be associated with generalized nodes or pyrexia, weight loss and lymphopaenia.

Treatment

If the otolaryngologist suspects AIDS, gloves should be worn and body fluids handled with care. The patient should be referred to a venereologist or physician. If surgery is required the same care for the safety of staff should be taken as is customary for hepatitis B infection.The patient should be treated with as much kindness and courtesy as any other (easily overlooked in the haste to take proper precautions).

Agranulocytosis

Aetiology and pathology

The condition is caused by susceptibility to drugs containing the benzene ring, especially amidopyrine (now obsolete), the sulphonamides, and more recently by cytotoxic agents. There is a marked reduction in the neutrophil polymorphs.

Clinical features

Agranulocytosis is a grave disorder and is nearly always fatal.
Local
1. *Sore throat* of sudden onset.
2. *Ulceration with false membrane formation* occurs on the tongue, buccal mucosa, and in the pharynx, usually on the faucial pillars first. This spreads, as a necrosis, to the tonsils and buccal mucosa.
3. *Moderate adenitis.*

General
1. *Pyrexia..* Up to 37.8°C (100°F).
2. *Headache.*
3. *Malaise.* Leading to marked prostration which may be terminal.

Diagnosis

Confirmed by the characteristic blood and bone-marrow picture.

Treatment

Immediate withdrawal of any possible causal drug.
Reverse isolation.
Systemic antibiotics. To counteract sepsis.
Blood transfusions and vitamin B$_{12}$ therapy are usually given.
Marrow transplantation has been used.

Leukaemia

Pathology

The *acute lymphatic* form is the commonest. It occurs most often in children. The earliest sign may be enlargement and bleeding of the gum margin which rapidly becomes worse, with severe ulceration. The pharyngeal lesion tends to imitate a severe 'simple' pharyngitis or tonsillitis. Leucocytosis may be up to 100 000 cells/ml. Immature cells are always present, often in relatively large numbers.

Chronic lymphatic leukaemia leads to enlargement of the tonsils and cervical lymph nodes, with mild sore throat and malaise in adults.

Chronic myeloid leukaemia is characterized by a huge spleen and bleeding from mucous surfaces, especially as epistaxis. Excess of granular cells may produce a leucocytosis up to 500 000 cells/ml.

Diagnosis

Made by the blood picture. The condition must be distinguished from acute pharyngitis and tonsillitis, Vincent's infection, diphtheria, syphilis, agranulocytosis and 'malignant ulceration'.

Treatment

Consists of steroids, cytotoxic agents and blood transfusions. Whole body radiation with marrow transfusion or transplantation is sometimes successful.

Oral and pharyngeal lesions associated with avitaminosis

Clinical features

Various lesions occur in the mouth and pharynx with certain vitamin deficiencies. *Deficiency of vitamin B$_{12}$ complex* is the commonest. Pellagra is caused by deficiencies of riboflavin and nicotinic acid, components of the B2 complex. This condition was common during the Second World War, in prisoner-of-war camps, and in old persons who live alone and neglect their diet and oral hygiene. The corners of the mouth become red, painful and cracked. The tongue becomes painfully inflamed and fissured. A chronic superficial ulceration may occur in the pharynx.

Deficiency of vitamin C (scurvy) is uncommon today in civilized countries. The gums may become hyperaemic and swollen, and haemorrhages and ulceration may occur.

Keratosis pharyngis

Clinical features

White or yellowish horny projections appear on the surface of lymphoid patches on the tonsils, pharyngeal wall and base of tongue. They are desquamated epithelium associated with leptothrix fungus. The excrescences cannot be wiped off. It is commonest in young adults and, although symptomless, the appearance alarms the patient.

Treatment

The condition may regress spontaneously and is therefore best left alone. Attention is given to oral hygiene and general health. Tonsillectomy may occasionally be justified.

Stylohyoid syndrome

Clinical features

Sharp pain is felt, lateralized to one side in the mouth or externally at hyoid level. The symptom, persistent over months or years, is aggravated by swallowing, and especially, by coughing, sneezing or straining. It may radiate towards the ear. Examination reveals tenderness at the attachment of the stylohyoid ligament to the hyoid bone. The aetiology is ossification of the ligament which can be seen on X-ray in some cases. Pressure on the glossopharyngeal nerve is assumed.

Treatment

Reassurance, may be followed by spontaneous remission. In severe and persistent cases injection of 2 ml Marcaine and Depomedrone into the point of maximum tenderness is often effective. Excision of an elongated styloid process via the tonsil fossa may be curative.

Globus pharyngis (*globus hystericus*)

Clinical features

Sensation of a 'lump in the throat' is the commonest complaint. There is no true dysphagia for either liquids or solids, and the symptom is often most noticeable when the patient is swallowing only saliva. Barium swallow and oesophagoscopy reveal no abnormality. The patient often admits to psychological stress or cancer phobia.

Differential diagnosis

Cricopharyngeal spasm, cervical osteophytosis, pharyngeal pouch, postcricoid carcinoma and thyroid adenoma must all be excluded. Hiatus hernia is a common problem and measuring the pH in the oesophagus is helpful.

Treatment

After careful exclusion of organic disease, an attempt should be made to offer insight into the nature of the problem. A history of friends or relatives with throat disease requires sympathetic probing. Recent bereavement is often relevant. It is important to request psychiatric attention for those who need it.

SLEEP APNOEA AND SNORING

Snoring is a sign of partial obstruction of the upper airway during sleep. Functional weakness of the soft palate, base of tongue or lateral pharyngeal walls during sleep is the commonest cause of snoring. Snoring is always present during obstructive type of sleep apnoea.

Sleep apnoea

Definition

Cessation of airflow at the mouth and nostrils lasting at least 10 seconds. The syndrome may be diagnosed if there at least 30 apnoeic episodes during both rapid eye movement and non-rapid eye movement sleep during a 7-hour period.

Central sleep apnoea

Rare. Due to a defect of the autonomic control of respiration in the medulla or peripheral chemoreceptors resulting in a failure of respiratory drive. When at its most severe this results in apnoea, however a milder form can exist with periods of hypoventilation.

Aetiology

Central sleep apnoea can occur with neural infections such as polio and encephalitis. Degenerative diseases and tumours involving the brainstem and anterolateral columns are other possible causes.

Obstructive sleep apnoea

Common. Due to obstruction of the upper respiratory passages in sleep.

Sites of obstruction

1. Nasal polypi and obstructing nasal tumours.
2. Deviated nasal septum.
3. Nasal packing.
4. Large tonsils and adenoids.
5. Nasopharyngeal tumours.
6. Retropharyngeal mass.
7. Macroglossia.
8. Micrognathia.
9. Lax pharyngeal musculature.
10. Obesity.
11. Acromegaly.
12. Myxoedema.
13. Tumours of tongue larynx and pharynx.
14. Laryngopharyngeal oedema.

Clinical features

Loud snoring interrupted by periods of apnoea. During the periods of apnoea respiratory efforts are observed. There may be restlessness in sleep. During the day there are often periods of somnolence. Poor concentration, headaches and lack of drive are common complaints from adults.

In children there may be feeding difficulties due to obstruction of oro- and nasopharynx. Examination and radiology usually reveal large obstructing tonsils and adenoids.

Adults may demonstrate an obvious obstructing problem but usually there is nothing obvious to find. They are often obese with a short thick neck.

Occasionally the referral may be to a neurologist or cardiologist. Right-sided heart failure or hypertension may be a presenting mode.

Investigations

1. Thorough ENT examination.
2. ECG, Chest radiograph and blood pressure monitoring.
3. Fibreoptic examination of the upper airway during sleep if necessary.
4. Lateral PNS and neck radiograph (particularly useful in children).
5. A screening observation of sleep by a trained observer with ECG and PO_2 monitoring.

These investigations will identify those children who require adenotonsillectomy. It should also identify those with significant cardiac abnormalities.

In those patients with suspected apnoea but no definite diagnosis a full sleep study may be useful. The stage of sleep is monitored with EEG, EMG and eye movement recordings. PO_2 is monitored and oral and nasal airflow recorded using oral and nasal thermistors. ECG is recorded.

Snoring

Although every sufferer of obstructive sleep apnoea snores most who snore do not have sleep apnoea. The oropharynx is the commonest site of the problem, however, the predominant source of noise can be from lax lateral pharyngeal walls, soft palate or tongue base. In planning surgical treatment it is important to identify the site of the problem. Fibreoptic examination and videofluoroscopy may be of value in doing this.

The older one gets, the more likely is one to snore. More than 50% are obese. Respiratory embarrassment may occur with night sedation or alcohol.

Prolonged severe snoring with periods of apnoea may lead to pulmonary hypertension, right heart failure with hypoxia. Arrhythmias can occur.

Daytime somnolence may lead to falling asleep while driving.

Treatment of sleep apnoea and snoring

Medical

Weight reduction. Avoidance of night sedation and alcohol. In central sleep apnoea acetazolamide and medroxyprogesterone are of value. Protriptyline works by reducing the amount of rapid eye movement sleep (during which the most severe episodes of hypoxia are likely to occur).

Continuous positive airway pressure

The patient wears a mask while sleeping which feeds air to the patient under pressure. The increased airway pressure hold the lax pharyngeal airway open. It is poorly tolerated by the patients in the long term but may be of value while a patient is losing weight.

Surgery

Avoid premedication prior to surgery as this may induce hypoxia.

Adenotonsillectomy is usually all that is required in children.

Nasal obstruction should be relieved.

The soft palate can be tightened up. Initially tonsillectomy with trimming of any redundant mucosa from the free edge of the soft palate was practised. Then punctate diathermy of the soft palate was introduced partially to scar the palate. Since 1981 uvulopalatopharyngoplasty has become more popular. There is a risk of developing hypernasal speech and even nasal regurgitation of food if the surgery is too enthusiastic.

Tracheostomy may be considered for those suffering from severe sleep apnoea.

Effective tongue base and hypopharyngeal surgery has now been developed for those cases where this is the main site of obstruction.

PART IV
The oesophagus

Chapter 14

Surgical anatomy and applied physiology

DEVELOPMENT OF THE OESOPHAGUS

The oesophagus is developed from that portion of the primitive foregut which succeeds the primitive pharynx.

The primitive oesophagus and trachea form a single structure up to the third week of fetal life.

Elongation occurs rapidly from the time of development of the lung buds.

The lateral septa

Two lateral septa develop in the tube during the third and fourth weeks. They grow to meet and fuse in the midline. Hence a partition is formed between the primitive trachea and oesophagus.

The fusion of the septa takes place from above downwards; the last part to be separated is at the level of the tracheal bifurcation.

Obliteration and recanalization

The oesophageal lumen thus established becomes closed by proliferation of its lining epithelium and recanalized later.

ANATOMY OF THE OESOPHAGUS

The oesophagus is a muscular tube 25 cm long in the adult. It extends from the lower border of the cricoid cartilage above at the level of the sixth cervical vertebra, to the cardiac orifice of the stomach below, at the level of the eleventh thoracic vertebra.

Direction

It descends almost vertically but inclines to the left:

1. From its origin to the root of the neck.
2. From the level of the seventh thoracic vertebra to the oesophageal opening in the diaphragm at the level of the tenth thoracic vertebra.

Constrictions

There are three constrictions:

1. 15 cm from the upper incisor teeth, at its commencement.
2. 25 cm from the upper incisor teeth, where it is crossed by the aortic arch and left main bronchus.
3. 40 cm from the upper incisor teeth, where it pierces the diaphragm.

Structure

The oesophagus has four coats:

1. *Mucous.* Lined by stratified squamous epithelium. It is thick and reddish above, pale below.
2. *Submucous.* Connects the mucous and muscular coats loosely.
3. *Muscular.* The upper third contains striped muscle only; the middle third striped and smooth; the lower third smooth only. There are two layers:
- *Internal circular.* Continuous above with the cricopharyngeal sphincter. It is thickened in its lower to form the cardiac sphincter.
- *External longitudinal.* Forms a complete investment except at its upper end posteriorly, where the fibres diverge in two longitudinal fasciculi. These pass forwards around the upper end of the tube, deep to the cricopharyngeal sphincter, to be inserted into the posterior surface of the cricoid lamina.
4. *Fibrous. Externally.* It is a loose investment.

Relations

Cervical part (Figure 14.1a)

In front. The trachea; left lobe of the thyroid gland.

Behind. Vertebral column; separated by the longus cervicis muscles and prevertebral facia.

On each side. The carotid sheath and its contents; lobe of the thyroid gland. The recurrent laryngeal nerves ascend in the groove between the oesophagus and trachea, or slightly in front of the groove.

Thoracic part (Figure 14.1b)

In front. Trachea; left main bronchus; pericardium and diaphragm.

Behind. Vertebral column; thoracic duct; azygos veins; and terminal parts of the hemiazygos veins. It rests on the front of the descending thoracic aorta below, near the diaphragm.

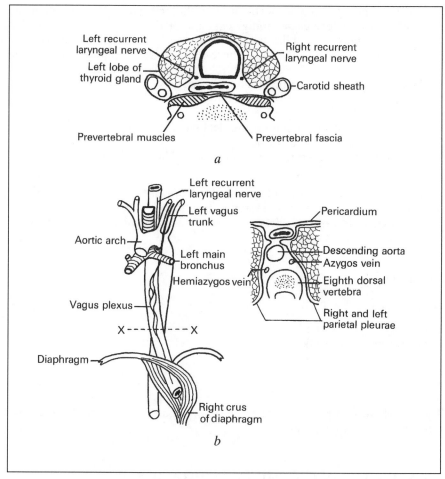

Figure 14.1 *a*, Relations of cervical oesophagus; *b*, relations of thoracic oesophagus. (*Inset:* Transverse section at level X–X)

On the left side. The aortic arch; left subclavian artery; thoracic duct and left pleura.

The *left recurrent laryngeal nerve* runs up in the groove between the oesophagus and trachea.

On the right side. Right pleura throughout its length; azygos vein.

The *vagus nerves* descend in close contact with the oesophagus, below the root of the lung; the right lies chiefly behind it, the left chiefly in front.

Blood supply

Arteries arise from:

1. The inferior thyroid artery, in the cervical part.

2. The descending thoracic aorta, in the thoracic part. The oesophageal branches of this artery each supply segments of the oesophagus. When the whole oesophagus is mobilized it is deprived of this blood supply and necrosis follows, down to the part where the left gastric supply ends, 25 cm above the cardia.

3. The left gastric artery, in the abdominal part.

Veins drain to:

1. The inferior thyroid vein, in the cervical part.
2. The azygos vein, in the thoracic part.
3. The left gastric vein, in the abdominal part. This vein is a tributary of the portal vein.

The lower end of the oesophagus is therefore one of the points at which the portal and systemic venous systems anastomose.

Varices occur in cases of portal obstruction as in Banti's disease or hepatic cirrhosis.

Nerve supply

Derived from:

1. The vagi – parasympathetic.
2. The sympathetic trunk.

Lymphatic drainage

The vessels form a plexus around the oesophagus. They drain into the posterior mediastinal lymph nodes.

EXAMINATION OF THE OESOPHAGUS

Radiography

Radiography of the chest and lateral views of the neck should always be done before the oesophagus is examined endoscopically. In most cases barium swallow examination is also indicated. If these precautions are not taken an unsuspected pharyngeal pouch may be entered and even pierced, or an aneurysm of the aorta perforated. Oesophageal obstruction from strictures, neoplasms, or other causes is also demonstrated. Videofluoroscopy can be useful in the diagnosis of neuromuscular derangements.

Endoscopy

Oesophageal speculum is used for examination of the upper end of the thoracic oesophagus, for removal of foreign bodies or obtaining biopsy specimens.

Oesophagoscope is used when the whole length of the oesophagus must be examined. The region of the arch of the aorta can be recognized by its pulsation. Below the cardiac sphincter the stomach is recognized by its redder, rugose mucosa.

Bronchoscopy should always be done in cases of oesophageal neoplasms. Erosion of the trachea or left main bronchus may be seen; or broadening of the carina may show evidence of enlargement of the mediastinal lymph nodes.

Flexible fibreoptic instruments have recently much enhanced the ease and value of these endoscopic procedures.

APPLIED PHYSIOLOGY OF THE OESOPHAGUS

Deglutition

Food enters the oesophagus at the beginning of the third stage of deglutition, by relaxation of the cricopharyngeal sphincter. Opening the mouth of the oesophagus is assisted by the simultaneous closure and elevation of the larynx, by virtue of the attachment of the longitudinal fasciculi to the cricoid cartilage which pull the oesophagus upwards over the bolus. This is assisted by gravity.

Dysphagia

Difficulty in swallowing may be caused by:

1. Mechanical obstruction to the oesophagus or lower pharynx.
2. Paralysis of the oesophageal or pharyngeal muscles, usually from lesions of the brainstem.

The various aetiological factors are discussed more fully with the individual causative conditions.

Chapter 15

Diseases of the oesophagus

CONGENITAL ABNORMALITIES OF THE OESOPHAGUS

Congenital atresia

Very rare but may account for some cases of infant deaths. It is caused by abnormalities in the development of the lateral septa between the primitive oesophagus and trachea and in the recanalization of the obliterated primitive oesophagus.

Pathology

There are two main types (Figure 15.1):

1. The upper part of the oesophagus ends blindly and is connected to the lower part by a fibrous band.

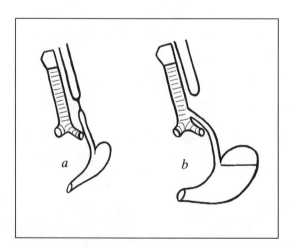

Figure 15.1 Congenital atresia of oesophagus. *a*, No connection with trachea (*stomach empty of gas*); *b*, with fistula between trachea and lower segment of oesophagus (*stomach contains gas*)

2. The upper part ends blindly but the lower part is connected with the trachea or a bronchus *(tracheo-oesophageal fistula)*. This is the commoner type. Meconium may be regurgitated into the trachea.

Clinical features

1. *Regurgitation of feeds usually becomes manifest on the second day of life.*
2. *Coughing is caused by 'spill-over' from the blind upper end of the oesophagus. Choking and asphyxia may ensue.*

Diagnosis

May be confirmed by:
 Hydramnios in the mother during the confinement should suggest the possibility of this defect.
 Passage of a catheter. A soft catheter fails to enter the stomach.
 Radiography. Bronchographic contrast is preferred to barium emulsion, to avoid pneumonia. The presence of air in the stomach indicates a fistula.

Treatment

Closure of fistula with end-to-end anastomosis must be performed immediately a diagnosis has been made (atresia with tracheo-oesophageal fistula). It is performed by a transthoracic approach.
 Gastrostomy should be performed in cases of simple atresia, without fistulae, but it tends to aggravate inhalation pneumonia when a fistula is present.

Congenital stricture

Rare. It may occur:

1. *At the cricopharyngeal sphincter,* where there may be a web, fold, or narrowing.
2. *In the thoracic oesophagus.* Usually in the lower third. A smooth circular lumen, often pin-hole in size, is seen. Dilatation above is considerable.

Clinical features

Dysphagia may not be evident until late adult life. Patients accommodate themselves to a 'small swallow' all their lives.

Treatment

Dilatation with bougies, from above, is usually successful.
 Gastrostomy with subsequent dilatation from below, may be indicated in some cases.
 Transcervical or transthoracic resection is sometimes necessary.

Congenital tracheo-oesophageal fistula (without atresia or stenosis)

Rare. May be very small, sometimes valvular. Causes coughing when fluids are swallowed, and recurring attacks of bronchitis or pneumonia.

Treatment

Surgical reconstruction of the viscera as soon as the diagnosis is made.

Congenital shortening

Associated with a thoracic stomach. The oesophagus usually ends at the level of the seventh thoracic vertebra.

Aetiology

The oesophagus is developed from the foregut. If elongation is prevented the diaphragm (which develops at a later date) comes into a more caudal relationship to the stomach. A portion of the stomach thus lies above the diaphragm, in the thorax.

Clinical features

There are no symptoms in many cases.
   Dysphagia results from narrowing at the lower end of the oesophagus.
   Discomfort caused by dilatation of the thoracic stomach.
   Vomiting. Sometimes.
   Pain may be caused by reflux oesophagitis.
   Loss of weight follows dysphagia.

Differential diagnosis

From strictures, carcinoma, oesophagectasia, hiatus hernia, anorexia nervosa, pharyngeal and oesophageal pouches, and lesions of the cardiac end of the stomach.

Treatment

Upright position affords greater comfort to the patient.
   Alkaline mixtures. Given by mouth to counteract the acid regurgitated from the stomach.
   Dilatation can be performed under direct vision, with bougies or hydrostatic bags.
   Transthoracic operations may be performed to mobilize the stomach. An anastomosis is sometimes made between the two parts of the stomach.
   Section of the left phrenic nerve has been performed with some success.

Hiatus hernia

The oesophagus becomes obstructed by pressure from the herniated stomach alongside it. *Discomfort on lying down* may not become evident until adult life.

Treatment

1. *Conservative* by assuming the upright position and maintaining it throughout the day and night; and by the administration of alkalis.
2. *Surgical* by reduction of the hernia and repair of the diaphragm.

Congenital diverticula

Rare. Such are usually small and situated near the lower end of the oesophagus. They are of the pulsion type and must be distinguished from the traction diverticula of acquired origin.

Dysphagia lusoria

Caused by compression of the oesophagus by an unusually located right subclavian artery (Figure 15.2). The term is used to include dysphagia caused by any aberrant great vessel. The condition is confined to the upper third of the oesophagus.

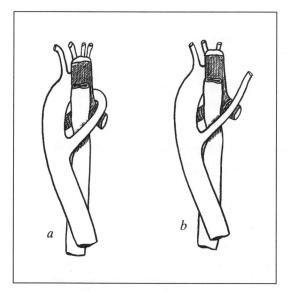

Figure 15.2 Dysphagia lusoria. *a*, Double aorta; *b*, abnormal subclavian artery (*seen from behind*)

TRAUMATIC CONDITIONS OF THE OESOPHAGUS

Spontaneous rupture

Rare and grave condition. Usually occurs in adults, most commonly in males of alcoholic disposition. Rupture occurs during violent vomiting, following a large meal.

Clinical features

Severe pain is felt in the lower chest and epigastrium, often radiating to the back.
Vomiting may continue for a short time after rupture.
Dyspnoea and collapse become marked.
Surgical emphysema may be apparent in the neck.
  Signs are those of an acute upper abdominal emergency.

Differential diagnosis

From perforated peptic ulcer, acute pancreatitis, coronary thrombosis, dissecting aneurysm, spontaneous pneumothorax and perforation from an unsuspected foreign body.
  Radiography of the chest should be done in every suspected case of acute upper abdominal emergency. In spontaneous rupture of the oesophagus, it shows the picture of a hydropneumothorax. Sometimes mediastinal emphysema is observed.

Treatment

By immediate open *thoracotomy with drainage.*
Actual repair is not often practicable.
Gastrostomy is essential.
Antibiotics are given intravenously.

Prognosis

Has improved with modern methods of early diagnosis and the use of antibiotics and drainage.

Direct injuries

Aetiology

1. Burns, scalds, and corrosive injuries.
2. Instrumentation for bouginage, removal of foreign bodies, or biopsy.
3. Foreign bodies.
4. Tears and wounds due to injuries of neck or chest.

Pathology

In minor degrees of trauma a localized oesophagitis occurs. In more severe degrees the oesophageal wall rapidly becomes necrosed, or may be actually *perforated* at the time of the injury. The pleural cavity or mediastinum becomes implicated, often fatally.

Clinical features

May be immediate or delayed in onset, depending on the nature and severity of the trauma and on the complications that follow.

Pain is usually severe and immediate in onset. It is supraclavicular in lesions of the cervical oesophagus; retrosternal in lesions of the thoracic portion and often radiates to the back or epigastrium.

Dysphagia usually marked at first, but may gradually disappear as feeding by mouth is stopped.

Shock is severe if rupture or perforation has occurred into the pleural cavity.

Dyspnoea becomes increasingly severe if a pneumothorax, empyema, or mediastinitis occurs.

The physical signs are those of either a cervical cellulitis or abscess, an intrathoracic lesion, or an acute upper abdominal condition with tenderness and rigidity.

Diagnosis

Plain radiographs should be taken at once and may show air in the neck or mediastinum, or a hydropneumothorax. An unsuspected foreign body may be demonstrated.

Barium swallow must not be performed for at least 3 or 4 days. It may then be needed to locate the site of trauma.

Endoscopic examination. Oesophagoscopy to locate the injury is hazardous. Some authorities advise endoscopy immediately before exploratory operation in very early cases in which there is a possibility of primary repair of the injured viscus.

Treatment

Shock must be treated.

Systemic antibiotics must be given in full dosage in all cases.

Steroid therapy. Advocated to inhibit fibrosis.

Dilute alkaline fluids may be taken by mouth in small amounts in minor degrees of oesophagitis without danger of perforation.

Nasogastric feeding tube should be inserted without delay.

Intravenous or rectal fluids. Given if there is acute dysphagia with danger of perforation. Fluids must be withheld by mouth for at least 4 days.

Gastrostomy. Necessary when perforation has occurred.

Cervical oesophagostomy is performed immediately by some surgeons. A small tube is passed into the stomach. This procedure is said to diminish the risk of stricture.

Transcervical and transthoracic drainage of the fascial spaces of the neck, mediastinum or pleural cavity is indicated when these spaces are infected.

Immediate repair of tears or ruptures may be attempted by an external operation, when diagnosis has been early. In cases of delayed diagnosis it is usually best simply to drain an abscess if it forms.

Complications

Immediate

1. *Para-oesophageal abscess, in the neck.*
2. *Infections of the mediastinum and pleural cavities.*
3. *Tracheo-oesophageal fistula, rarely.*

Delayed

Stricture is the commonest complication.

Foreign bodies

The impaction of a foreign body depends chiefly on its size and shape.

Sharp or pointed articles may stick in any part of the oesophagus.

A large article or bolus of food may become impacted in a normal oesophagus, especially if swallowed hurriedly or accidentally. Insane or inebriated persons are especially at risk.

Small articles may be impacted at a site of normal narrowing or spasm.

In contrast to those in the trachea and bronchi, non-vegetable foreign bodies (and especially sharp ones) are the most dangerous.

The commonest objects are coins in children, fish or meat bones in adults.

Site

Objects which pass through the upper part of the oesophagus will usually traverse the whole intestinal tract without trouble, except in the case of sharp objects.

The thoracic inlet. The commonest site of impaction, just below the cricopharyngeal sphincter. Large coins may, however, be arrested by the sphincter itself.

The cardia. Relatively few objects are held up at the cardia.

Clinical features

Symptoms are usually complained of immediately, but some objects (such as coins or other smooth articles) may be impacted for weeks or even months before symptoms occur. There may be no obvious history of the swallowing of a foreign body, especially in children. A piece of glass may be contained in custard, jam, or milk.

Pain is the predominant symptom. It is frequently retrosternal and/or in the back.

Dysphagia. A sense of obstruction is usual. It may be impossible to swallow even saliva.

A persistent assertion of the above symptoms demands careful investigation.

Excessive saliva collects in the pyriform fossa.

Regurgitation of food. Occasionally.

Dyspnoea and hoarseness may occur if the foreign body is impacted high up, near the cricopharyngeal sphincter. They are due to swelling of the laryngeal mucosa. Dyspnoea occurs, especially in small children, when the trachea itself may be compressed by the object in the oesophagus. Actual asphyxia has been recorded.

Localized tenderness in the lower part of the neck, especially on manipulation of the larynx, with loss of laryngeal crepitus due to mucosal oedema.

Localized swelling may occur in the supraclavicular region, more commonly on the left side, when a para-oesophageal abscess is formed.

Diagnosis

Radiography. Plain X-ray films should be taken, with anteroposterior, lateral and oblique views. Opaque flat objects are shown lying in the coronal plane, e.g. coins. They appear larger than their actual size. Fish bones may be translucent. Non-opaque objects may be localized with a very small amount of barium swallowed with a few shreds of cotton-wool. A persistent air-bubble in the oesophagus may indicate the presence and level of a non-opaque foreign body.

Endoscopic examination under general anaesthetic. With the oesophageal speculum or oesophagoscope. Indicated when symptoms are marked in spite of negative radiographic findings.

Treatment

In uncertain cases justifiable to delay endoscopy, at least for several hours.

Endoscopic removal

Some objects, such as brooches in children or dental plates in adults, may have to be cut with shears. Open safety-pins should be closed, or the point engaged in the endoscope, when the point is directed upwards.

External cervical or transthoracic oesophagotomy

Occasionally indicated in difficult cases. It sometimes is helpful to anchor the foreign body with endoscopic forceps during open removal.

Although it is nearly always possible to remove foreign bodies from the oesophagus by one or other of the above methods, it is occasionally wiser to push an object (e.g. a safety-pin open point upwards) into the stomach and to remove it from there.

Complications

Are life-threatening. They include:

1. Para-oesophageal emphysema, cellulitis, or abscess in the neck.
2. Mediastinal emphysema, mediastinitis, or localized mediastinal abscess (para-oesophageal) in the thorax.
3. Pneumothorax, pleurisy, or empyema.
4. Oedema of the larynx.
5. Tracheal compression.
6. Septicaemia.
7. Perforation of the aorta.
8. Stricture.
9. Tracheo-oesophageal fistula.

INFLAMMATION AND ULCERATION OF THE OESOPHAGUS

Acute oesophagitis

This is uncommon, except as a complication of traumatic conditions. It is occasionally seen as a result of thrush especially in infants, when it is associated with infection in the mouth.

A relatively mild degree of oesophagitis occurs in many cases of dilatation of the oesophagus. The wall above the stricture or obstruction is oedematous.

A 'reflux' oesophagitis occurs with certain types of short oesophagus and with certain lesions of the cardiac end of the stomach. Fungal oesophagitis may complicate broad-spectrum antibiotic therapy.

Ulceration of the oesophagus

Peptic

Areas of heterotopic peptic tissue are rarely found in the lower third of the oesophagus, and even in the upper third. A typical peptic ulcer may occur. *Pain* is present. Haemorrhages, perforation and malignant changes are recorded. Stricture formation is the commonest complication. This may lead to acquired shortening of the oesophagus.

Bacterial infections

Ulceration may follow diphtheria, scarlet fever and typhoid. Tuberculous and syphilitic ulcers have been recorded. Healing leads to fibrous strictures.

Superficial erosions

May be of a simple inflammatory type, often associated with a 'dyspepsia'. They are usually multiple. They may cause localized spasm and may possibly initiate the radiological changes described as 'corkscrew oesophagus'.

Mild dysphagia with retrosternal discomfort ('heart-burn') is the usual symptom.

NEOPLASMS OF THE OESOPHAGUS

Benign growths are rare, primary carcinoma common. Carcinoma is the only malignant neoplasm of practical concern in the oesophagus. Sarcoma is extremely rare. Secondary malignant invasion is much less frequent than the primary disease and usually results from spread from bronchial carcinoma or its lymphatic metastases, less commonly from the stomach, laryngopharynx or thyroid gland. Despite more successful results from radical surgery, prognosis remains poor as the disease has almost always passed the confines of the oesophagus when the patient is first seen.

Benign neoplasms

All Are extremely rare but leiomyoma, papilloma, adenoma, fibroma, angiofibroma, lipoma and other tumours have been recorded. They are usually polypoid, so that some are removed by endoscopic methods. The upper end of the oesophagus appears to be the usual site. Occasionally there may be a long stalk, and they may even appear in the mouth. True dysphagia is generally absent, and there is merely a sensation of 'lump in the throat'. The 'angioma' (varix) is not a true neoplasm and is described later.

Carcinoma of the oesophagus

Aetiology

Unknown. It is associated with cigarette smoking and a high alcohol consumption. A pre-existing abnormality of the oesophagus such as achalasia predisposes to the development of carcinoma. Tylosis (genetically determined thickening of the skin of the palms of the hand and soles of the feet) is associated with the development of carcinoma in males.

Incidence

Age

Seventy-five per cent occur over the age of 50, most often in the sixties. Few occur under 40.

Sex

Over 80% are in males.

Site

Probably one-half are in the middle third of the oesophagus. In men the middle and lower thirds are most often affected; in women, the upper third.

Pathology

Squamous-cell carcinoma occurs in all grades, from keratinized to undifferentiated forms. *Adenocarcinoma* is much less common and almost always occurs near the lower end of the oesophagus. Lympho-epithelioma is not found. Spread in the oesophagus may be either annular (causing stenosis) or longitudinal (causing relatively little obstruction). The neoplasm may be be infiltrating, ulcerative, or proliferative, the latter fungating into the lumen. Outcropping from submucosal lymphatic spread can produce 'satellite' growths at some distance from the primary.

Direct spread

Trachea, bronchi, pleura, spine and recurrent laryngeal nerves are sometimes invaded.

Lymphatic spread

Metastases occur early in the mediastinal nodes. Cervical nodes are invaded from growths in the upper oesophagus, the upper abdominal nodes from lower growths.

Haematogenous spread

Blood-borne metastases are seen in the liver, lungs and brain.

Clinical features

Discomfort is usually the earliest symptom. Insidious in onset and fairly well localized by the patient.

Dysphagia at first for solids only. This increases until complete obstruction occurs. Sudden impaction of food is sometimes the first indication of an oesophageal growth. The lumen may be reduced by half before symptoms present, and several months of valuable time are thus lost. High growths give rise to symptoms sooner than others.

Cough may rarely herald the disease. Caused by tracheal invasion.

Cachexia. Once obstruction is present the general condition rapidly deteriorates.

Pain is a late and infrequent symptom.

Diagnosis

Marked dysphagia is usually a late sign, so that any abnormal sensation on swallowing (however slight) calls for investigation. A history of more than one year almost excludes carcinoma except in those cases where it arises in association with chronic hypopharyngitis in women, a pharyngeal pouch, or oesophagectasia. Examination of the cervical and abdominal lymph nodes and the larynx must not be neglected.

Radiography

A barium swallow will usually show an irregular and notched filling defect (Figure 15.3). Diverticula and oesophagectasia can be excluded. Benign stricture and peptic ulceration may be difficult to differentiate on radiological evidence alone.

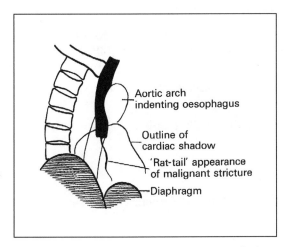

Figure 15.3 Carcinoma of oesophagus as seen on barium swallow in the right anterior oblique position

Oesophagoscopy

The endoscopic appearances are varied. Usually there is a hard fixed stricture with ulcerated and bleeding margins. Sometimes it may present as an indurated plaque or as a fungating and almost pedunculated mass. The essential biopsy is generally easy and conclusive.

Treatment

1. Oesophagectomy

Transpleural excision of the growth and all of the oesophagus below it, with anastomosis of the stomach or intestine to the severed oesophagus above, offers the best chance of survival. Colon transplantation is increasingly successfully used in both excisional and by-pass (palliative) operations. Operation, however, often reveals unsuspected metastases and spread of the disease. Nevertheless, it is occasionally justified as a palliative procedure. Some high growths must be excised from the neck and continuity restored by colon transplantation or by mobilization of the stomach which can be brought up to a high level in the neck. Injury to the recurrent laryngeal nerves may result. If very high the growth may involve the back of the larynx, so that pharyngo-oesophago-laryngectomy becomes necessary.

2. Radiotherapy

This is the best form of palliation, particularly for growths of the upper oesophagus. Newer techniques offer some hope of occasional cures. These include the use of 'computer-tracking' teletherapy which can follow the dimensions of the larger tumours with extreme accuracy.

3. Palliative intubation of the stricture

Dilatation of the stricture and insertion of Celestin's or Mousseau-Barbin tubes relieve obstruction in growths of the middle or lower thirds.

4. Palliative gastro-oesophageal, jejuno-oesophageal, or colon by-pass anastomosis

This may be possible in growths of the cardia and is preferable to gastrostomy in such cases.

5. Gastrostomy

This is rarely justifiable. In most cases it merely prolongs misery.

6. Neodymium YAG laser

This can be used endoscopically to burn a passage through the tumour thus giving temporary relief of the dysphagia.

MISCELLANEOUS CONDITIONS OF THE OESOPHAGUS

Stricture

Aetiology

Benign strictures are fibrous in nature. Causes include:

1. *Congenital.* These are rare. They are usually single and found most often in the lower third.
2. *Post-traumatic.* The commonest type.
- *Corrosives* may be swallowed. They include phenol or lye, used in many countries for cleaning and soap-making and often left in unlabelled wine and beverage bottles. Corrosive strictures are usually multiple, leading to a tortuous oesophageal lumen.
- *Foreign bodies* or instrumentation for their removal, may cause ulceration and subsequent stricture formation.

Post-inflammatory. These follow ulceration, of which the commonest cause is reflux oesophagitis, usually in association with hiatus hernia ('sliding' type).

Clinical features

1. *Dysphagia.* First for solids only, later for fluids also.
2. *Regurgitation of food.*
3. *Loss of weight.*
4. *Cough.*

Diagnosis

Made by X-rays with barium and confirmed by oesophagoscopy. Strictures must be differentiated from all other causes of dysphagia, and in particular carcinoma, foreign body, oesophagectasia and pharyngeal pouch.

Treatment

Dilatation by one of several techniques. In all, great care must be taken not to rupture the oesophageal wall. In the common type of partial occlusion, bougies can be passed carefully through the stricture under direct vision, at frequent intervals over a considerable period of time. Dilatation may also be achieved by the hydrostatic bag. With traumatic conditions most surgeons prefer to delay bouginage until 2 weeks after the accident, to allow subsidence of the oedema. In children a cervical oesophagostomy may be established to facilitate frequent bouginage. Patients with partial occlusion who cannot feed adequately must have either a small indwelling nasogastric tube passed through the stricture or a gastrostomy.

Gastrostomy must be performed when obstruction is severe. A small lead shot on a thread may be swallowed and, in nearly every case, will eventually work its way through the stricture. Threaded olive bougies of increasing size are then passed down the stricture and removed through the gastrostomy. Retrograde bouginage is sometimes indicated.

Thoracotomy may be required for resection, anastomosis, or plastic procedures when the above measures fail.

Achalasia of the cardia (oesophagectasia)

Pathology

There is a marked dilatation of the lower two-thirds of the oesophagus. The lumen may be as much as 7.5 cm in diameter. The muscular walls may be hypertrophied but there is no special hypertrophy of the cardiac sphincter.

Aetiology

Uncertain.

Hurst postulated a failure of relaxation of the cardiac orifice (achalasia), from degeneration of Auerbach's plexus.

Chevalier Jackson suggested an abnormal 'pinchcock' action of the right crus of the diaphragm.

Many surgeons have postulated an actual spasm at the cardia, but none is apparent on oesophagoscopy.

Aerophagy (air-swallowing) may play a part in dilating the oesophagus.

In many respects oesophagectasia resembles Hirschsprung's disease of the colon (i.e. a primary dilatation).

Clinical features

The condition affects young persons of both sexes. Symptoms usually develop insidiously but in rare instances the onset is relatively sudden, after a nervous shock or childbirth.

Fullness after meals is the main symptom. It is retrosternal or epigastric.

Dysphagia follows later and is more marked for fluids than for solids. The epigastric discomfort is, however, sometimes relieved by drinking more fluids.

Regurgitation of undigested food, sometimes taken the day before.

Loss of weight may occur but is rarely severe. There may be remissions of symptoms over periods of years. The patient rarely becomes ill or cachectic unless inhalation pneumonia or carcinoma of the oesophagus supervene.

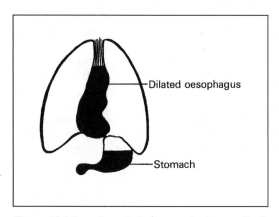

Figure 15.4 Oesophagectasia (seen on barium swallow)

Diagnosis

Radiography

The appearances on a barium swallow are typical (Figure 15.4). There is marked or enormous dilatation with a smooth rounded lower border at the cardia. There is usually a fluid level in the oesophagus about 20 cm from the cardia. The condition can usually be differentiated from carcinoma of the oesophagus and stricture.

Oesophagoscopy

This is essential to exclude carcinoma unless enormous dilatation and prolonged history make this diagnosis unlikely. Carcinoma may complicate the disease.

It must be differentiated from Chagas disease.

Treatment

1. *Lavage* with a stomach tube, is useful as a preliminary to other forms of treatment.
2. *Amyl or octyl nitrite* inhaled from capsules before meals, may give relaxation and allow comfortable swallowing.
3. *Dilatation of the lower end* is done under direct vision with bougies and then a hydrostatic bag.
   Repeated dilatation may have to be done, even by the patient himself, using Hurst's mercury bougies. This simple practice has lost favour in recent years and operation is preferred in obstinate cases.
4. *Cardioplasty (Heller's operation)* is the operation of choice. The cardiac sphincter is incised down to mucosa (cf. Ramstedt's operation for infantile pyloric stenosis).
5. *Anastomotic operations.* Anastomosis between stomach and oesophagus may be indicated when the oesophagus is grossly lengthened and kinked.

Acquired diverticulum

This is a *traction pouch*. It usually occurs at the level of the bifurcation of the trachea and is usually the result of tuberculosis of the tracheobronchial lymph nodes. Rarely, the pouch may be large, from spontaneous rupture of a mediastinal abscess or cyst into the oesophagus. It is generally symptomless but there may be vague 'dyspepsia' or dysphagia. It can occur at any age. The diverticulum is difficult to see on oesophagoscopy.

Acquired tracheo-oesophageal fistula

Aetiology

1. *Carcinoma of the oesophagus.* The commonest cause.
2. *Rupture of a para-oesophageal abscess.*
3. *Perichondritis of the tracheal rings.* Rarely.
4. *Trauma from foreign bodies.*
5. *Direct or indirect trauma.* From external violence (e.g. crushed chest) or penetrating wounds. Pressure necrosis from an unsuitable tracheostomy tube.

Clinical features

Cough is marked, especially on taking food or fluids. Expectoration of food or fluid may be slight or marked. Bronchopneumonia develops early.

Treatment

Stomach tube should be passed if possible.
   Gastrostomy must be performed if the tube cannot be passed.
   Repair is attempted in traumatic cases. This may be done with skin flaps in the cervical region but great difficulties are encountered in the thorax.

Acquired hiatus hernia

Types

(a) Sliding

The cardiac part of the stomach follows the oesophagus in line through the diaphragm. Occurs in middle-aged and elderly patients. Probably due to increased abdominal pressure, e.g. obesity, constipation, and rarely traumatic compression of abdominal wall.

(b) Para-oesophageal

The cardia retains its normal position while the fundus of the stomach herniates into the thorax alongside the oesophagus. Congenital and acquired cases may not be easy to differentiate.

Symptoms

Heartburn and *pain* are due to acid reflux into oesophagus. Both are aggravated by lying down, relieved by alkalis, and occur more usually in the sliding type in which the cardiac sphincter mechanism is ineffective. Bleeding *(haematemesis* or *melaena)* is due to oesophagitis in sliding hernias, or peptic ulcer in the thoracic stomach in para-oesophageal hernias. *Dyspnoea* is caused by distension after meals.

Diagnosis

Confirmed by barium swallow and oesophagoscopy. Carcinoma must be carefully excluded, especially in cases complicated by oesophagitis, spasm, and stricture formation.

Treatment

In most cases weight reduction, alkalis by mouth, and sleeping propped up with pillows will give some relief. Surgical operation with replacement of the stomach in the abdomen and repair of the diaphragm is usually reserved for severe cases in which medical treatment has failed.

PART V
The Larynx

Chapter 16

Surgical anatomy

DEVELOPMENT OF THE LARYNX

The *hypobranchial eminence* or *copula* (see Figure 1.1) is formed in the floor of the primitive pharynx between the ventral ends of the fourth, third and second visceral arches.

The *tracheobronchial groove* appears caudal to the hypobranchial eminence. It is from this groove that the primitive larynx, bronchi and lungs develop, as an outpouching from the floor of the pharynx in the third week of intrauterine life. The groove soon becomes converted into a *tracheo-bronchial tube*. The tube is lined with entoderm, from which the lower respiratory epithelium is developed. The cephalic end of the groove is the first rudiment of the larynx.

Laryngeal inlet

The upper aperture of the larynx is at first a vertical slit. It is converted into a T-shaped cleft by enlargement of the arytenoid swellings. The vertical limb of the T lies between the arytenoid swellings, the horizontal limb between them and the epiglottis. The epithelial walls of the cleft adhere to each other soon after its appearance and the aperture becomes occluded. The lumen is re-established in the third fetal month.

Laryngeal cartilages

These develop during the first and second months of intra-uterine life. They appear in the mesoderm surrounding the upper part of the tracheobronchial groove.

Thyroid cartilage is developed from the ventral ends of the fourth visceral arch in the first fetal month. Chondrification has progressed considerably by the end of the sixth week. The fifth arch disappears.

Cricoid cartilage appears in the sixth arch during the sixth week. The whole ring is chondrified at the end of the second month.

Arytenoid cartilages are derived from the skeletal elements of the sixth visceral arch.

Epiglottis develops from the fourth arch.

Laryngeal muscles

Sphincter and dilator muscles. Arise from mesoderm of the sixth visceral arch. Both groups are derived from the inner constrictor layer of the primitive pharynx.

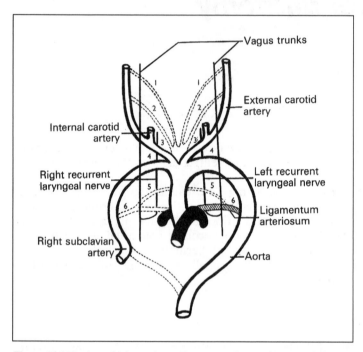

Figure 16.1 The branchial arteries and recurrent laryngeal nerves (after Grant)

Tensor muscles. The paired cricothyroid muscles are derived from the outer ring of musculature surrounding the primitive pharynx.

Laryngeal nerves

The branchial nerves of the fourth and sixth arches supply the larynx (Figure 16.1). These are the superior and inferior (recurrent) laryngeal nerves. Each visceral arch is traversed by an artery (aortic arch). Each aortic arch connects the ventral and dorsal aortae of its own visceral arch. The primitive recurrent laryngeal nerve enters the sixth visceral arch, on each side, caudal to the sixth aortic arch.

On the left side it retains this position as the ductus arteriosus and is found on the left side of (i.e. caudal to) the ligamentum arteriosum in the adult.

On the right side the dorsal part of the sixth aortic arch and the whole of the fifth disappear. The nerve is therefore found on the caudal aspect of the fourth aortic arch, which becomes the subclavian artery.

Infantile larynx

Size. The larynx is both absolutely and relatively smaller in infants than in adults. The lumen is therefore disproportionately narrower.

Shape. The infantile larynx is more funnel-shaped. Its narrowest part is at the junction of the subglottic larynx with the trachea. A very slight swelling of the lax mucosa at this point may produce a serious obstruction to breathing.

Consistency. The laryngeal cartilages are much softer in the infant. They therefore collapse more easily in forced inspiratory efforts or oedematous conditions.

Position. The infantile larynx lies high up under the tongue, but with development assumes an increasingly lower position. The plane of its inlet is less oblique and the axis of air entry is straighter than in the adult.

ANATOMY OF THE LARYNX

The larynx is situated in the midline of the neck at the meeting of the digestive and respiratory passages. It lies in front of the laryngopharynx from the level of the third to the sixth cervical vertebrae. It consists of a framework of cartilages, connected by ligaments and membranes, lined by a mucous membrane and moved by muscles. The male larynx increases in size at puberty. All the cartilages enlarge and the projection of the thyroid cartilage produces the 'Adam's apple'. The hyoid bone is a structure pertaining to the tongue.

Laryngeal cartilages

Form the main framework of the larynx.

Unpaired cartilages

There are three:

Thyroid cartilage

The largest (Figure 16.2). Each half consists of:

1. *Ala (lamina):* an almost square plate of cartilage. It begins to ossify at the age of 25 and may be completely converted to bone by 65.

The two alae meet in the midline, forming an angle of about 90° in men, about 120° in women. The laryngeal prominence is formed in men by this more acute angle.

Medially the anterior portion is related to the glottis, the posterior portion forms the lateral boundary of the pyriform fossa. The point of junction of the upper borders of the alae is indented by the V-shaped *thyroid notch.* An *oblique line,* the site of muscular attachments, runs downwards and forwards on the outer surface of each lamina.

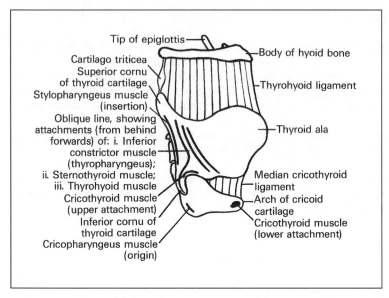

Figure 16.2 Cartilages of larynx and hyoid bone – lateral view

2. *Superior cornu.* Arises from the posterosuperior angle of the ala.
3. *Inferior cornu.* Arises from the posterio-inferior angle of the ala. There is a small oval facet on its inner surface, for articulation with the cricoid cartilage.

Cricoid cartilage (Figure 16.3)

Thicker and stronger than the thyroid cartilage. It resembles a signet ring, narrow in front, broad behind. Ossification begins at the age of 30 and may be complete by 65. It consists of:

1. *Lamina.* Posteriorly. This is flat and quadrate in shape. Its posterior surface is marked by a vertical ridge in the midline, with a shallow depression on each side. The upper fibres of the oesophagus are attached to the upper part of the ridge. There is a smooth oval facet on each side of the upper border of the lamina, for articulation with the arytenoid cartilage.
2. *Arch.* Anteriorly. This is narrow in front and expands posteriorly to the lamina. The upper border passes obliquely upwards and backwards. The lower border is straight and almost horizontal. There is a rounded facet at the junction of the arch with the lamina on each side, for articulation with the inferior cornu of the thyroid cartilage.
3. *Cartilage of epiglottis.* Rises up behind the tongue. It is a thin leaf-like sheet of elastic fibrocartilage. The stem, directed downwards, is long and thin and is attached to the posterior surface of the thyroid alae at their junction. The free border, directed upwards, is broad and rounded from side to side.

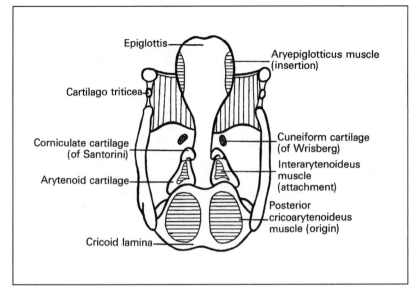

Figure 16.3 Laryngeal cartilages and hyoid bone – posterior view

The *anterior surface* is free in its upper part but is separated from the hyoid bone and thyrohyoid membrane by some fatty tissue in its lower part (pre-epiglottic space).

The *posterior surface* is indented by several small pits, in which mucous glands are embedded.

The *tubercle* of the epiglottis projects backwards in its lower part.

Paired cartilages

There are three pairs:

1. Arytenoid cartilages

These are the largest. They are pyramidal in shape.
- *Posterior surface* is triangular and concave. It extends laterally into a *muscular process*.
- *Anterolateral surface* is convex. It extends forward into a *vocal process*.
- *Medial surface* is narrow, smooth' and flat.
- *Inferior surface* or base, is concave. It articulates with the cricoid cartilage.
- *Apex* curves backwards to articulate with the corniculate cartilage.

2. Corniculate cartilages

The cartilages of Santorini. These are small. They articulate with the apices of the arytenoid cartilages and prolong them backwards and medially. They give attachment to the upper fibres of the oesophagus.

3. Cuneiform cartilages

The cartilages of Wrisberg. These are small bars of yellow elastic cartilage. There is one in each ary-epiglottic fold, where it acts as a passive prop. They do not articulate with any other cartilage.

Laryngeal joints

The two important joints of the larynx on each side are:

1. Cricothyroid joint

Between the inferior cornu of the thyroid cartilage and the facet on the cricoid cartilage at the junction of arch with lamina. It is a synovial joint with a capsular ligament. Two movements occur:
- *Rotation*, through a transverse axis.
- *Gliding*, slightly.

2. Crico-arytenoid joint

Between the base of the arytenoid cartilage and the facet on the upper border of the lamina of the cricoid cartilage. It also is a synovial joint with a capsular ligament. Two movements occur:
- *Rotation*. Of the arytenoid, on a vertical axis. The vocal process moves medially or laterally.
- *Gliding*. The arytenoids move towards or away from each other.

A strong posterior *crico-arytenoid ligament* prevents excessive movements of the arytenoid on the cricoid.

Laryngeal ligaments and membranes

These are of two types:

1. Intrinsic

Uniting the cartilages of the larynx to one another (Figure 16.4).

The elastic membrane of larynx is the fibrous framework of the larynx. It lies beneath the laryngeal mucosa and is divided into upper and lower parts by the ventricle of the larynx.
- *The upper part* contributes to the support of the aryepiglottic and ventricular folds. The *ventricular ligament* is a thickening of the free edge.
- *The lower part* is called the conus elasticus or cricovocal membrane. It is composed mainly of yellow elastic tissue. Below it is attached to the superior border of the cricoid cartilage. Above it is attached:
(a) In front to the deep surface of the angle of the thyroid cartilage.

The *median cricothyroid ligament* is formed by the thickened anterior part of the conus. It broadens out from its upper attachment to the lower border of the thyroid cartilage towards its lower attachment to the upper border of the cricoid cartilage.

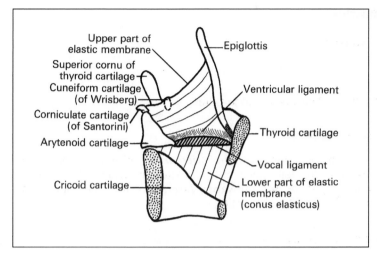

Figure 16.4 Sagittal section of larynx, to show intrinsic ligaments

(b) Behind to the vocal process of the arytenoid cartilage. The *vocal ligament* is the free upper edge of the conus between these points of attachment.
● *Thyro-epiglottic ligament* attaches the epiglottis to the thyroid cartilage.

2. Extrinsic

Uniting the cartilages of the larynx to the skeletal structures outside the larynx.
● *Thyrohyoid membrane* is a broad sheet of fibro-elastic tissue.
   Below it is attached to the thyroid cartilage at:
(a) Upper border of alae.
(b) Front of superior cornua.
Above it is attached to the hyoid bone at:
(c) Upper margin of posterior surface of body.
(d) Upper margin of greater horns.
   The *subhyoid bursa* separates the membrane from the posterior surface of the body. Upward movement of the larynx during deglutition is facilitated by the bursa.
   The membrane is pierced on each side by: (i) superior laryngeal vessels; (ii) internal branch of superior laryngeal nerve.
● *Median thyrohyoid ligament* is the thickened median portion of the thyrohyoid membrane.
● *Lateral thyrohyoid ligaments* form the thickened posterior border of the thyrohyoid membrane. They are attached on each side: below to the tips of the superior cornua of the thyroid cartilage; above to the posterior ends of the greater horns of the hyoid bone. The *cartilago triticea* is a small cartilage often found in each ligament.
● *Cricotracheal membrane* is attached: *below* to the first ring of the trachea; *above* to the lower border of the cricoid cartilage.
● *Hyo-epiglottic ligament* attaches the epiglottis to the hyoid bone.

Laryngeal muscles

These are of two types:

1. Intrinsic

Between one laryngeal cartilage and another.

Abductors of the vocal cords

There is only one on each side. *Posterior crico-arytenoid muscle.* Opens the glottis. *Origin* – from the depression on the posterior surface of the cricoid lamina. *Direction* – upwards and outwards. *Insertion* – into the back of the muscular process of the arytenoid cartilage.

Adductors of the vocal cords

There are three on each side:
- *Lateral crico-arytenoid muscle: Origin* – from the upper border of the arch of the cricoid cartilage. *Direction* – upwards and backwards. *Insertion* – into the front of the muscular process of the arytenoid cartilage.
- *Transverse portion of interarytenoid muscle.* A single muscle. *Origin* – from the back of the muscular process and lateral border of one arytenoid cartilage. *Insertion* – into the corresponding portion of the other.
- *External portion of thyro-arytenoid muscle.* Forms a thin sheet which lies outside the vocal cord, ventricle and saccule of the larynx. *Origin* – anteriorly, from the lower half of the angle of the thyroid cartilage and from the cricothyroid ligament. *Direction* – backwards, upwards and outwards. *Insertion* – into the anterolateral surface of the arytenoid cartilage. Its upper part forms the ventricular band.

Tensors of the vocal cords

There are two on each side:
- *Cricothyroid muscle. Origin* – from the front and lateral part of the outer surface of the cricoid cartilage. *Direction* – backwards, upwards and outwards. *Insertion* – into the lower border of the ala and the anterior border of the inferior cornu of the thyroid cartilage. It is known as the 'external tensor'.
- *Internal portion of thyro-arytenoid (vocalis) muscle* is a specialized portion of the lower and deeper fibres of the thyro-arytenoid muscle. It forms a triangular bundle inserted into the lateral surface of the vocal process and anterolateral surface of the arytenoid cartilage. Some of its fibres gain attachment to the vocal ligament. It is known as the 'internal tensor'.

Opener of the laryngeal inlet

Thyro-epiglottic muscle is a part of the thyro-arytenoid muscles whose fibres are prolonged into the aryepiglottic fold. Some of these reach the margin of the epiglottis.

Closers of the laryngeal inlet

- *Oblique portion of interarytenoid muscle* is superficial to the transverse portion. The two bundles of fibres cross each other. *Origin* – from the back of the muscular process of one arytenoid cartilage. *Insertion* – into the apex of the other.
- *Aryepiglottic muscle* is a prolongation of the oblique fibres of the interarytenoid muscle into the aryepiglottic fold.

2. Extrinsic

Between the larynx and neighbouring structures. There are two main groups:

'Strap' muscles of the neck

- *Sternothyroid muscle. Origin* – from the posterior surface of the manubrium sterni and the first costal cartilage. *Direction* – upwards. *Insertion* – into the oblique line on the thyroid ala. *Action* – draws the larynx downwards.
- *Thyrohyoid muscle. Origin* – from the oblique line on the thyroid ala. *Direction* – upwards. *Insertion* – into the lower border of the greater horn of the hyoid bone. *Action*–raises the larynx if the hyoid is fixed. Depresses the hyoid if the larynx is fixed.

Pharyngeal muscles

A few of these have minor insertions into the laryngeal skeleton.
- *Stylopharyngeus. Origin* – from the base of the styloid process of the temporal bone. *Insertion* – (few fibres) into the posterior border of the thyroid cartilage. *Action* – assists in raising the larynx.
- *Palatopharyngeus.* Contained in the posterior pillars of the fauces. *Insertion* – some fibres are inserted into the posterior border of the thyroid cartilage. *Action* – helps to tilt the larynx forwards during deglutition.
- *Inferior constrictor muscle.* The origin and insertion have been described in the anatomy of the pharynx. It has no effect on the movements of the larynx.

Cavity of the larynx

Extends from the inlet of the larynx where it opens into the laryngopharynx, to the lower border of the cricoid cartilage, where it is continuous with the trachea. It is divided into three parts by two folds of mucous membrane:

1. False vocal cords

These are the ventricular bands, which are formed by the mucous membrane covering the ventricular ligament and the upper part of the external portion of the thyro-arytenoid muscle.

2. True vocal cords

Project further into the cavity than the false cords and lie at a lower level. Parts of them can therefore be seen by inspection from above. The covering epithelium is closely bound down to the underlying vocal ligament and the blood supply is poor; hence the pearly white appearance of the vocal cords in life.

The mucosal folds divide the cavity into the following parts:

1. Vestibule

Lies between the inlet and the edges of the false cords. It is deeper in front than behind. It is bounded by:
- Posterior surface of epiglottis in front. The *pre-epiglottic space* is a wedge-shaped space lying in front of the epiglottis and bounded anteriorly by the thyrohyoid membrane and hyoid bone. Bounded above by a deep layer of fascia connecting the epiglottis to the hyoid bone (hyo-epiglottic ligament).
- Interval between the arytenoid cartilages behind.
- Inner surface of the ary-epiglottic folds and upper surfaces of the false cords on each side.

2. Ventricle of larynx

A recess between the false and true vocal cords. It is lined by a mucous membrane which is covered externally by the thyro-arytenoid muscle.

The *saccule* is a conical pouch which ascends from the anterior part of the ventricle. It lies between the inner surface of the thyroid cartilage and the false cord. Numerous mucous glands open on to the surface of its lining mucosa.

The *glottis* (rima glottidis) is the interval between: (i) the true vocal cords in its anterior three-fifths; (ii) the vocal processes of the arytenoid cartilages in its posterior two-fifths. Its average length in the adult male is about 2.5 cm, in the adult female about 1.6 cm.

3. Subglottic space

Lies between the true vocal cords and the lower border of the cricoid cartilage.

Mucous membrane of the larynx

This lines the whole cavity. It is continuous above with that of the mouth and laryngopharynx, below with that of the trachea. It is closely attached to the walls over the true vocal cords, the epiglottis, and the cartilages of Santorini and Wrisberg. Elsewhere it is loosely attached and therefore liable to become swollen from effusion.

Reinke's layer of connective tissue lies immediately under the epithelium of the larynx and superficial to the elastic layer. There are no glands beneath it and no lymph vessels in it.

Stratified squamous epithelium is found over:

1. Vocal cords.
2. Upper part of vestibule of larynx.

Ciliated columnar epithelium lines the remainder of the cavity.
Mucous glands are plentiful on:

1. Ventricles and saccules.
2. Posterior surface of epiglottis.
3. Margins of aryepiglottic folds. There are none on the free edges of the vocal cords.

Blood supply of the larynx

The larynx is supplied by:

1. *Laryngeal branches of superior thyroid artery.* Pierce the posterior inferior part of the thyrohyoid membrane on each side, deep to the thyrohyoid muscle.
2. *Laryngeal branches of inferior thyroid artery.* Accompany the recurrent laryngeal nerves. The relationship is variable.
3. *Cricothyroid branches of superior thyroid artery.* Cross the midline at the upper part of the cricothyroid membrane. The branches of the two sides anastomose freely with one another. Veins accompany the arteries.

Nerve supply of the larynx

The larynx is supplied by branches of the vagus nerve.
Superior laryngeal nerve has two laryngeal branches:

1. *Internal branch.* Entirely *sensory*. It pierces the thyrohyoid membrane with the superior laryngeal artery and vein. It supplies the cavity of the larynx as far down as the level of the vocal cords.
2. *External branch.* Travels down on the inferior constrictor muscle of the pharynx. It supplies the cricothyroid muscle and part of the anterior subglottis.

Recurrent (inferior) laryngeal nerve has a much longer course on the left side than on the right. On the left side it turns round the arch of the aorta. On the right side it turns round the subclavian artery. In the neck it lies between the trachea and oesophagus as it approaches the larynx. Its terminal part passes upwards, under cover of the ala of the thyroid cartilage, immediately behind the inferior cricothyroid joint. It then divides into:

1. *An anterolateral (motor) branch* which supplies all the intrinsic muscles of the larynx except the cricothyroid muscle. No fibres cross the midline and there is no spatial differentiation between those supplying abductors and those supplying adductors.
2. *Posteromedial (sensory) branch* which supplies the cavity of the larynx below the level of the vocal cords. The loop of Galen is formed by nerve

fibres which pass between the posteromedial branch of the recurrent laryngeal nerve and the internal branch of the superior laryngeal nerve.

Lymphatic drainage of the larynx

The edges of the vocal cords divide the lymphatic system of the larynx into two parts:

1. *Supraglottic* above the vocal cords. The vessels drain into:
- *Pre-epiglottic nodes.*
- *Upper deep cervical nodes.* After piercing the thyrohyoid membrane the vessels passing to these nodes accompany the superior thyroid artery.
2. *Subglottic* below the vocal cords. The vessels drain to:
- *Prelaryngeal and pretracheal nodes.* After piercing the cricothyroid ligament.
- *Lower deep cervical nodes.* After emerging from below the cricoid cartilage.

The vocal cords themselves have practically no lymphatic vessels, hence malignant tumours limited to them do not spread readily.

PHYSICAL EXAMINATION OF THE LARYNX

External examination

Information may be obtained by:

1. Inspection

For position and movements of the larynx. The larynx moves upwards on deglutition and sometimes on singing high notes. It moves downwards during inspiration in cases of laryngeal stenosis but is immobile in tracheal stenosis.

2. Palpation

For broadening and tenderness, as in perichondritis. The regional lymph nodes should always be examined.

3. Indirect laryngoscopy

Examination of the larynx from above by a laryngeal mirror. The various structures must be examined methodically:

Epiglottis

Usually presents a slightly curved and regular upper edge but this is sometimes acutely curved and conical ('infantile' type). It may hang backwards and obscure a view of the vocal cords in the relaxed state, or forwards to hide the valleculae. It rises upwards and forwards during phonation.

Ary-epiglottic folds

Must be inspected for swelling or ulceration.

Interarytenoid area

May be thickened or mammillated.

False cords

May show swelling or ulceration.

Vocal cords

Must be examined for:

1. *Colour.* The normal vocal cord is pearly white.
2. *Movement.* Examined at rest, during phonation and forced inspiration and on coughing. It may be restricted in abductor and adductor pareses, or by infiltration with growth. Arthritis of the crico-arytenoid joint also limits movement.
3. *Surface.* May be intact or ulcerated.
4. *Edge.* May be irregular.

The *anterior commissure* is not always easy to see.

Subglottic space

Difficult to examine but swellings may be seen below the level of the vocal cords.

Fibreoptic laryngeal examination

May be very useful in patients with sensitive throats or difficult anatomy.

Direct laryngoscopy

Endoscopic examination of the larynx with the laryngoscope. The head must be extended on the neck, the neck flexed on the chest. The larynx does not appear foreshortened as in indirect laryngoscopy. Direct laryngoscopy is necessary for examination in most children and for biopsy or endoscopic treatment at all ages. A specially designed laryngoscope is available for examination of the anterior commissure.

The use of the operating microscope greatly facilitates inspection and instrumentation of the larynx in anaesthetized patients.

Stroboscopy and video recording

Have been used for the analysis of cord movements.

RADIOGRAPHIC EXAMINATION OF THE LARYNX

General considerations

Radiographic examination is most commonly requested in established new growths to determine the lower limit and the degree of spread.

Views

1. Lateral soft-tissue view

Shows the air spaces well. The normal ventricle is seen as a clear horizontal area. Encroachment on the normal cavity may be seen and the lower limit of a growth determined.

2. Tomography

Of great value in assessing the presence and degree of a subglottic carcinoma. Infiltration of surrounding structures, such as the ventricles, may also be demonstrated.

3. Contrast laryngography

After topical anaesthesia, medium is introduced to outline the normal and diseased contours. The extent of tumours may be seen, especially if combined with cineradiography or videotape recording.

4. CT scan (Figure 16.5)

This demonstrates well the soft tissues as well as skeletal structures. The airways can be accurately assessed.

5. MRI

This appears to have significant advantages in demonstrating the extent of laryngeal neoplasms because of its tissue differentiation characteristics and ability to produce pictures in any plane.

ANATOMICAL PRINCIPLES OF LARYNGEAL SURGERY

Direct laryngoscopy

Apart from its value as a method of examination the direct laryngoscope can be used for:
1. *Biopsy,* which must always be performed in suspected neoplasia.

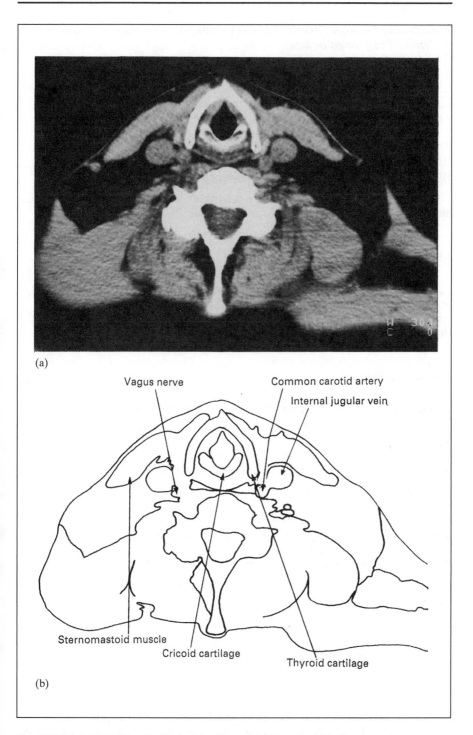

Figure 16.5 (a) Axial CT at the level of the fifth cervical vertebra; (b) diagrammatic representation

2. *Removal of benign tumours* such as papillomas, fibromas, or polypi.
3. *Removal of foreign bodies.*
4. Diathermy.
5. *Cryosurgery.*
6. Laser surgery.
7. Injection of sclerosing fluids (as in 'haemangioma' of the larynx) or of *Teflon paste* (as for cord palsies).
8. *Removal of membrane* in diphtheritic laryngitis, now rare.
9. *Insertion of endotracheal anaesthetic tubes,* usually with a modified form of laryngoscope.
10. *As a preliminary to bronchoscopy,* especially in children.

All these procedures are greatly facilitated by the use of the operating microscope, which is mandatory for laser work.

Laryngotomy

For sudden severe laryngeal obstruction, especially for impacted foreign bodies. A *transverse stab* is made through the *cricothyroid membrane* to insert a tube flattened in its transverse axis. It is the operation of choice for the less experienced surgeon, in an emergency.

Laryngofissure

A splitting of the larynx in the midline through an external incision.

Indications

The interior of the larynx may be exposed by this route for:

1. *Removal of small intralaryngeal tumours.* Particularly early glottic carcinoma.
2. *Excision of webs or strictures.*
3. *Submucous excision of one vocal cord.* In cases of bilateral laryngeal paralysis. This is now rarely practiced.
4. *Removal of impacted foreign body.*

Anatomical stages

Tracheostomy

With insertion of a cuffed tracheostomy tube.

Incision

Usually a midline vertical one from the hyoid bone to a point below the lower border of the cricoid cartilage. A transverse incision is preferred by some.

Entry to larynx

Entry is gained by a horizontal incision in the cricothyroid membrane. Through this opening packing must be inserted down to the tracheostomy tube unless an inflatable cuffed anaesthetic tube is used.

Fissure

The cartilage is divided in the midline or slightly to one side of it, and the halves are separated by retractors. Partial laryngectomy utilizes this approach.

Total laryngectomy

Indicated in certain advanced carcinomas of the larynx. Preliminary tracheostomy is sometimes considered advisable.

Incision

Several are in common use, particularly:

1. U-*flap*.
2. I-*flap*.

Skeletonizing the larynx

The 'strap' muscles are divided and the thyroid isthmus severed.

Ligature of superior laryngeal vessels

One of the most important steps of the operation. The superior laryngeal vessels and nerves are sought as they pierce the thyrohyoid membrane, just above the upper border of the thyroid ala and just in front of the superior cornu. They are ligatured and divided on each side.

Excision of larynx

From above downwards, allows inspection of the growth before removal. Three stages can be described.

1. *Exposure of pharynx*. An incision may be made through the thyrohyoid membrane just above the ala and is carried back to the superior cornu, thus exposing the epiglottis, but most surgeons prefer to open the pharynx above the hyoid bone and to remove it with the larynx. This allows for removal of the pre-epiglottic space and makes subsequent closure of the pharynx easier.
2. *Separation of larynx from pharynx*. The inferior constrictor muscle of the pharynx is divided along the posterior border of the thyroid ala. Scissor cuts from above downwards divide the mucosa of the lateral walls of the pyriform fossa. This division is continued across the back of the cricoid cartilage.

3. *Separation of larynx from trachea.* Made as high as possible. Enough of the trachea must be removed to give free clearance of any subglottic extension of the growth.

Anchoring of trachea

The trachea can be brought out through a separate transverse skin incision above the sternum or anchored in the original incision.

Closure of pharynx

The pharynx is closed, usually over an oesophageal feeding tube, by at least two layers of sutures. The inferior constrictor muscles are sutured to each other to protect the mucosal repair before the skin incision is closed.

Partial laryngectomy

May be indicated for the removal of certain tumours, especially when it is desirable to preserve the vocal function of the larynx. The main types are:

1. *Lateral partial laryngectomy* (by laryngofissure). For limited cordal tumours.
2. *Frontolateral partial laryngectomy.* For glottic tumours which cross the anterior commissure to involve the anterior third of the opposite cord, without reduction of mobility. This may be extended to include the whole ventricular band and arytenoid cartilage.
3. *Supraglottic partial laryngectomy.* For lesions of the infrahyoid epiglottis and adnexae, to spare the vocal cords.

Arytenoidectomy and fixation of cord

In bilateral vocal cord paralysis there is now a choice of endoscopic operations. Lateralization of the vocal cord by an external approach using the Woodman technique is now rarely used.

Endoscopic arytenoidectomy

This can be performed using microlaryngeal surgical instruments or the CO_2 laser. A cordectomy can be performed as an adjunct if necessary.

Suture lateralization

Via a small neck incision, large bore needles are passed into the lumen of the larynx above and below the vocal process of one arytenoid. A non-absorbable suture is passed through the inferior needle. An endoscopist grabs the suture and passes it back out of the larynx through the superior needle. Both needles are then withdrawn and the suture tied thus lateralizing the cord.

'Block' dissection of the neck

Indicated in some cases of head and neck cancer if the primary is considered to be cured or curable and may, in the case of pharyngeal or laryngeal tumours, be done in continuity with the removal of the primary disease. Technique may be the classic 'total' clearance of the contents of the anterior and posterior triangles together with removal of the sternomastoid muscle and internal jugular vein (Crile's operation). Only the carotid vessels are left on the exposed prevertebral fascia. Less radical methods aim to conserve the accessory nerve, sometimes the sternomastoid, and, if the procedure is bilateral, the internal jugular vein on the less diseased side.

A so-called suprahyoid 'block' is sometimes combined with excision of tongue and mouth cancers.

Chapter 17

Applied physiology of the larynx

FUNCTIONS OF THE LARYNX

Protection of the lower air passages

The most important function of the larynx, and is the earliest one to develop phylogenetically. Several mechanisms are involved:

1. Closure of the laryngeal inlet

When food is swallowed the laryngeal inlet closes. The aryepiglottic folds move towards one another and close the inlet. In many cases the epiglottis appears to lie over the closed inlet and to divert the food stream into the lateral channels, but it has been surgically removed without any adverse effects.

2. Closure of the glottis

Accompanies closure of the inlet. This normal reflex is present from the time of birth.

3. Cessation of respiration

Automatic. The IXth cranial nerve forms the afferent pathway of the reflex which is initiated by the contact of food with the posterior pharyngeal wall and base of tongue, which are supplied by this nerve.

4. Cough reflex

Should any particles enter the trachea and bronchi the act of coughing will usually dislodge them. Forced expiration is made against a closed larynx. Chevalier Jackson called the larynx the 'watchdog of the lungs'. The rarity with which foreign bodies gain entrance to the lower air passages, even in early infancy, is perhaps the highest testimony to the efficiency of the larynx in performing this function.

Phonation

Develops later in the evolution of the larynx. *Voice* is produced by vibration of the vocal cords. The sound so produced is amplified selectively by the resonating chambers of the mouth, pharynx, nose and chest.

1. Pitch

The vibrations of the cords cut the air column into puffs and the frequency of the puffs determines the pitch produced. The larynx is therefore a wind instrument. The average individual human voice can produce a frequency range of two octaves in singing.

2. 'Volume'

The intensity of sound produced by the larynx depends on the air pressure generated in the lungs by contraction of the abdominal and thoracic muscles.

Respiration

The larynx plays a part in the mechanism of respiration by reflex adjustments of the glottic aperture. These movements of abduction during inspiration and adduction during expiration also contribute to the regulation of acid-base balance in the body by influencing the carbon dioxide tension of the blood.

Fixation of the chest

When the larynx is closed the thoracic cage becomes fixed permitting climbing or digging. Since the ribs cannot rise freely a fixed support is given to the pectoral muscles.

Laryngeal sphincters

The larynx has been described as a three-tiered sphincter (Figure 17.1).

True vocal cords

This sphincter opens readily but in a controlled fashion when pressure is exerted on the cords from below. This allows the passage of air from below and results in sound-producing vibrations. The true vocal cords, however resist pressure from above.

False vocal cords

Resist pressure from below. When they are closed they become valves capable of trapping air below the level of the larynx. This is necessary for

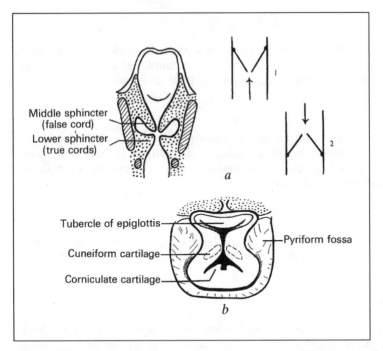

Figure 17.1 Sphincters of the larynx. a, Coronal section. (Inset 1 indicates valvular resitance to upward pressure at the middle shincter. Inset 2 indicates valvular resistance to downward pressure at the lower sphincter); b, upper sphincter in contraction (seen from above). (After Pressman)

producing increased intrathoracic pressure (required in coughing) or increased intra-abdominal pressure (produced in such acts as defaecation, urination and parturition). The closure of this valve is comparable to the simple circular form of muscle closure of the primitive larynx.

Aryepiglottic sphincter

Perhaps the most important of all, for it protects the lower air passages by preventing the invasion of foreign material. The tubercle of the epiglottis fills an anterior dehiscence between the aryepiglottic folds when the sphincter is closed. The cartilages of Wrisberg are sited in the aryepiglottic folds as sesamoid cartilages and serve a stiffeners for these folds. The sphincter is active in retching, gagging, swallowing and vomiting, or when threatened by a foreign body.

MECHANICS OF LARYNGEAL MOVEMENTS

Abduction of the vocal cords

There is only one abductor of the vocal cords. This is the *posterior crico-arytenoid muscle*. Contraction of the muscle causes the muscular process of the arytenoid cartilage to be rotated backwards, round a vertical axis (Figure 17.2). Hence the vocal process, together with the posterior end of the vocal cords, moves outwards. There is at the same time a backward bracing of the arytenoid cartilages.

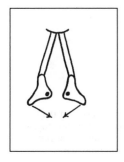

Figure 17.2 Movements of the vocal cords – abduction. Posterior cricoarytenoid muscles

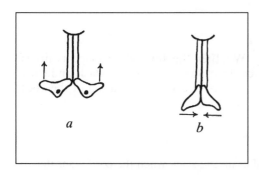

a

b

Figure 17.3 Movements of the vocal cords – adduction. a, Lateral cricoarytenoid muscles; b, interarytenoid muscles

Adduction of the vocal cords

Three muscles contribute to the closure of the glottis (Figure 17.3):

1. Lateral crico-arytenoid muscle

Contraction of this muscle rotates the muscular process of the arytenoid cartilage forwards and so turns the vocal process medially.

2. Transverse portion of the interarytenoid muscle

Contraction approximates the arytenoid cartilages of the two sides. This closes the posterior part of the glottis.

3. Thyro-arytenoid muscle

Promotes glottic closure by medial rotation of the arytenoid cartilages, and it partially controls the length and tension of the vocal cord, as an antagonist to the cricothyroid muscle.

Tension of the vocal cords

Two muscles are responsible:

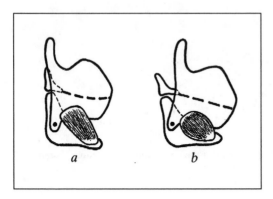

a   *b*

Figure 17.4 Movements of the vocal cords – tension. a, The cricothyroid muscle (external tensor) at rest; b, the cricothyroid muscle in contraction

1. Cricothyroid muscle

The external tensor (Figure 17.4). Whether the thyroid cartilage is drawn downwards and forwards or the cricoid cartilage is drawn upwards and backwards, contraction of the cricothyroid muscle causes elongation of the vocal cords with increase in tension.

2. Vocalis muscle

The internal tensor contracts and takes up the slack when the cord is shortened.

Opening of the laryngeal inlet

Produced by the thyro-epiglottic muscle. Contraction of the muscle pulls the aryepiglottic folds outwards.

Closure of the laryngeal inlet

Effected by two muscles:

1. Oblique portion of interarytenoid muscle

Contraction of these fibres brings the ary-epiglottic folds together with a 'scissor' action.

2. Aryepiglottic muscle

Contraction brings the arytenoids closer to the epiglottis.

Raising and lowering of the larynx

These movements are brought about by the attachment of the larynx to the hyoid bone. The mylohyoid, geniohyoid and stylohyoid muscles raise the hyoid bone and hence the larynx. The sternohyoid and omohyoid muscles depress the hyoid bone and hence the larynx. The actions of the stylopharyngeus and palatopharyngeus muscles and the 'strap' muscles of the neck have been described on p. 297.

Chapter 18

Diseases of the larynx

CONGENITAL ABNORMALITIES OF THE LARYNX

Laryngomalacia (congenital laryngeal stridor)

The larynx is of an *exaggerated infantile type (Figure 18.1)*. The *epiglottis* is long and narrow and folded backwards at each lateral edge. This converts the epiglottis into an omega shaped incomplete cylinder. The *aryepiglottic folds* are also approximated. The laryngeal inlet is therefore reduced to a cruciate slit, the edges of which are sucked together by each inspiration.

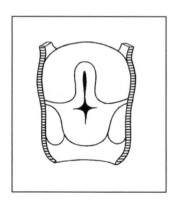

Figure 18.1 Exaggerated infantile type of laryngeal inlet

Clinical features

Stridor is the only symptom and appears at or soon after birth. It is *croaking* in character and mainly *inspiratory* in phase. It is diminished by rest, responsive to changes of posture but increased by exertion. It disappears between the second and fifth years of life.

Cyanosis is rare and the *voice* is unchanged.

Exaggerated infantile type of larynx can be seen on direct laryngoscopy. The edges of the laryngeal inlet are seen to be drawn in with inspiration.

Diagnosis

Can be made by a careful history and examination.

Inspiratory stridor without hoarseness is always suggestive when occurring at, or soon after, birth.

Flexible fibrescopic examination, or direct laryngoscopy, will distinguish this condition from those below.

Treatment

Reassurance is usually all that is necessary. Tracheostomy may rarely have to be performed in very severe cases. It should be avoided whenever possible as it carries a 5–10% mortality.

Prognosis

Should be guarded but is mostly good. Death in the first year of life, usually from pneumonia, occurs occasionally.

Subglottic stenosis

Most cases are acquired from intubation trauma in premature infants, few cases are spontaneous. Inspiratory *stridor* is partially relieved by rest and worsened by exertion but *unaffected by posture.* The voice is normal. Feeding is difficult because there is little time to spare for swallowing. The work of respiration is considerably increased and *failure to thrive* occurs in severe cases.

Diagnosis and treatment

Direct laryngoscopy and broncoscopy is required. The subglottis should be measured. If the infant fails to thrive a *tracheostomy* is required. Growth of the subglottis allows *decannulation after some years* of tracheostomy life in most cases. If a *laser* is available to vaporize the stenosis, long-term tracheostomy can sometimes be avoided. There is a 5–10% mortality rate from both the condition and tracheostomy at home. Mother *must* be able to change the tube.

Subglottic haemangioma

This condition is clinically indistinguishable from subglottic stenosis and the diagnosis and management are the same. Laser treatment is particularly effective.

Laryngotracheal cleft

This is the least manifestation of failure of the lateral septa of the primitive oesophagus to fuse in the midline. Minor clefts present with stridor, more severe ones with aspiration of milk and pneumonia.

Diagnosis and treatment

The diagnosis is made by barium swallow followed by direct laryngoscopy. Particular care must be taken to probe between the arytenoids in all cases of congenital stridor because the cleft is not usually visible. Clefts of the cricoid at or above the cords are treated conservatively, clefts below the cords cause aspiration and require open surgical repair with a preliminary tracheostomy. The mortality of cases which aspirate is 50%.

Laryngeal cyst

Small cysts present with hoarseness or a muffled cry, larger ones cause *inspiratory stridor*. Direct laryngoscopy is required to evacuate and *uncap* a cyst but the diagnosis may be made with a fibreoptic flexible laryngoscope in the clinic. Treatment may need to be repeated.

Laryngeal web

Aetiology and pathology

The web is due to an arrest in development and consists of a fibrous tissue stroma covered by epithelium, in the anterior half of the glottis. Atresia may be complete. This causes stillbirth and may be overlooked at autopsy.

Clinical features

The symptoms vary with the size of the web.

Hoarseness is usually present.

Inspiratory stridor occurs in severe cases. It may be accompanied by dyspnoea on exertion.

Web can be seen by direct or fibroscopic laryngoscopy (Figure 18.2). It may be white or pink, thin or very dense. The posterior border is sharp and curved.

Differential diagnosis

A congenital web must be distinguished from an acquired web due to:

1. *Trauma.* Accidental or surgical, especially after cordectomy.

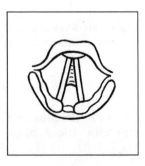

Figure 18.2 Congenital web of the larynx

2. *Acute specfic infections.* As in healed diphtheria or typhoid fever.
3. *Chronic specfic infections.* Such as tuberculosis, syphilis or scleroma.

Treatment

No treatment. In the milder forms. Hoarseness is not relieved by operation and recurrence of a thick fibrous band may follow.
    Laser excision.
    Tracheostomy. Essential when stridor and dyspnoea are severe.
    Excision by laryngofissure. May be advised later, but it should be postponed if possible until the larynx has developed fully. The larynx is split in the midline, the web excised, and the laryngeal lumen maintained by a plastic triangular tube. The tube is surrounded by a Thiersch graft and transfixed through the thyroid cartilage by wires.

Vocal cord palsy

Often overlooked as a cause of inspiratory stridor and hoarseness in a neonate. Even direct laryngoscopy under general anaesthetic *fails to reveal* the condition unless the surgeon watches the cords patiently as the anaesthetic wears off and the larynx comes to life. Fibreoptic laryngoscopy is the most appropriate technique. Caused by damage to the recurrent laryngeal nerve in neck or chest usually from birth trauma. Treatment is expectant.

TRAUMATIC CONDITIONS OF THE LARYNX

Direct injuries

Compression (closed) injuries

As in blows and strangulation.

Pathology

The changes resulting from compression injuries may be extralaryngeal or intralaryngeal and may involve the cartilages themselves.

1. *Bruising of skin* may occur but superficial changes may be slight or absent.
2. *Surgical emphysema* involves the tissues of the neck in the first instance. It may spread to the face, chest, abdomen and upper limbs.
3. *Submucosal haemorrhage* can involve any part of the interior of the larynx.
4. *Adhesions* may develop between the opposed surfaces of an abraded or lacerated laryngeal mucosa.
5. *Stenosis* follows in some cases. Its onset may be sudden or gradual, immediate or delayed.
6. *Perichondritis* results if infection supervenes.

7. *Fracture of the laryngeal cartilages* may accompany these changes.
- The *thyroid cartilage* is more commonly involved because of its more exposed situation.
- Fracture of the *cricoid cartilage* leads quickly to subglottic swelling. Nearly all recorded cases have been fatal.

Clinical features

The most important symptoms are those caused by interference with respiration.

1. *Dyspnoea* may be marked and of sudden onset. Asphyxia will follow if relief is not immediate. It is caused by:
- *Submucosal infiltration* or soft-tissue displacement.
- *Mediastinal emphysema.*
2. Hoarseness or weakness of the voice, is common.
3. *Dysphagia* is a frequent symptom.
4. *Haemoptysis* is usually slight.
5. *Pain* is variable.
6. *Tenderness* may be elicited by palpation.
7. *Crepitus* is difficult to detect. It must not be confused with the grating sensation produced by movements of the normal larynx against the vertebral column.
8. *External swelling* may result from surgical emphysema or haematoma.
9. *External bruises* are sometimes seen.
10. *Submucosal haemorrhages* can be seen on indirect laryngoscopy.

Diagnosis

The history and physical signs usually allow a diagnosis to be made.

Plain X-rays or CT scan may confirm the presence of a fracture in a cartilage.

Treatment

The chief danger of these injuries is interference with respiration.

1. *Tracheostomy* or laryngotomy, may be urgently required.
2. *Systemic antibiotics* should be given prophylactically in every case. They must be continued if perichondritis threatens or supervenes.
3. *Incision and drainage* are needed for abscess formation.
4. *Laryngofissure* may be required later for the treatment of:
- *Fractures of the thyroid cartilage: To hold the displaced fragments outwards.*
- *Subsequent stenosis.*

Penetrating (open) wounds

Usually fatal. They are caused by gunshot injuries, stabs or cuts.

Pathology

The laryngeal injuries are generally accompanied by damage to vital structures. These depend upon the direction of the injury.

1. *Oblique wounds* usually involve the great vessels of the neck.
2. *Anteroposterior wounds* may cause death from involvement of the cervical spine.
3. *Transverse wounds* may involve the larynx only. Survival is rare even in this type.

Clinical features

Dominated by respiratory obstruction and haemorrhage.

1. *Dyspnoea* results from several different causes, separately or combined:
- *Haemorrhage into the larynx and tracheobronchial tree:* Usually from branches of the thyroid vessels.
- *Swelling of the soft tissues of the larynx:* by oedema, submucosal haemorrhage or displacement of the soft tissues.
- *Displacement of fractured cartilages:* most commonly the thyroid cartilage.
- *Mediastinal emphysema*
- *Perichondritis and/or stenosis:* subsequently.
2. *Haemorrhage* may be massive and rapidly fatal.

Treatment

Must be immediate.

1. *Clamping and ligature* of divided vessels.
2. *Intubation* through the open wound may prevent asphyxia.
3. *Tracheostomy* should be performed as soon as facilities permit.
4. *Removal of foreign bodies* with excision of devitalized tissues and suturing of the mucosa.
5. *Systemic antibiotics.*
6. Laryngofissure at a later date if stenosis occurs.
7. *Fluids intravenously or by nasogastric tube.* No food must be given by mouth for at least 24 hours.

Burns and scalds

Aetiology

These rare injuries may follow:

1. Inhalation of irritant fumes or gases.
2. Swallowing of corrosive fluids.
3. Inhalation of steam.

Pathology

Oedema of the structures of the laryngeal inlet and vestibule is the usual finding. The term 'oedema of the glottis' usually applied to the condition is a misnomer, for the glottis itself is usually spared.

Clinical features

Dyspnoea is the presenting symptom. Pain and dysphagia are usual.

Treatment

Usually conservative.

1. *Rest* must be enforced by confinement to bed, strict rest of the voice, and sedative drugs.
2. *Steroids* should be given by intravenous or intramuscular injection.
3. *Antibiotics* to prevent secondary infection.
4. *Analgesic drugs.*
5. *Tracheostomy or laryngotomy* must be performed if the airway is compromised.
6. *Local treatment* is unnecessary unless stenosis follows.

Radiotherapy reactions

Severe local reactions in the larynx may follow radical irradiation. The radiotherapist monitors the reaction throughout treatment as the total dose given may well be determined by this reaction. Reactions will be exacerbated by smoking, the drinking of spirits, and local infections, including the common cold.

Dyspnoea of acute onset can occur following the initial treatment of advanced laryngeal tumours. In these cases the initial daily dosage should be gradually increased and where necessary 'cover' with dexamethasone should be used.

Discomfort on swallowing may result from 'membrane reaction' or oedema of the mucosa in the region of the arytenoid 'mound' and aryepiglottic fold. The presence of dry, tenacious mucus increases the discomfort.

Pain results from perichondritis or cartilage necrosis. It may be referred to the ear.

Treatment

Preventive or curative.

1. *Elimination of oral sepsis* should be ensured before radiotherapy is begun.
2. *Tracheostomy* is rarely necessary but should not be delayed in the presence of dyspnoea.
3. *Systemic antibiotics* when perichondritis is present or threatening.
4. *Aspirin mucilage* or a similar analgesic preparation, lessens the pain and discomfort of swallowing.
5. *Laryngectomy* in severe intractable cases where necrosis is present.

Inhaled foreign bodies

Foreign bodies in the larynx are rare. Most foreign bodies entering through the mouth or nose are either held up in the upper part of the cervical oesophagus or pass through the glottis into the bronchi, but sharp foreign bodies, such as pins or glass, may be impacted in the larynx. Large foreign bodies, such as boluses of food, are almost immediately fatal when impacted in the larynx.

Clinical features

Smaller foreign bodies may be compatible with life.
Dyspnoea may be urgent.
Cough. A violent bout of coughing may be followed by a quiescent phase. This applies to small objects such as pins.
Hoarseness or aphonia may appear immediately or later from oedema.
Perichondritis and stenosis follow when the foreign body is retained or causes severe trauma.

Treatment

A *'bear hug'* (Heimlich's manoeuvre) from behind with hands clasped just below the xiphisternum may expel the object with a gust of air.
Removal by direct laryngoscopy as soon as possible. Very rarely removal by *laryngofissure* is necessary.
Tracheostomy or laryngotomy may be necessary in an emergency. Suitable instruments are often not available for removal of the foreign body. Tracheostomy is always preferable to laryngotomy if time and available skills permit. A catheter or any suitable substitute may be used instead of a tracheostomy tube if the latter is not at hand. The tracheostomy must be kept open until all danger from oedema has passed.
Systemic antibiotics should be given to prevent bronchopulmonary infection.

Intubation injuries

Aetiology

These injuries mostly occur in patients having prolonged respiration in Intensive Care Units, and are caused by:

1. Rough intubation, particularly when it is blind. The use of relaxant drugs has diminished the incidence of these injuries.
2. The prolonged presence of the tube between the vocal cords.
3. The use of too large a tube.

Pathology

1. *Superficial abrasions.*
2. *Granulomatous formation.* Usually occurs over the vocal processes of the

arytenoid cartilages. It is much more common in women than in men (4:1) and is bilateral in one-half of the cases.
3. *Subglottic oedema.* In children, rarely in adults.

Clinical features

Hoarseness
   Dyspnoea. Sometimes.

Prevention

Consists of avoidance of blind intubation, particularly in the presence of an upper respiratory infection. Tracheostomy (to permit removal of endotracheal tube) should not be too long delayed if assisted respiration is required for periods of more than a few days.

Treatment

Voice rest may suffice.
   Endoscopic removal of granulomas becomes necessary when the condition persists.
   Tracheostomy for dyspnoea.

Acute submucosal haemorrhages on the vocal cords (acute haemorrhagic laryngitis)

Aetiology

The haemorrhages are due to sudden violent and forceful approximation of the vocal cords. They are seen after coughing, shouting, weight-lifting and injuries to the larynx.

Clinical features

Hoarseness occurs suddenly after a vocal strain. *Pain* may occur. The *haemorrhages* may be single or multiple and the remainder of the cords may be injected. Rarely the whole of one cord is involved. The haemorrhages may organize into the granulomatous or fibrous nodules requiring endoscopic removal.

Differential diagnosis

From acute laryngitis, external injury, leukaemia, purpura and carcinoma.

Treatment

Vocal rest. The most important part of the treatment.

'Singer's nodes'; vocal nodules

Definition

A condition occurring in persons who use the voice excessively, with straining or faulty production.

Aetiology

Singers (especially sopranos and tenors), actors, teachers, mothers of young children and persons talking to the deaf are most frequently affected. It is more common in women and in singers who use the 'coup de glotte' or sing above their natural tessitura (range).

Pathology

Localized hyperkeratosis. The site is constant, at the junction of the anterior third and posterior two-thirds of the free edge of one or both vocal cords. The nodules never become neoplastic.

Clinical features

Increasing hoarseness. Appears either quite suddenly after one episode of strain, or slowly and insidiously over a period of weeks or months.

Vocal fatigue is noticed.

Nodules are more commonly bilateral and symmetrical (Figure 18.3). They vary in size from that of a minute pinhead to that of a grape-pip. An adherent blob of mucus may obscure or mimic a node.

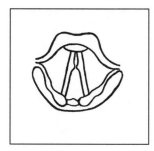

Figure 18.3 Singer's nodes

Treatment

Vocal rest is essential and may cure some of the recent and small nodules.

Elimination of focal sepsis. Particularly in teeth, tonsils and sinuses.

Removal by direct laryngoscopy with operating microscope is indicated if the condition persists. Precise removal is possible without damage to the voice.

Speech therapy helps to re-educate voice production.

Contact 'ulcer'

Aetiology

An uncommon condition which occurs almost exclusively in male adults. It occurs in singers and street vendors and results from the hammering of one vocal process of the arytenoid cartilage against the other.

Vocal abuse is an important contributory factor.

Coughing is always detrimental.

Pathology

Thickening of the tissues around the vocal process usually on one side only.

A saucer-shaped depression may occur over one vocal process. The epithelium is not broken so it is not a true ulcer.

Clinical features

Discomfort in the throat may be slight or severe.

Huskiness may also be slight, or severe and persistent.

Vocal fatigue occurs easily.

Referred otalgia may occur, when ulceration is present.

'Kiss ulcer' is the common finding on indirect laryngoscopy, the granuloma of one side fitting into the 'ulcer' crater of the other.

Treatment

Vocal rest is the most important part of the treatment. Total abstinence for 2 or 3 weeks may be necessary.

Steroids have proved successful, given systemically in some cases.

Removal of thickened epithelium by microlaryngoscopy.

Vocal rehabilitation is essential after the lesions have healed, or recurrence will almost certainly occur.

INFLAMMATIONS OF THE LARYNX

Acute non-specific laryngitis

Acute simple laryngitis in adults

An acute superficial inflammation of the laryngeal mucous membrane.

Aetiology

1. *Infection.* Laryngitis occurs either as a part of a generalized upper respiratory infection, or as a sudden localized laryngitis. These forms are commonly viral.

It is more common in winter and early spring and often occurs each year. Patients suffering from sinusitis, nasal obstruction from any cause, overuse of the voice, and indulgence in alcohol or tobacco are more prone. It is often associated with the common infectious diseases.

2. *Trauma* due to vocal abuse and/or endoscopic manipulation.

3. *Irritation* from inhaled fumes or gas, including tobacco smoke.

Pathology

1. *Infection of the mucosa* is at first slight and generalized, and the vocal cords themselves may escape in the early stages. Later they become reddened.

2. *Oedema* follows and the whole laryngeal mucosa is usually symmetrically involved.

3. *Sticky mucopurulent exudate* may cover the surface.

4. *Slight abrasions* are sometimes seen, but deep ulceration does not occur.

5. *Purulent exudation* occurs in the very severe forms with marked injection and oedema ('septic laryngitis').

6. *Fibrinous laryngitis* occurs in influenza, or in certain coccal infections. There are white deposits or plaques on the surfaces of the cords and upper laryngeal inlet. Minute erosions may be found; they heal in a few days.

7. *Perichondritis* may follow the purulent form. The causal organism is usually the haemolytic streptococcus.

Clinical features

1. *Hoarseness.* The patient may speak in a gruff or falsetto voice, or become quite aphonic.

2. *Discomfort in the throat* is common.

3. *Pain* is slight or absent except in very severe cases.

4. *Dysphagia* is usually slight, unless the epiglottis or arytenoids are markedly involved as after swallowing hot fluids.

5. *Dyspnoea* is absent, unless oedema occurs in severe cases.

6. *Cough.* If present is dry and irritating.

7. *Generalized symptoms.* Malaise and fever often occur before the local symptoms appear. Severe toxaemia is rare.

8. *Symmetrical redness and/or sticky secretions* on both vocal cords, at indirect laryngoscopy.

Progress

The inflammation usually resolves in a few days. The hoarseness may persist for as long as 2 weeks after apparent resolution. A functional aphonia may follow a simple acute laryngitis, especially in women. In severe cases the inflammation may spread throughout the lungs, more commonly in aged patients.

Treatment

1. *Local*
- *Vocal rest* is essential. A quiet (unforced) whisper is allowed.
- *Steam inhalations* with Tinct. Benzoin Co. or menthol, help to loosen viscid secretions.

- *Aspirin for its anti-inflammatory effect* may be soothing.
- *Warm applications* to the neck.
- *Codeine to suppress dry cough* is comforting.
2. *General*
- *Rest.* In a room with an equable temperature. Sedatives may help.
- *Avoidance of alcohol and tobacco*
- *Systemic antibiotics in cases of* infective origin.

Acute simple laryngitis in children

Acute laryngitis is a more serious condition in children than in adults. The main reasons for this have been discussed under the 'Infantile larynx', in the section on anatomy. The lymphatic drainage of the larynx is richer in the child and the submucosa is therefore more likely to swell. The neuromuscular mechanism is also more easily upset and spasm more easily provoked. Finally, the child is less able to expel the secretions by coughing.

Aetiology

1. *Any upper respiratory infection.* Viral or bacterial, may lead to an acute laryngitis. It is often associated with the common infectious diseases.
2. *Trauma.* To the pharyngeal or laryngeal mucosa may institute an attack.

Clinical features

The onset is usually preceded by a simple sore throat, with slight fever and irritating cough.

1. *Cough.* A laryngeal spasm ('false croup') develops suddenly.
2. *Dyspnoea, cyanosis and stridor.* From laryngeal spasm and mucosal oedema, the latter sometimes extending to the subglottic space.
    '*Laryngitis stridulosa*' is the name given to the condition when stridor is present. It is inspiratory and indrawing of the supra- and infra-clavicular fossae may be present during the paroxysms of stridor.
3. *Hoarseness.* The voice is hoarse but strong unless the condition is very severe and exhausting, when it becomes weak.

Differential diagnosis

1. *Laryngeal diphtheria* in which the child is usually more ill but less febrile; the characteristic membrane can usually be seen; and the organism can be identified on culture.
2. *Impacted foreign body in the larynx.*
3. *Inhaled foreign body in the bronchus* in which general disturbance and infection are absent in the early stages.
4. *Congenital laryngeal stridor, webs, cysts.*
5. *Spasmodic laryngitis (spasmodic croup).*
6. *Laryngeal oedema from steam or corrosives.*
7. *'Allergic' laryngitis* (Quincke's oedema). Rarely.
8. *Laryngeal papillomatosis.*

Treatment

1. *Rest in bed* is essential. A sitting position should be adopted.
2. *Systemic antibiotics.* Antibiotics are given in full doses to ill children and especially to infants.
3. *Systemic steroids* in all severe cases.
4. *Humidification* is helpful for the first day or two.
5. *Oxygen.* May be essential; 80% helium 20% oxygen quarters the work of breathing.
6. *Nasotracheal tube* may be inserted.
7. *Tracheostomy* is indicated when the obstruction is severe. It is better done too early than too late. Cardiac insufficiency may develop suddenly though it is less common than in diphtheria.
8. *Laryngotomy* is quicker to perform and may thus be life-saving. It must be replaced by a tracheostomy as soon as possible.
9. *Intravenous fluids* are sometimes necessary to combat dehydration.

After the acute phase has subsided it is necessary to attend to the general health and to remove infected tonsils, adenoids, or teeth.

Acute epiglottitis

Definition

Special form of acute laryngitis, in which the inflammatory changes affect mainly the loosely attached mucosa of the epiglottis.

Pathology

Localized oedema may obstruct the airway, especially in children. *H. influenzae* is the usual causal organism, B Haemolytic streptococci rarely. Submucosal abscesses may form.

Clinical features

1. *Dyspnoea* may be progressive and alarming, especially in children, in whom death may occur within a few hours of onset.
2. *Pain on swallowing* is commoner than respiratory obstruction in adults.

Treatment

1. *Constant supervision* in hospital, when stridor is present.
2. *Throat swab and blood cultures before antibiotics are started. Septicaemia accompanies the laryngeal infection.*
3. *Intravenous antibiotics* in high doses chosen to kill *H. influenzae.* type B which also causes the concomitant septicaemia
4. *Endotracheal intubation.* May prove extremely difficult.
5. *Tracheostomy* may become urgently necessary, especially in children.

Acute laryngotracheobronchitis

Aetiology

Affects infants and young children. Causative organism is usually parain-
fluenza virus type 1 or similar which shows seasonal and epidemic tendencies.
Secondary bacterial infection by the third day of symptoms is common and
makes the condition worse.

Clinical features

Are those of an acute simple laryngitis as it occurs in children, but are much
more severe.

1. *Hard, dry, croupy cough and hoarseness.* Occur after a cold or influenza.
2. *Pyrexia.* May be very high.
3. *Dyspnoea and cyanosis.* Often marked, from involvement of the trachea
and bronchi.
4. *Tenacious exudation and crusting.* Characteristic.
5. *Oedema of the larynx.* Seen on laryngoscopy.
6. *Atelectasis.* Caused by occlusion of the bronchi.

Differential diagnosis

1. *Acute simple laryngitis* which is less severe and produces no physical signs
in the chest.
2. *Diphtheria* which can be distinguished by bacteriological examination.
There is no bleeding when the crusts are removed in cases of acute laryngotracheobronchitis.
3. *Bronchopneumonia* in which there is usually no crusting.
4. *Bronchial foreign bodies* especially those of a vegetable nature.

Treatment

Should be in hospital.

1. *Rest and reassurance* are important.
2. *Systemic antibiotics and anti-pyretics* must be started immediately. Each
degree Celsius rise in body temperature causes an obligatory 10% rise in
metabolic rate.
3. *Humidification* of inspired air.
4. *Oxygen* may have to be given, preferably in a tent. Heliox (see above) may
be given also.
5. *Fluids* must be given by mouth or intravenously to prevent dehydration.
6. *Nasotracheal tube or tracheostomy* may be necessary.
7. *Removal of secretions* may be effected by:
● *Bronchoscopy* with removal by suction or forceps.
● *Tracheostomy* followed by intermittent suction. This is preferred to
repeated peroral endoscopy.

Diphtheritic laryngitis

Laryngeal diphtheria is usually an extension of a faucial infection. It is difficult to diagnose when it is primarily laryngeal. It is the true 'croup' of pre-microbic days.

Aetiology

Infection is due to the *Corynebacterium diphtheriae.* The incidence is greater in children under 10 years of age, but occasionally affects young adults in camps. It has been less frequent since universal immunization and is now rare in the UK.

Clinical features

The onset is usually insidious and undramatic.

Cough of a hoarse, croupy nature is the first symptom.

Stridor. Inspiratory in phase, soon follows. It is accompanied by cyanosis and recession of the chest wall. The cough becomes weak and muffled.

Pyrexia is rarely above 37.8°C (100°F).

Weak and rapid pulse accompanies the pyrexia. The stridor is rarely marked in adults, but a child may become prostrated rapidly.

Greyish-white membrane appears on the affected parts. Bleeding may accompany its separation.

Diagnosis

Established by identifying the specific organism in swabs from the membrane. These may have to be obtained by direct laryngoscopy when the pharynx is not involved. Diphtheria must be differentiated from:

1. Acute laryngotracheobronchitis.
2. Inhaled vegetable foreign body.
3. Acute simple laryngitis associated with an exanthematous fever.
4. Spasmodic laryngitis (spasmodic croup).

Treatment

1. *Antitoxin injections* by the intramuscular or intravenous route, should by given whenever there is any suspicion of diphtheritic infection, while awaiting confirmation of the diagnosis. The dosage varies from 20 000 to 100 000 units according to age.
2. *Systemic penicillin*
3. *Oxygen* is essential in severe cases.
4. *Tracheostomy* may have to be performed and should be done before signs of cardiac failure appear.

Herpes zoster of the larynx

Rare condition due to a neurotrophic virus. The superior laryngeal branch of the vagus nerve and the pharyngeal plexus may be involved, especially in debilitated persons.

Clinical features

Pain in the throat is the main local symptom.
   Dysphagia accompanies it.
   Fever and malaise
   Vesicles are found on the epiglottis, arytenoid 'mound', and ventricular bands. They are usually unilateral.
   Palsies of the vocal cords occasionally result from involvement of the motor branch to the cricothyroid muscle or of the recurrent laryngeal nerve.

Treatment

Oral Acyclovir 800 mg five times daily for a week if a *painful cord palsy* is diagnosed within the first 3 days of onset. Cranial nerve palsies due to *zoster* have a poor prognosis and should be treated aggressively. If seen late, symptomatic treatment with rest in bed and local applications to relieve pain.

Pemphigus of the larynx

Rare vesicular condition of unknown aetiology. Most common in elderly debilitated persons.

Clinical features

There are two clinical types:

Acute type. A very serious and lethal condition.
1. Headache.
2. Malaise.
3. Fever.
4. Dysphagia.
5. Hoarseness.
Chronic type. In which the patient feels well and has no fever.
1. A burning sensation in the throat.
2. Skin lesions are usually present, often in the form of a vesicle of the umbilicus.

   The larynx is rarely involved alone; the mouth, gums and pharynx are commonly affected also. In the larynx the *epiglottis* is the common site; the arytenoids may be affected. The local lesion is a *vesicle* which bursts to leave a whitish membrane. This may disappear and then recur at intervals; it rarely leaves any adhesion or stenosis as it may in the pharynx or nose.

Differential diagnosis

Mainly from diphtheria and syphilis.

Prognosis

Must be guarded. The disease may resolve completely in the less severe forms but death may occur within 2 years in more severe cases.

Treatment

Mainly by steroids. Secondary infection must be dealt with and pain must be relieved by analgesics.

Chronic non-specific laryngitis

This may follow an acute attack, but more often it arises insidiously due to:

1. *Faulty use of the voice,* overstraining or excessive force, is the most important factor.
2. *Infection in teeth, tonsils and sinuses* especially when they result in excessive hawking or coughing.
3. *Excessive alcohol or tobacco.*
4. *Dust or irritant fumes.*

Pathology

Hyperaemia of the vocal cords is generally marked.
   Oedema may also be present even in the absence of hyperaemia.
   Myositis occurs in the intrinsic muscles.
   Excessive viscid secretions result from increased activity of the mucous glands.
   The hyperaemic and oedematous stage often passes to a granular hypertrophic one, rarely to an atrophic one.

Clinical features

Hoarseness is intermittent at first and may become less marked after use of the voice.
   Cough may be present. It is only slight and is dry and irritating, with constant hawking and clearing of the throat.
   Soreness in the throat is a common complaint.

Laryngeal appearances

There are three types of chronic simple laryngitis:

1. *Hyperaemic* in which the cords are injected or dull pink and stiffened in appearance. There may be some loss of adduction due to myositis. Flecks of viscid mucus may lie on the cords and in the interarytenoid space. In severe cases the cords are deep red in colour and appear rounded and 'sausage-like'.
2. *Hypertrophic* in which there is thickening of the tissues of the cords and also of the ventricular bands, arytenoids, interarytenoid space, and sometimes of the subglottic region (Figure 18.4).
3. *Oedematous* in which the true cords are swollen and pale. The condition may be of long standing.

   In all types the larynx is nearly always affected *bilaterally* and *symmetrically.*

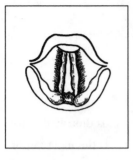

Figure 18.4 Chronic hypertrophic laryngitis

Treatment

Vocal rest
   Speech therapy may supplement it and correct faulty use.
   Systemic antibiotics. When swabs show a significant growth of organisms the appropriate antibiotic is chosen.
   Elimination of irritating factors, such as dust, and tobacco-smoking.
   Carbocisteine (a mucolytic) may give symptomatic benefit when secretions are thick and tenacious on the cords.
   Stripping of the vocal cords is performed endoscopically in resistant cases of chronic oedematous laryngitis.

Hyperkeratosis of the larynx (keratosis)

Definition

A localized form of epithelial hyperplasia characterized by white 'leucoplakic' raised patches on the vocal cords.

Aetiology

The condition is rare and occurs more commonly in men. Although its causation is often obscure, it is included in this section because of its clinical resemblance to and association with some chronic inflammations of the larynx.

Pathology

There is a hyperplastic change in the epithelium, leading to excessive cornification, together with extension of the papillae into the corium, the basement membrane remaining intact.

Clinical features

Hoarseness of gradual onset, is persistent.
   White raised patches appear on one or both vocal cords. The anterior and middle thirds are usually involved. Mobility of the cords is not impaired.

Prognosis

The condition must be considered precancerous and carcinoma in situ frequently supervenes. It tends to persist in spite of conservative treatment.

Treatment

Septic foci in the mouth, throat and nose must be treated, but response is uncertain. Biopsy of suspicious areas is essential, and may require repetition.

Constant supervision is essential to detect early malignant change, demanding radical removal or radiotherapy.

Stripping of the cords can sometimes be done through a direct laryngoscope but recurrence is usual.

Removal of the affected cord(s) by laryngofissure is possible in advanced and prolonged cases. Skin-grafting may be necessary.

Radiotherapy is not indicated.

Pachydermia laryngis

Definition

A form of chronic hypertrophic laryngitis affecting the epithelium and subepithelium of the posterior part of the larynx, i.e. the posterior halves of the cords, the vocal processes, and the interarytenoid region. The ventricular bands may occasionally be affected.

Aetiology

A rare condition, more common in men. Often no known causes, but aggravating factors include excessive alcohol and tobacco.

Pathology

Hypertrophy occurs both in the epithelium and in subepithelial connective tissue. An inflammatory reaction may be seen. Neoplastic change does not occur.

Clinical features

Hoarseness. The voice is usually husky but may occasionally be normal.

Irritation or discomfort. Sometimes.

'Granular' or papilliferous appearance The heaping-up of the mucosa occurs in the posterior sites and is bilateral and symmetrical. Any unilateral condition must be regarded as neoplastic until proved otherwise.

Treatment

Similar to that for simple chronic laryngitis. Surgical removal and diathermy of the masses give little relief and are inadvisable.

Atrophic laryngitis (laryngitis sicca)

An uncommon type of chronic laryngitis, usually associated with atrophic rhinitis and pharyngitis.

Aetiology

Aggravating factors include dusty atmospheres, industrial fumes and chronic infection in the paranasal sinuses. It appears to be more common in women.

Clinical features

Hoarseness and irritation in the throat both of which are improved temporarily by hawking and coughing up the crusts.

Dyspnoea may be caused by large obstructing crusts.

Dry and atrophic mucosa over the whole of the interior of the larynx.

Crusts of varying sizes lie over the mucosa which may be excoriated when they are removed. They have a foul odour. The crusting usually extends into the trachea.

Treatment

Eradication of associated lesions in the nose and paranasal sinuses.

Change of atmospheric conditions may be beneficial.

Removal of crusts will afford some local relief. This is aided by:

1. *Inhalations* of menthol, or oil of pine.
2. *Carbocisteine* by mouth.
3. *Laryngeal sprays* e.g. Benadryl, 05% or solutions of sodium bicarbonate.
4. *Hormones.* Local applications of hormones in oils have been tried, with uncertain results.

Tuberculous laryngitis

1. Acute miliary tuberculosis of the larynx

The rare laryngeal lesions are accompanied by lesions in the pharynx. Tubercles appear on the swollen mucosa of the epiglottis and arytenoids. These break down and form confluent greyish *ulcers*. Great *pain* is usually present. The prognosis is serious and the treatment is that of the general infection.

2. Chronic tuberculosis of the larynx; laryngeal phthisis

Aetiology

Infection in the larynx is almost always secondary to a pulmonary lesion. Reports of primary infection are very rare and increasingly so with improved methods of diagnosis. Most infections are *sputogenic,* a few are haematogenous and a very small number are carried by the lymph stream. The incidence has fallen dramatically from about 25% of all cases of pulmonary tuberculosis to less than 2.5%. The sexes are equally affected. Persons between 20 and 40 years of age are most often affected though it may occur in children and elderly persons.

Pathology

With the common sputogenic type of infection the tubercle bacillus can infect the intact laryngeal mucosa, especially that in the posterior third of the larynx. Infected sputum lies in the interarytenoid region.

The submucosal layer becomes infected and small round-cell *infiltration* follows. Before infiltration is marked there may be considerable myositis with resulting weakness of the intralaryngeal muscles. One or more surface *nodules* soon appear which *caseate* and lead to *ulceration* which gradually extends. Progress of the disease leads to masses of *granulation tissue* and also to cellular swelling *(a pseudo-oedema)* Lesions are usually *asymmetrical,* except with interarytenoid granulations and the turban-like pseudo-oedema which involves the epiglottis, aryepiglottic folds, arytenoids, and ventricular bands.

The posterior half of the larynx is most frequently involved, but often one whole cord may be affected or the epiglottis, or the mucosa of the ventricle. At a later stage there is *perichondritis* and *cartilage necrosis,* together with true oedema. A 'simple' laryngitis is common in patients with pulmonary disease.

Clinical features

1. *Weakness of the voice* with periods of aphonia, is sometimes the earliest symptom.
2. *Hoarseness* becomes evident in varying degrees. Even minimal lesions can cause marked voice changes, leading to an erroneous diagnosis of a functional condition. Complete aphonia is rare. Occasionally large lesions produce little hoarseness.
3. *Cough* is a prominent symptom.
4. *Pain on swallowing* is present if the laryngeal inlet is involved. It is a common symptom in advanced lesions and it may be severe.
5. *Referred otalgia* is common.
6. *Dyspnoea* is rare unless perichondritis causes marked oedema.
7. *Localized tenderness* is rare unless perichondritis is present. A 'cold' abscess may point externally.
8. *Laryngoscopic appearances*
- *Slight impairment of adduction* may be an early sign and is caused by a myositis.
- *Marked injection of one vocal cord* may involve the whole of the cord or the posterior part of it.
- *Ulceration of the edge of the cord* giving the appearance of having been 'mouse-nibbled' (Figure 18.5).
- *Granulations in the interarytenoid region* or on the vocal process of the arytenoid cartilage. This is the commonest tuberculous lesion and is often accompanied by a hidden shallow indolent ulceration. In older patients this may resemble a carcinoma very closely.

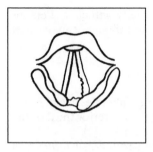

Figure 18.5 Tuberculous laryngitis, showing 'mouse-nibbled' cord and heaping-up of posterior commissure

- *Oedema of the mucosa of the ventricle* causing swelling which mimics a prolapse.
- *Pseudo-oedema of the epiglottis and arytenoids* ("turban larynx') of a pale sausage-like appearance, with occasional small bluish superficial ulcers.
- *Subglottic infiltration* with ulceration and granulation, is uncommon.
- *Tuberculoma* is a very rare manifestation and presents as a small grey 'tumour', often associated with ulceration of the base of the epiglottis.
- *Perichondritis and cartilage necrosis* leads to erosions of the epiglottis, laryngeal stenosis, or vocal cord fixation from ankylosis of the crico-arytenoid joint.
- *Vocal cord paralysis* may occur from apical pulmonary disease, with thickening of the pleura. This affects the right side more commonly than the left.

Diagnosis

Early manifestations may need careful investigation. Later manifestations can mimic or coexist with syphilis or carcinoma.

Chest radiographs must always be taken when there are persistent laryngeal symptoms from any cause, to exclude TB of the lungs.

Sputum will usually contain tubercle bacilli.

Biopsy is essential when any doubt exists about the nature of any laryngeal lesion occurring in a tuberculous patient. The lesions most often confused with tuberculous laryngitis are carcinoma, ulcerative type of syphilis, lupus, pachydermia and chronic simple laryngitis.

Treatment

The most important of all is that of the primary lung disease.

Antituberculous chemotherapy. Rifampicin, ethambutol, INAH, streptomycin, and PAS are used. A dramatic response in the local laryngeal lesions results.

Vocal rest is still necessary. Complete silence is difficult to enforce and a forced whisper is deleterious. A quiet whisper all the time or a normal voice for short periods two or three times a day is therefore advocated. Smoking should be stopped and any nasal infection should be treated.

3. Lupus of the larynx

Rare and is usually secondary to disease in the nose and pharynx. It appears to be more common in young females. The epiglottis is involved first, then the aryepiglottic folds. The vocal cords may be involved much later. Reddish, nodular *granulations* are seen on a pale mucosal base. Areas of *ulceration* and *scarring* coexist. The epiglottis may be notched in the form of a V. *Stenosis* may be a late result.

Clinical features

Symptoms are few. The laryngeal condition is often symptomless and discovered only on examination in cases of nasal lupus.
   Vague discomfort in the throat.
   Hoarseness. Present only in late cases, and if the cords are involved.
   Dyspnoea. Follows rarely when stenosis is marked.

Prognosis

Good.

Treatment

Antituberculous chemotherapy.
Calciferol (Vitamin D_2). In massive doses, i.e. 150 000 i.u. daily for 3–6 months. Two pints of milk per day should be taken with the calciferol.
   Attention to general health
   Tracheostomy has been performed in cases with marked stenosis.

Syphilitic laryngitis

Congenital syphilis

Rarely affects the larynx. Organism is the spirochaete *Treponema pallidum.*

1. Early form

Occurs in the first few months of life. *Perichondritis* is the main lesion. *Acute laryngeal obstruchon* may be caused by the resulting oedema. Other luetic lesions are usually present.

2. Late form

Occurs between the ages of 2 and 10. Mucosal *hyperplasia with granulations* is the commonest lesion. *Ulceration* and *necrosis* follow. The epiglottis is the commonest site and may be completely eroded. The cords may be extensively ulcerated. *Stenosis* may follow. *Hoarseness* in a child must lead to suspicion of a luetic infection. *Stridor* may occur.

Acquired syphilis

The secondary stage is rarely observed in the larynx, but the tertiary forms are met with frequently enough to cause diagnostic problems.

1. *Gumma.* The commonest lesion and is most frequently seen on the *epiglottis.* The ventricular bands are sometimes involved. There is marked swelling of a dark red hue, with areas of *'wash-leather' ulceration.*
2. *Diffuse infiltration.* Without ulceration, is common and affects any part or all of the larynx. It resembles a chronic simple hyperplastic laryngitis but may also simulate a carcinoma or tuberculous laryngitis when nodular.
3. *Ulceration.* Occurs in one of two forms:
- *Small superficial ulcers* on the epiglottis or arytenoids (Chancre).
- *Deep serpiginous or punched-out ulcers* usually on the epiglottis, as the result of a gumma. Necrosis, scarring and atrophy follow. The ulcers are commonly painless.
4. *Perichondritis.* Result of extension of the above lesions. It leads to oedema and sequestration of cartilage.
5. *Scar tissue and adhesions.* The results of the above inflammatory changes and may lead to laryngeal stenosis.

Clinical features

Vary with the nature and the site of the lesion.
   Hoarseness. The usual complaint.
   Dyspnoea and stridor may occur.

Diagnosis

Syphilis can mimic all other laryngeal diseases.

Treatment

1. *Systemic penicillin.*
2. *Tracheostomy.* May be needed for laryngeal obstruction.
3. *Reconstructive plastic operations.* Can be carried out safely in inactive late cases of severe stenosis.

Leprosy of the larynx

Leprosy is rarely seen in Britain. It affects the larynx in about 10% of cases. The laryngeal infection is always associated with that of the skin and nose or pharynx.

Pathology

Diffuse nodular infiltration affects chiefly the epiglottis, arytenoids and ventricular bands.
   Deformity of the laryngeal inlet results from contraction and destruction of its tissues. The vocal cords usually remain free until a late stage of the disease.

Clinical features

Dyspnoea. May be marked.
   Hoarseness. Present only in the later stages.

Laryngoscopic appearances. The laryngeal mirror may show a small hook or knob-like epiglottis over a 'buttonhole' glottic chink. Leprous nodules may be seen anywhere in the larynx. They vary in size from that of a pinhead to that of a walnut. They have an analgesic surface.

Treatment

Chiefly for the general disease, by chemotherapy with clofazimine, rifampicin and dapsone.
Tracheostomy. Seldom necessary.

Scleroma of the larynx

Aetiology

Has been discussed under Rhinoscleroma. It is endemic in Central and Eastern Europe and also in Central and South America.

Pathology

Subglottic region is most commonly affected. The typical lesion is a gross subepithelial infiltration with resultant swelling of the subglottic tissues. This produces pale pinkish swellings on either side below the vocal cords.

Clinical features

The condition tends to spread down to the trachea and bronchi, causing: *hoarseness, cough and increasing dyspnoea*

Differential diagnosis

From syphilis, carcinoma and chronic subglottic laryngitis. The complement fixation test is positive in 90% of cases. Biopsy may be necessary.

Treatment

1. *Systemic antibiotics.* Streptomycin and the tetracyclines offer most hope of cure or at least amelioration.
2. *Steroids* may prevent fibrosis in the active stage.
3. *Tracheostomy* is often needed. Removal of obstructing masses by laryngofissure has been advocated. If all activity has ceased reconstructive plastic operations can be done for severe stenosis.

Wegener's ('malignant') granuloma of the larynx (non-healing granuloma)

Rare, and affects the glottic and subglottic regions, threatening asphyxia, though insidious in its development. Tracheostomy may become necessary. The pathology and treatment are described on p. 227.

Mycoses of the larynx

Apart from Candida, fungus infections are extremely rare in the larynx. They include:

Actinomycosis

Characterized by yellowish infiltration, which breaks down soon into a suppurative mass. Lymphadenitis occurs early.

Hoarseness and cough with an offensive sputum, occur. The pus contains the ray fungus.

Potassium iodide in massive doses, together with systemic penicillin may effect a cure in early cases.

Blastomycosis

Occurring primarily in the larynx. Occurs mainly in grain workers in South America and is caused by the yeast fungus. Starting as a chronic granuloma with giant cells, it breaks down to form ulcers with soft, granular bases.

Hoarseness and cough occur early.

Dyspnoea and dysphagia are later symptoms.

The differential diagnosis is from tuberculosis, syphilis and carcinoma and is made by microscopic examination of the tissues or sputum. Treatment is by antifungal agents, e.g. amphotericin B.

Perichondritis of the larynx

Definition

An inflammation of the perichondrium of the laryngeal cartilages.

Aetiology

There are several causes:

1. *Inflammatory.* From tuberculous and syphilitic infections; acute septic laryngitis, as in the exanthemas, typhoid fever and diphtheria; or from spread of infection from sepsis in the mouth.
2. *Traumatic.* From cut-throat wounds; impacted foreign bodies and high tracheostomy tubes. Perichondritis may follow radiotherapy.
3. *Neoplastic.* From advanced carcinoma with secondary infection.
4. *Ionizing radiation* usually during treatment of advanced laryngeal tumours.

Pathology

The perichondrium, becomes infected and separates from the cartilage. *Exudates occur leading to subperichondrial* abscess and *necrosis* of areas of cartilage. Pointing of the abscess and sequestration of cartilage follows. *Oedema* of the overlying mucosa is marked. Subsequent resolution leads to deformity and stenosis from fibrous tissue formation. Fixation of the crico-arytenoid joints may occur.

Clinical features

The condition may be of sudden or insidious onset.

Malaise, fever and even rigors occur in the acute form.

Local pain is always present and often radiates to the ears.

Tenderness.

Enlargement of the laryngeal contour can be elicited by inspection and palpation.

Swelling of the neck is caused by an abscess. This may burst to form a sinus or fistula.

Cough.

Hoarseness.

Dysphagia.

Dyspnoea which increases.

Prognosis

Depends chiefly on the condition causing the perichondritis. Laryngeal obstruction, inhalation pneumonia, or abscess and septicaemia are the common immediate dangers. Laryngeal stenosis and permanent hoarseness are late results.

Differential diagnosis

From conditions causing oedema without perichondritis. Syphilis and malignant disease may need careful investigation and treatment before differentiation is possible. An unsuspected foreign body must be excluded.

Treatment

Absolute rest both general and local in the acute stage.

Systemic antibiotics.

Laryngeal sprays of ephedrine 0.5% and cocaine 2% are sometimes useful in the early stages.

Tracheostomy is indicated when dyspnoea is marked and should be made as low as possible.

Incision of an abscess, either externally or internally, is necessary when pointing is seen. Fragments of necrotic cartilage are removed.

Laryngofissure with skin grafting if airway is inadequate.

Laryngectomy is indicated when marked necrosis has occurred, especially following radiotherapy. It must be considered when pain or spill-over of food leads to a gradual deterioration in the general condition.

NEOPLASMS AND CYSTS OF THE LARYNX

Epithelial neoplasms of the larynx, both benign and malignant, are far more common than those derived from connective tissue. Malignant glottic tumours cause hoarseness at a very early stage so that early diagnosis and high cure rates are possible.

Benign neoplasms of the larynx

Epithelial tumours

Single papilloma of the larynx

This is the common type in adults, but is rare in children. It may be sessile or pedunculated. The usual site is the region of the anterior commissure and the anterior half of the vocal cord. Less often the ventricular band is involved. It is twice as common in men as in women. *Hoarseness* is present when the glottis is involved. A pedunculated papilloma may be sucked down between the cords during inspiration and then blown up again to rest on the cords during phonation.

Treatment is by *endoscopic forceps* removal. When large, *laryngofissure* may be necessary. Histological examination is obligatory to confirm the clinical diagnosis of benignity, especially in recurrent cases which tend ultimately towards malignant change.

Multiple papillomas of the larynx

These are the usual type in infants and young children, but are rare in adults. A virus may be responsible. The vocal cords and ventricular bands are the usual sites but spread may occur to the epiglottis, trachea and bronchi. *Hoarseness* is always present when the cord is affected. *Dyspnoea* may result from obstruction by the papillomas, especially in infants.

Treatment is by *endoscopic removal* with the CO_2 laser of each papilloma, care being taken not to cause submucosal scarring. Recurrence is usual so that operation may have to be repeated several times. In children recurrence does not lead to malignant change. *Tracheostomy* may be needed to relieve dyspnoea and the tube may have to be worn until the spontaneous disappearance of the papillomas, which is alleged to occur at puberty. *Radiotherapy* has been employed but may damage the laryngeal cartilages in the young. It may also be followed by malignant change many years later and is not advised owing to risk of postoperative stenosis. Very rarely laryngectomy is necessary.

Connective-tissue tumours

Fibroma of the vocal cord

Most of the tumours diagnosed clinically as fibromas result either from the organization of a submucosal haematoma of the cord or are of inflammatory origin and thus are not true neoplasms. Rarely, a laryngeal neurofibroma is seen in generalized neurofibromatosis. *Hoarseness* is produced early by fibromas situated on the edge of the vocal cord. The tumour is rarely large enough to cause dyspnoea.

Treatment is by *endoscopic removal* under the operating microscope.

Chondroma

More common in males. This generally arises from the cricoid but sometimes it is attached to other cartilages. The posterior cricoid plate is the usual site. Hoarseness is caused by encroachment on the laryngeal lumen. *Dyspnoea* follows later. *Tracheostomy* may be required. *Removal by open operation* is feasible in some cases, and some form of *laryngectomy* may be required for very large tumours.

'Angioma'

By a strict pathological classification these tumours should be regarded as malformations and not as neoplasms. There are two types:

1. *Telangiectases.* Often familial.
2. *Varices.* These lie submucosally and are usually extensions from the oropharynx or pyriform fossa. A *purplish swelling* appears in the laryngeal vestibule.

   Treatment is required only when obstruction or haemorrhage occurs. It is then similar to that of pharyngeal 'angiomas' (p. 000).

Other benign connective-tissue tumours

Include: *lipoma. rhabdomyoma and leiomyoma.*

Malignant neoplasms of the larynx

Epithelial tumours

For practical purposes all malignant tumours of the larynx are squamous-cell carcinomas. Adenocarcinoma, cylindroma, basal-cell carcinoma, and the connective-tissue malignant tumours are all extremely rare.

Squamous-cell carcinoma

Pathologically these tumours range from highly keratinized types to anaplastic types. Biopsy is always necessary, both for diagnosis and to ascertain the degree of differentiation; the latter assists in the choice of treatment. Clinically the growth may be ulcerative or proliferative. The topographical types are shown in Figure 18.6.

1. *Supraglottic carcinoma* (Figure 18.7). Two regional subdivisons of this group are distinguished:
   - *Those arising in the upper part of the vestibule,* which is bounded above by the line of closure of the aryepiglottic sphincter and is limited below by a level immediately above the ventricular band. The intralaryngeal aspects of the infrahyoid portion of the epiglottis, the aryepiglottic folds, the arytenoids, and the interarytenoid membrane form the walls of this part of the vestibule. Growths usually arise from the anterior half of this area. These are sometimes included in the adjacent superior group of laryngopharyngeal growths which they resemble in their symptomatology and

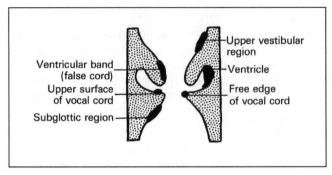

Figure 18.6 Sites of laryngeal carcinoma (coronal section of larynx)

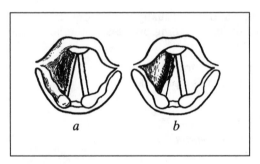

Figure 18.7 Supraglottic carcinoma. a, Upper vestibular; b, ventricular

treatment. Limited growths of this region, however, can be treated by removal of the affected part, on one or both sides of the larynx (partial laryngectomy).

● *Those arising on the ventricular band itself and in its underlying ventricle and saccule.* *Hoarseness* may be relatively late and is preceded by a sense of discomfort in the larynx. Those arising in the ventricle or saccule may present difficulty in diagnosis when they cause the ventricular band to be swollen but not ulcerated. In such cases it may be necessary to pierce the band deeply to reach the tumour when taking a biopsy specimen. *Tomography* and laryngography with opaque contrast medium help to define these tumours. The growth may project through the laryngeal sinus and lie over the cord to resemble a cordal cancer. Direct spread to the pre-epiglottic space may be surprisingly early and extensive. The rich lymphatic drainage of this area makes metastases in the upper deep cervical glands a frequent accompaniment (40%).

2. *Glottic carcinoma.* Carcinoma of the cord is the commonest form of intralaryngeal growth (Figure 18.8). All degrees of differentiation are encountered. The majority show keratinization. Occasionally the carcinomatous change is confined to the surface epithelium without invasion of the supporting connective tissue (*'carcinoma-in-situ'*). Carcinomatous change may supervene on a hyperkeratosis.

Site. The site of origin of a cordal carcinoma may be the free edge or the flat upper surface of the cord, usually in its central portion or its anterior half.

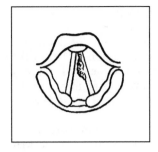

Figure 18.8 Glottic carcinoma

Direct spread. Forwards to the anterior commissure and backwards to the vocal process, is usual and may occur early. From the anterior commissure it may spread across the midline to the anterior end of the opposite cord and upwards to the pre-epiglottic space. Spread upwards into the ventricular band is late as is backward spread beyond the vocal process. Downward spread occurs into the subglottic space on the same side or below the anterior commissure. It may reach the trachea.

Lymphatic spread. Owing to the paucity of lymphatics the early growths limited to the cord do not show lymphatic metastases in more than 4%.

Clinical features. Patients are most commonly seen in the fifth and sixth decades. *Hoarseness,* gradually increasing, is the earliest and the only sign until stridor occurs from the increased size of the growth and accompanying oedema. *A nodular or generalized swelling of the cord* may be seen on indirect laryngoscopy. Other clinical types include a *white papilliferous excrescence* or an *ulcerated area* or a *plaque. Impaired movement* of the affected cord results from infiltration. *Fixation* is regarded as a late sign. *Pain (often referred to the ear), dyspnoea,* and *dysphagia* are caused by perichondritis as the disease advances. Metastasis in the lymphatic glands of the neck appears as a hard painless mass beneath the sternomastoid.

3. *Subglottic carcinoma.* The incidence is midway between that of glottic and supraglottic cancer. The primary site is usually the subglottic surface of the cord, but sometimes it is immediately below the anterior commissure (Figure 18.9).

Direct spread:
- Upwards to the cord edge. This may be late.
- Downwards to the trachea.
- Circumferential spread. The posterior wall is attacked last.

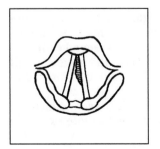

Figure 18.9 Subglottic carcinoma

Lymphatic spread. Metastases occur in the lower deep cervical, cricothyroid, paratracheal and mediastinal lymph nodes.

Clinical features. The growth may not be readily seen in the laryngeal mirror until it has reached the edge of the cord or formed a tumour below the anterior commissure. *Hoarseness* results from infiltration of the cord and may therefore be late in appearing. *Immobility of the cord* results from neoplastic infiltration or from paralysis of the nearby recurrent laryngeal nerve. *Stridor* presents as the growth increases in size.

Diagnosis. Established by endoscopy with the anterior commissure laryngoscope passed between the cords. Radiography, particularly CT or MR scanning, assists in delineating the tumour.

Summary of UICC classification

Glottis
T1   Limited/mobile.
　　　a. One cord.
　　　b. Both cords.
T2   Extension to supra- or sub- glottis/mobile.
T3   Fixation of cord(s).
T4   Extension beyond the larynx.
Supra- and sub-glottis
T1   Limited/mobile.
T2   Extension to glottis/mobile.
T3   Fixation of cord(s).
T4   Extension beyond the larynx.
All regions
N1   Homolateral movable.
N2   Contra- or bilateral movable.
N3   Fixed.

Treatment

1. Radiotherapy

Usually delivered by the cobalt unit or by megavoltage therapy.
　　Radiotherapy is indicated in:
● Anaplastic tumours.
● Early cordal growths, in preference to partial laryngectomy (cordectomy).
● Tumours which only slightly exceed the limitations demanded by partial laryngectomy.

A slightly higher rate of cure in early cordal growths is obtained by radiotherapy than by surgery and the voice after treatment may be perfect. Failure of radiotherapy may demand total laryngectomy; a second course of radiotherapy should never be given. In general growths in the posterior half of the larynx and those involving cartilage are less suitable for radiotherapy.

In some centres radiotherapy combined with hyperbaric oxygen to increase the cancericidal effects is proving successful with some of the more extensive growths.

2. Chemotherapy

Cytotoxic drugs are now used intravenously (systemically) in advanced cases:
- In combination with radiotherapy, bleomycin and methotrexate act synergistically.

The role of adjuvant chemotherapy has not been fully evaluated. As a definitive treatment in advanced cases, chemotherapy appears neither to improve the length of life nor its quality. It appears to have no role in the management of cases that have failed to be controlled by surgery and radiation.

3. Surgery

After failure of radiotherapy, or in some circumstances as primary curative treatment, excision of the tumour may require:
- *Total laryngectomy.* The larynx is removed *in toto* and the resultant gap in the pharyngeal wall is closed. The hyoid bone must be removed with the rest of the larynx in cases in which the anterior commissure is involved, so as to include the pre-epiglottic space which is often invaded. The resulting permanent tracheostomy does not exclude a working life. This operation is indicated in cases which have advanced so far as to preclude laryngofissure and in cases which have recurred after radiotherapy. It is sometimes indicated as a palliative measure in advanced cases with fungation, infection, and pain. When involvement of lymph nodes is present a *monoblock dissection* is made to include the larynx together with the thyroid lobe, sternomastoid muscle, internal jugular vein and nodes on the same side as the lesion. Simultaneous bilateral block dissection has been performed but retention of the jugular vein on the side less likely to be involved is advisable. Alternatively, there can be a 3-week interval between the full block dissections on the first and second sides. Bilateral cervical metastases, however, generally constitute a contraindication to radical surgery. *Tube feeding* (as described for pharyngolaryngectomy) is usual for 10–12 days, although fluids have been swallowed naturally the day after the operation without ill effect. One or two lessons in swallowing air and belching it up to produce sounds are given before operation. As soon as possible after operation the patient starts speaking with this *'oesophageal' voice,* preferably under group instruction. Rarely an external vibrator may be necessary. Recently an artificial larynx has been devised with respiratory valves and vibrating reed. Its lower end fits the tracheostome, and its upper end communicates with the pharynx through a surgically created skin-lined fistula.
- *Partial laryngectomy (see* p. 434). Such operations preserve function but carry higher risks of incomplete removal of growth, and postoperative chest infections. It is essential to ensure by radiography and endoscopy that the growth is resectable by the technique envisaged. If there is persistent doubt, or if the patient is frail, very old, or has impaired pulmonary function, total laryngectomy is preferable. *In all cases* the patient must give prior consent for total laryngectomy, if at operation the growth is found to be too extensive for partial laryngectomy. A tracheostomy should always be made to safeguard the airway as the first stage of any of

these operations. It can be decannulated and allowed to close during the second postoperative week as soon as swallowing without spillover and an adequate airway are secure. Nasogastric tube-feeding is also essential through this period.

After cordectomy dense inert scar tissue replaces the excised cord and the voice is rough but serviceable.

(a) Lateral partial laryngectomy (laryngofissure with cordectomy). The larynx is split in the midline and the affected cord is excised with a *wide margin of healthy tissue* around the growth. Suitable for small carcinomas in the anterior part of the cord.

(b) Frontolateral partial laryngectomy. Used for more extensive growths, anteriorly placed and involving both cords. After the thyroid cartilage has been split and partially removed, the larynx is entered on both sides well behind the limits of the growth. Only possible if the resulting shortened glottis is adequate for respiration.

(c) Supraglottic partial laryngectomy is occasionally appropriate for aryepiglottic, epiglottic, or even false cord tumours. Meticulous preoperative assessment of resectability and planning of technique are essential. Cricopharyngeal sphincterotomy is necessary to assist rehabilitation of swallowing.

Management of cervical lymph-node metastases

1. *Observation.* In cancers limited to one vocal cord neither planned irradiation of the lymphatic areas nor prophylactic block dissection is undertaken in the absence of metastases, whether the primary growth be treated surgically or by radiotherapy. Continued strict and regular observation, however, is essential if metastases are to be detected early.

2. *Presentation.* Palpable nodes in the neck at presentation should be treated by block neck dissection unless the patient is unfit, or the extent of the disease indicates that the outlook is poor.

3. *Prophylactic treatment.* Radiotherapy of the more advanced cancers of the larynx should include the lymphatic areas.

4. *Treatment of postoperative and post-irradiational lymph-node metastases.* Metastases after radiotherapy or surgery should be treated by block dissection. The appearance of metastases after block dissection demands irradiation, provided that it has not been given previously. Even if the nodes do not disappear they may remain clinically controlled for a long period after irradiation.

Connective-tissue tumours

All extremely rare though most forms of sarcoma have been recorded. Fibrosarcoma is said to attack the cords most often, while others, e.g. malignant lymphoma, leiomyosarcoma or plasmacytoma, may be found in the vestibule.

The presence of a rapidly growing tumour, especially if not ulcerated, will arouse suspicion. Diagnosis depends on biopsy. Treatment is by irradiation in the radiosensitive types, by laryngectomy in the insensitive. Chemotherapy will be appropriate in sarcomas.

Cysts and allied conditions of the larynx

Cysts of the larynx

Developmental cysts

Infants. Rarely, cysts in close connection with the saccule may obstruct the larynx.

Adults. These cysts are derived from portions of a *laryngocele* that have become disconnected from the larynx by inflammatory adhesions and subsequently distended with gelatinous or milky fluid. They may occasionally become actively infected.

Acquired cysts

Mucous retention cysts. Usually seen on the epiglottis, the ventricular band, and the upper part of the vestibule.

Subhyoid bursa is due to an enlargement of the normal bursa, probably of inflammatory origin.

Cysts resulting from degenerative changes.

1. In a haematoma or 'fibroma' of the cord.
2. In a polypus (localized oedema of the larynx).

Treatment

Small cysts projecting into the laryngeal cavity may be opened or removed endoscopically. Those outside the cavity require an external approach through the neck.

Polypus of the larynx

A smooth, sessile or pedunculated, tumour of the vocal cord. It probably represents a localized area of chronic oedema in the lax tissues of Reinke's space. It is easily stripped off endoscopically with forceps.

Prolapse of the ventricle

Probably not a true eversion of the ventricle and saccule, but a protrusion of an oedematous and hypertrophied portion of the ventriculosaccular lining. It is rarely secondary to neoplastic change and must be differentiated from a tuberculous lesion. A rare familial tendency has been noted. The condition is sometimes bilateral. Removal is usually possibly by endoscopic methods, but occasionally laryngofissure is preferred for large ones.

Laryngocele

A bulbous air-containing prolongation of the laryngeal ventricle and saccule. It is sometimes bilateral and may be homologous with the air sacs of monkeys. Expiration against resistance, as in trumpeters and glassblowers, was at one time thought to be an aetiological factor but no longer. It is more common in

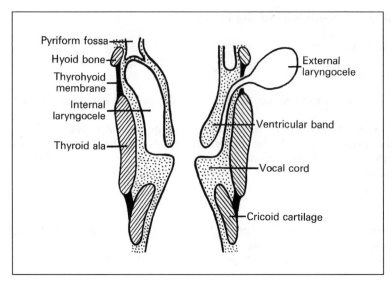

Figure 18.10 Laryngoceles

men with a peak incidence between 50 and 60 years. External laryngoceles can be found in 16% of laryngectomy specimens for laryngeal carcinoma.

Types (Figure 18.10)

1. *Internal.* This is confined to the interior of the laryngeal framework and presents under the mucosa of the valleculae and pharyngo-epiglottic fold and enters the pre-epiglottic space. The cyst can be 'uncapped' or evacuated endoscopically

2. *External.* The enlarging herniation finds its way outside the laryngeal structures by passing round the lateral margins of the thyrohyoid membrane, or by traversing it at the point where the internal branch of the superior laryngeal nerve and the superior laryngeal artery pierce it. It then passes through the gap between the inferior and middle constrictor muscles.

3. *Combined internal and external.* The external type presents as a swelling in the thyrohyoid region which expands on coughing and empties on digital pressure. The internal type is seen as a smooth submucosal swelling in the vallecula and obliterating the pharyngo-epiglottic fold. A muffled and hoarse voice is present. Radiographic examination delineates the air space during forcible Valsalva expiration. Treatment by excision is required to relieve voice changes, dyspnoea, dysphagia, or external swelling.

MISCELLANEOUS CONDITIONS OF THE LARYNX

Oedema of the larynx

This term refers to an oedema of the laryngeal mucosa, almost always above or below the true vocal cords but often erroneously called 'oedema of the glottis'. Although it is usually subglottic in children and supraglottic in adults, an infective oedema of the supraglottis (acute epiglottitis) may occur in infants and young children which can be rapid and dangerous.

Aetiology

Oedema is a complication of many laryngeal conditions:

1. *Infection.* Due to:
- *Laryngitis, especially streptococcal or diphtheritic.*
- *Spread of infection from the oropharynx and laryngopharynx and their surrounding fascial spaces, as in quinsy, Ludwig's angina and retropharyngeal abscess.*
2. *Trauma.* From wounds, foreign bodies, intubation, endoscopy, or inhalation of steam and corrosives.
3. *Neoplasms.* The commonest cause in patients over 50. Radiotherapy reactions may be included here.
4. *Perichondritis.* Especially from cancer, syphilis and tuberculosis.
5. *Allergy* ('Quincke's oedema' or angioneurotic oedema.) Brought on by mental excitement or idiosyncrasy to foods or drugs (especially iodine and aspirin).
6. *Intrathoracic diseases.* By causing venous stasis in the neck.
7. *Generalized diseases.* Such as cardiac failure and renal disease. It may be a presenting sign in myxoedema.

Pathology

Marked oedema occurs in the lax submucosa of the arytenoids, aryepiglottic folds, and ventricular bands, often of the valleculae also. The subglottic submucosa may be involved, especially in children.

Clinical features

1. *Dyspnoea* sometimes with cyanosis.
2. *Stridor* which is inspiratory in phase. There is evidence of increasing respiratory obstruction when the condition is progressive.
3. *Hoarseness.*
4. *Oedema of the lax laryngeal tissues* is readily seen on indirect laryngoscopy.

Treatment

Rest in the sitting position. This may be all that is required to give relief in less severe cases.

Nebulized adrenaline is helpful.

Steam inhalations are soothing.

Oxygen is often essential. A mixture of oxygen and helium reduces the work of breathing.

Injections.

1. *Hydrocortisone (100 mg)* or *Phenergan* intravenously.

2. *Adrenaline* (1:1000) in doses of 0.5 ml for adults, 0.1 ml in children, subcutaneously. It can be repeated if necessary or given as an intravenous drip (1:100 000 thirty drops per minute). Extreme care to avoid overdosage must be taken.

Tracheostomy or laryngotomy must be performed for respiratory distress before cardiac failure supervenes. Unless temporary, laryngotomy is liable to lead to stenosis and should only be used in times of great urgency.

Arthritis of the crico-arytenoid joint

Aetiology

Acute form occurs in:

1. Rheumatic fever where there is an acute streptococcal infection.
2. Gonococcal infection.
3. Injuries to the larynx.
4. Perichondritis of the larynx.

   Chronic form follows:

1. The acute form, which may have been relatively mild.
2. The insidious type of perichondritis of the larynx.
3. Ulcerations of the laryngeal mucosa, especially in syphilis.
4. Rheumatoid arthritis.

Clinical features

Hoarseness varies in degree according to the degree of abduction.

Redness and swelling of the arytenoid is seen on the affected side in the acute form, especially at its base. There is *no active or passive movement.*

Ankylosis of the arytenoid occurs in the chronic form. The cord is usually near the midline.

Dyspnoea occurs if both arytenoids are fixed in or near the midline position of the cord.

Differential diagnosis

From paralysis of the recurrent laryngeal nerve. With fixation of the joint the aryepiglottic fold may appear lengthened, with the tip of the arytenoid cartilage leaning backwards. With paralysis the affected arytenoid leans forwards and the cord appears shortened.

Differentiation is made by:

1. *Direct laryngoscopy* to test mobility with forceps.
2. *Electromyography* in which muscle contractions without joint movement are recorded.

Treatment

Vocal rest and systemic antibiotics are needed for the acute form.

Salicylates or cortisone should be given in acute rheumatic disease.

Tracheostomy is necessary if bilateral fixation in adduction occurs.

Arytenoidectomy and cordopexy may be indicated later in bilateral cases to enlarge the glottic aperture.

Laryngismus stridulus

Definition

Episodes of apyrexial laryngeal stridor in young children (first decade), usually in boys. It commonly begins in the winter, about the fourth year of life.

Aetiology

The condition was more frequent when *ill health* and *under-nourishment* were prevalent among children. *Rickets, whooping-cough, and sepsis or irritation in the upper respiratory and digestive tracts* are possible factors. The stridor has been regarded as due to:

1. *Spasm.* In which the condition is a manifestation of *tetany*. The calcium deficiency is due to *vitamin D or parathyroid insufficiency.*
2. *Passive obstruction.* The flabby soft tissues of the larynx are passively sucked inwards during inspiration and eventually obstruct until active dilatation (abduction) results from the rising carbon dioxide content of the blood.

Clinical features

Crowing stridor. The child, free from laryngeal symptoms by day, wakes at night with a crowing stridor. This increases into violent and convulsive efforts at inspiration.

Cyanosis is usual.

Carpopedal spasm is frequent.

After a minute or so the attack suddenly ceases with a long inspiration. The child then sleeps but another attack may occur later. Death has very rarely followed the 'breath-holding'.

Prognosis

The condition usually recovers spontaneously.

Treatment

During the attack. Respiration can be stimulated by splashing with cold water and by pulling the tongue forwards.

General. Attention to diet and regular exercise. Vitamins should be given in prophylactic doses if necessary. Any upper airway obstruction must be treated, particularly obstructive tonsils or adenoids.

Paralysis of the larynx

Paralysis of motor nerves

Aetiology

Paralysis of the motor nerves may be caused by:

1. *Lesions in the central nervous system.* Which are of two types:
- *Upper motor neurone lesions:* since the larynx is represented on both sides of the motor area of the cortex an upper motor neurone paralysis can occur only when a cortical lesion is large enough to involve the laryngeal centres on both sides.
- *Lower motor neurone lesions.* involvement of the nucleus ambiguus in diseases affecting the medulla may produce a bilateral or less often a unilateral paralysis. It is usually accompanied by other signs of the causal disease as described in the Neurological Section. Tracheostomy may be needed to relieve the dyspnoea.
2. *Lesions of the peripheral motor nerves to the larynx.* These nerves are the vagus trunk and the superior and recurrent laryngeal nerves. The condition is usually unilateral, the left side being more often affected owing to the longer course of the left recurrent laryngeal nerve. The cause lies in the skull, at the exit of the nerves from the skull, in the neck or in the thorax on the left side. In about one-quarter of the total the cause remains unknown (idiopathic group). Paralysis of these nerves results from:
- *Pressure or stretching* due to contiguous disease.
- *Injury,* usually surgical.
- *Malignant disease,* e.g. of thyroid, oesophagus, bronchial tree, nasopharynx, lymph nodes.
- *Peripheral neuritis* of infective or toxic form. It may be caused by:
(a) Chemical toxins e.g. lead and perhaps some other metallic poisons.
(b) Infective toxins as from diphtheria and typhoid fever; streptococcal infections associated with severe tonsillitis; possibly influenzal and herpetic types of virus infection.
(c) Avitaminosis e.g. the polyneuritis of beriberi.

Clinical features

1. *Effect on voice and respiration*
- *Unilateral recurrent laryngeal nerve paralysis.* Respiration is unaffected. The *voice remains acceptable* if the paralysed cord is *median* and taut. The active cord makes good approximation and compensation occurs.
  Hoarseness results if the paralysed cord is not in the midline and the active cord fails to compensate.
- *Bilateral recurrent laryngeal nerve paralysis. Severe dyspnoea* is produced by exertion and a laryngitis can precipitate an urgent state if the cords are *median.* Sudden onset of the paralysis is associated with urgent dyspnoea, but a gradual onset allows adaptation to the obstruction. Quiet respiration occurs through the chink afforded by the absence of the bracing action of the posticus muscle. The voice is good if the cords are paramedian.

- *Superior laryngeal nerve paralysis.* A slack wavy cord is said to result; the condition rarely occurs without a recurrent laryngeal nerve paralysis; it may be unilateral or bilateral. May follow carotid endarterectomy. *The voice is rough and tires quickly* but respiration is unaffected. When combined with a recurrent laryngeal nerve paralysis the wide immobile 'cadaveric' position of the glottis makes the voice very feeble and hoarse in unilateral cases, almost non-existent in bilateral cases. *Inhalation of food* is a marked feature, especially in bilateral cases, probably from associated sensory loss.

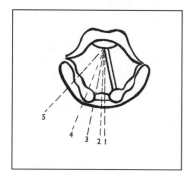

Figure 18.11 Positions of vocal cords. 1, Median; 2, paramedian; 3, cadaveric; 4, moderate abduction; 5, full abduction

2. Position of the cord (Figure 18.11)

- *Combined paralysis of superior and recurrent laryngeal nerves.* The nerve to the cricothyroid (external laryngeal nerve) and the recurrent laryngeal nerve may be paralysed either by separate lesions in the respective nerves or by a lesion of the vagus above the level at which its superior laryngeal branch is given off. The *vocal cord* lies in a position intermediate between that of phonation *(midline)* and that of quiet inspiration *(moderate abduction)*. This is termed the *cadaveric position* because every muscle is inactive as in death.
- *Paralysis of the recurrent laryngeal nerve alone.* The cricothyroid muscle is still active. The *vocal cord* assumes a position nearer the midline than in the higher vagal lesion. There are greater number of faster conducting large diameter myelinated nerves on the left compared with the right side. This explains why the cords work in unison (even in giraffes) although the left nerve has a longer course.

3. Other changes in the larynx

- *Paralysed cord is often at a lower level* than the unaffected cord. This is caused by absence of the backward-bracing action of the crico-arytenoideus posticus muscle, thus allowing the arytenoid cartilage to fall forwards.
- *Cartilage of Wrisberg and the aryepiglottic fold may lean inwards*
- *Subsequent fibrosis and contractures* in the muscles and the capsule of the crico-arytenoid joint may affect the position, tension and thickness of the paralysed cord.

Treatment

Indicated when dyspnoea is present, as in cases of bilateral recurrent laryngeal nerve paralysis.

Tracheostomy is indicated:

1. In bedridden cases or patients with malignant disease. When the tracheostomy is to be permanent a speaking valve is used.
2. As a preliminary to further surgical treatment which should not be undertaken for at least 12 months after the onset of paralysis, because delayed spontaneous recovery may occur.

Extralaryngeal arytenoidectomy and cordopexy is preferred in many patients in whom an active life is anticipated.

Endoscopic arytenoidectomy may be performed as an alternative to the extralaryngeal operation. The CO_2 laser is useful. Abduction of the cord follows from cicatrization.

Other procedures. Various operations have been used to improve the voice in unilateral cases if speech therapy fails. The concave or flabby edge of a cord may be stiffened by injection of *Teflon paste* , this is ideal for cases due to *bronchial carcinoma* where voice recovery is not expected; alternatively, the arytenoid cartilage has been displaced inwards towards the active cord. It must be remembered that cords paralysed by unknown factors have recovered, sometimes 2 years after the onset of the paralysis.

Myasthenia of the larynx (phonasthenia)

A disorder of the phonatory muscles. Usually a paresis due to *vocal misuse* or *laryngitis* but is sometimes seen as the first sign of laryngeal *tuberculosis*. *Myasthenia gravis* and *myotonia atrophica* are rare causes.

Internal tensors are most often affected. The cords come together on phonation but leave an elliptical space between them. A weak voice results, with air escape.

Interarytenoideus muscle is less often affected. The cords approximate on phonation but a triangular space is seen in the posterior commissure. There is only slight voice change.

Internal tensors and interarytenoideus may be affected together. A characteristic keyhole-shaped glottis appears on phonation.

Adductors (lateral crico-arytenoid muscles) may fail to approximate the cords completely, so that a poor voice ensues.

Treatment

That of the cause, e.g. vocal rest in cases due to overuse. Any superadded psychological element must be recognized and eliminated.

Functional paralysis (hysterical aphonia)

Functional paralysis of the adductors during phonation occurs most often in emotionally unstable individuals, particularly in young women.

Clinical features

Aphonia is sometimes complete but more often the voice is reduced to a whisper. Onset and recovery are usually sudden.

Laryngeal paraesthesia is occasionally present.

Cords fail to meet on attempted phonation. Sometimes they nearly close but no sound is produced. It is sometimes noticed during indirect laryngoscopy that the pharyngeal reflexes are strikingly insensitive. *Cough is normal,* when the glottis may be seen to close.

Treatment

Persuasion will cause the voice to return in many cases but relapse is likely unless the underlying psychogenic cause is removed. Speech therapy can be of great value.

Faradic stimulation should not be used for fear of fixing the neurosis.

Dysphonia plicae ventricularis

Aetiology

Ventricular band voice is produced by the apposition of the false cords in phonation.

This may be part of an attempt to compensate for myasthenia or other vocal disabilities. Commonly, however, the condition is psychogenic.

Clinical features

The voice is unpleasant, producing a low rough sound.

Treatment

Vocal rest is essential.
Speech therapy may help.

ASPIRATION

The larynx as a sphincter

The primary function of the larynx is to prevent food and drink entering the trachea. Because the airway lies open at rest only muscular activity stands between life, and death by aspiration. Three paired sensory branches of cranial nerves IX and X and three paired motor branches of cranial nerves X and XI are vital to laryngeal competence. Where medical treatment has failed surgical management of established aspiration is possible but depends upon knowing the pathological process and the exact anatomical site of the lesion.

History

Onset, progress, voice, swallow, and weight loss are considered. As a general rule chronic dysphagia for liquids is neurological, that for solids is due to a mass and painful dysphagia is peptic, except where malignancy is far advanced. Dysphagia due to stroke is usually fairly straight forward to diagnose due to its sudden onset, coincidental vascular disease and the presence of other neurological abnormality.

Examination

Pay special attention to the functions of the last four cranial nerves. Sensory function is difficult to assess, except where probing the tonsil finds an anaesthetic area (loss of IX). It is safe to assume a unilateral pharyngeal sensory loss if palate and vocal cord of the same side are paralysed (loss of X).

Sensory loss is minimal in upper motor neurone lesions (damage in the motor cortex) and profound in lower motor neurone lesions (brain stem or nerve fibre damage).

Indirect laryngoscopy

Shows weakness of vocal cords. If the area is anaesthetic saliva will be seen washing in and out of the laryngeal inlet with each breath. A sip of water will result in a spasm of coughing.

Investigations

A chest X-ray is needed to see if food and drink have already reached the lungs. A large volume barium swallow is contraindicated as barium is often aspirated. The definitive radiograph is a cine or video swallow using a tiny quantity of dense contrast medium. The loop of film is then viewed repeatedly with the radiologist until faults in the three phases of swallowing can be defined.

Videofluoroscopy has major advantages in clarifying the situation concerning muscle coordination and movement without significant risk to the patient.

In general a Horner's syndrome indicates extracranial disease and long tract signs intracranial disease. Once a diagnosis has been made and definitive treatment completed established palsies still require management.

Mixed palsies

Brainstem infarcts, tumours, demyelination and skull base tumours threaten a patient's life by thirst, starvation or aspiration. Where some function survives the swallow can be improved by:

1. *Supraglottic 'grip'*. Holding breath and trying to exhale against a closed glottis (Valsalva manoeuvre) produces maximum sphincter action at the level of false cords. When practised during swallowing entry of liquid into trachea can often be prevented, whereas a simple swallow provokes a spasm of coughing.
2. *Building up* the patients strength and correcting electrolyte and nutitional deficit by nasogastric tube feeding as a preliminary to:
3. *Cricopharyngeal myotomy*. The muscle is divided down to the mucosa to encourage free drainage of fluid from the hypopharynx.

4. *Epiglottopexy*. The epiglottis is sutured down over the laryngeal inlet, leaving a small airway. A lateral pharyngotomy gives access and the tracheostomy can be removed after a week. The voice is muffled.

5. *Ventral suspension of the larynx*. The larynx rises in a normal swallow, pulling it up close against the posterior third of the tongue within the arch of the hyoid. When this componant of swallow is seen to have been lost on video or cine swallow it may be restored by hitching up the laryngeal cartilages to the hyoid by non-absorbable sutures.

6. *Combination of these techniques* may produce a 'swallow without a cough'.

7. *Laryngectomy*. As a last resort, for patients who have no voice to lose. Aspiration is impossible except by dribbling, immersion or a fistula. Prolongs the life of a patient with motor neurone disease by about a year.

Incompetence of the larynx combined with severe neuromuscular incoordination of swallowing may coexist with a useful voice. In this situation pneumonia may be an ever present risk. The presence of a nasogastric tube for feeding can promote aspiration of saliva and thus be a unsatisfactory means of management. In this situation a feeding gastrostomy may be a suitable alternative if accepted by the patient, though a laryngectomy may turn out to be the only long-term solution to the protection of the lower respiratory tract.

Table of palsies and surgical remedies

Palsy	Consequences	Remedy
Unilateral IX	Numb tonsil/1/3 tongue	None required
Unilateral Sup. laryngeal	Numb hemi supraglottis Episodes of laryngospasm	None possible
Bilateral Sup. laryngeal	Numb supraglottis. Weak voice	None required
Unilateral Rec. laryngeal	Husky voice	Teflon injection
Bilateral Recurrent Laryngeal	Dyspnoea on exertion	Cordopexy, arytenoidectomy, tracheostomy
Unilateral total X	Husky voice Episodes of laryngospasm	Teflon improves voice and swallow
Bilateral X	Gaping cords Numb throat Aspiration	Tracheostomy, NG tube epiglottopexy, laryngectomy
Bilateral XII	Atrophy of tongue No aspiration	None possible Liquid diet only.

Chapter 19

Surgical anatomy

DEVELOPMENT OF THE TRACHEA AND BRONCHI

Median tracheobronchial groove

Appears in the ventral wall of the primitive pharynx during the third week of fetal life.

Tracheobronchial tube

The groove deepens and becomes converted into the tracheobronchial tube by the formation and eventual fusion of two lateral septa in the primitive oesophagus. By the end of the fifth week the respiratory tube communicates with the foregut by a narrow opening, the *primitive laryngeal inlet*. The *trachea* is formed by the cranial end of the tube.

Lung buds

The caudal end divides into two lateral outgrowths which form the right and left lung buds. They grow out into those parts of the coelom which become the primitive pleural cavities. They are covered with splanchnic mesoderm, from which the connective tissues of the bronchi and lungs develop.

Lobules

The lung buds divide into lobules: three on the right side, two on the left. These give rise to the definitive lobes of the lungs.

ANATOMY OF THE TRACHEA

The trachea is a membrano-cartilaginous tube between 10 and 11.5 cm in length in the adult. Rather less than one-half lies in the neck and rather more than one-half in the chest. It extends from the level of the sixth cervical vertebra above to the fifth thoracic vertebra below. Here it divides into right and left main bronchi, a little to the right of the median plane.

Structure

Cartilages

The trachea comprises incomplete rings of cartilage joined by fibrous tissue and smooth muscle fibres. The number varies from 16 to 20, the upper 6 or 7 being in the neck. The cartilages are deficient behind, where the tube is flattened. The cartilaginous portion occupies roughly the anterior two-thirds of the circumference. They calcify in old age.

Fibrous membrane

Encloses the cartilages in two layers, one outside the rings and one inside. The layers are joined to each other above and below each ring, and where the rings are deficient posteriorly they enclose some muscle fibres ('trachealis' muscle).

Mucosa

Has a ciliated columnar epithelium.

Relations of cervical trachea

In front

It is covered with skin, superficial and deep fasciae.

1. *Jugular arch* connecting the anterior jugular veins of the two sides.
2. *Sternohyoid and sternothyroid muscles* lying beneath the skin and fasciae. The muscles of the two sides approach one another in the midline.
3. *Isthmus of the thyroid gland* crossing the second, third and fourth rings of the trachea. In infancy the isthmus lies at a higher level.
4. *Anastomosing vessel* between the two superior thyroid arteries, passing immediately above the isthmus.
5. *Left brachiocephalic vein and artery* cross obliquely in front of the trachea, the vein is superficial, the artery deep at or just above the upper border of the manubrium sterni in children. In adults they cross at a lower level. The vein is at risk during tracheostomy, the artery may be eroded by the tip of an ill fitting tube.
6. *Thymus gland* lies in front of the trachea, in infants at the root of the neck.

Behind

1. *Oesophagus* separating it from the vertebral column.
2. *Recurrent laryngeal nerves lying in the groove between trachea and oesophagus or just in front of the groove.*

On each side

1. *Lobe of the thyroid gland* descending to the level of the sixth ring.
2. *Common carotid artery and internal jugular vein.*
3. *Inferior thyroid artery.*
4. *Vagus nerves.*

Blood supply

The arterial supply is derived mainly from the inferior thyroid artery. The veins drain into the thyroid venous plexus.

Nerve supply

From the *vagi*, the *recurrent laryngeal nerves* and the *sympathetic trunk.*

Lymphatic drainage

To the *pretracheal* and *paratracheal nodes.*

ENDOSCOPIC ANATOMY OF THE TRACHEOBRONCHIAL TREE

The branches of the tracheobronchial tree are illustrated in Figure 19.1 as seen endoscopically.

Bifurcation of the trachea

The bifurcation is at the level of the upper border of the fifth thoracic vertebra. It is about 25 cm from the incisor teeth in an adult. The *carina* is a keel-like spur produced by the lowest ring of the trachea at the point of separation into the two main bronchi.

Right main bronchus

This has a greater diameter and is shorter and more vertical than the left. Foreign bodies therefore have a tendency to enter the right rather than the left main bronchus. It has the following branches:

1. Right upper-lobe bronchus

Passes upwards and laterally from the parent bronchus. It then divides into three main segmental bronchi:

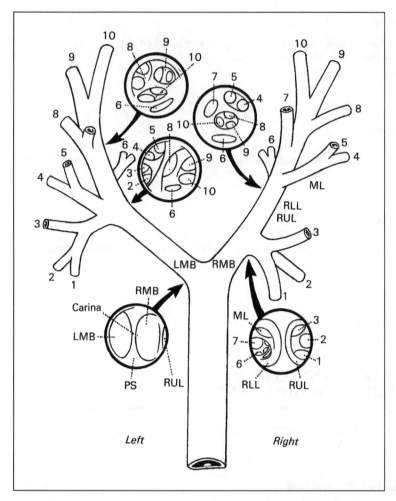

Figure 19.1 Endoscopic anatomy of tracheobronchial tree. *Left*: LMB, Left main bronchus; PS, posterior spur of carina; 1, apical; 2, posterior; 3, anterior; 4, superior lingular; 5, inferior lingular; 6, apical of lower lobe; 8, anterior basal; 9, lateral basal; 10, posterior basal. *Right*: RMB, Right main bronchus; RUL, right upper lobe bronchus; RLL, right lowr lobe bronchus; ML, middle lobe bronchus; 1, apical; 2, posterior; 3, anterior; 4, lateral of middle lobe; 6, apical of inferior lobe; 7, medial basal; 9, lateral basal; 10, posterior basal

Apical bronchus

Passes upwards and laterally.

Posterior bronchus

Passes backwards and laterally.

Anterior bronchus

Runs downwards, forwards and medially.

2. Middle-lobe bronchus

Arises from the anterior aspect of the main bronchus, about 2.5 cm below the orifice of the upper-lobe bronchus. It passes forwards and downwards and subdivides into:

Lateral branch

Runs downwards and more laterally.

Medial branch

Runs downwards and forwards.

3. Right lower-lobe bronchus

Almost immediately sends off:

Apical bronchus

Passes directly backwards.

Medial basal (cardiac) bronchus

Given off from the medial side of the lower-lobe bronchus about 1.5 cm below the apical bronchus.

Subapical bronchus

Sometimes present. It arises from the posterior aspect of the lower-lobe bronchus, just below the medial basal bronchus.

Three basal bronchi

Given off from the lower-lobe bronchus about 0.5 cm below the origin of the medial basal bronchus.
- *Posterior basal bronchus*
- *Lateral basal bronchus*
- *Anterior basal bronchus*

Left main bronchus

Narrower, longer and more horizontal than the right. It has the following branches:

1. Left upper-lobe bronchus

Arises as a bifurcation of the main bronchus and divides into:

Apical bronchus

Posterior bronchus

Anterior bronchus

Lingular bronchus

2. Left lower-lobe bronchus

Passes downwards, backwards, and laterally. Divides into:

Apical bronchus

Arises from the posterior wall, rather less than 1 cm below the origin of the lower-lobe bronchus.

Subapical bronchus

May be present about 1 cm below the orifice of the apical bronchus.

Three basal bronchi

Arise from the lower-lobe bronchus rather more than 1.5–2.0 cm below the apical bronchus.
● *Anterior basal bronchus.*
● *Lateral basal bronchus.*
● *Posterior basal bronchus.*
  The main bronchi are known alternatively as primary bronchi. Subsequent divisions and subdivisions are known as secondary, tertiary and quaternary bronchi.

Bronchopulmonary segments

The segmental bronchi supply definite segments of the lungs. A segment of the lung with its segmental bronchus is known as a bronchopulmonary segment. These segments bear the same names as the bronchi by which they are ventilated.

Tracheobronchial lymph nodes

The tracheal and bronchial lymph nodes lie mainly in the paratracheal, tracheobronchial and hilar regions.

EXAMINATION OF THE TRACHEA AND BRONCHI

Indirect tracheoscopy

The upper 2.5 cm or so of the trachea can often be seen well with a laryngeal mirror. Occasionally even the carina is visible.

Radiography

Examination of the lower respiratory system must include:

1. *Plain chest radiographs.* Anteroposterior, lateral and oblique views.
2. *Tomography and CT scan.* Widely used and adds invaluable information.
3. *Bronchography.* Dilatation or narrowing of the bronchial tree can be demonstrated by the introduction of radiopaque media, followed by an X-ray. *Iodized oil* is usually employed and is instilled through the glottis by cannula or through the cricothyroid membrane by injection.

Direct endoscopy

The parts of the tracheobronchial tree described under Endoscopic anatomy can be examined with a bronchoscope. Straight or retrograde telescopes may be required; the latter are needed to visualize the divisions of the right and left upper-lobe bronchi. The Neodinium YAG laser may be used theraputically via a rigid or a flexible fibreoptic endoscope.

The *fibreoptic flexible bronchoscope* has greatly facilitated the endoscopic examination of the tracheobronchial tree but obstructs the airway in infants for whom a ventilating bronchoscope is required.

Cytological examination of endobronchial washings, brushings, and histology of pinch biopsies are all essential diagnostic aids.

Mediastinoscopy

Through a suprasternal incision, may be used to inspect the outside of the trachea and the paratracheal nodes.

LARYNGOTOMY AND TRACHEOSTOMY

Laryngotomy

Definition

An opening through cricothyroid membrane.

Indications

Sudden laryngeal obstruction when intubation is impossible and facilities or experience for tracheostomy are not available. Impaction of a foreign body in the larynx is the commonest indication.

Technique

Performed without any anaesthetic. Any available sharp knife or even scissors are used, though preferably a combined knife and laryngotomy tube if available. A small transverse incision is made and deepened to open the cricothyroid membrane; bleeding is minimal. Any available tube, even the barrel of a ball-point pen, or rotation of the knife-blade, allows an airway. If for any reason an opening cannot be attempted, oxygen may be given through a wide-bore needle inserted through the cricothyroid membrane and connected to an inflating bag.

An elective tracheostomy is performed within a few hours if the obstruction is still present.

Tracheostomy

Indications

1. *Relief of respiratory obstruction.* Above upper tracheal level, due to the following causes:

Congenital

- *Bilateral choanal atresia.*
- *Laryngeal web or cyst.*
- *Upper tracheal stenosis.*
- *Tracheo-oesophageal anomalies.*

Traumatic

- *External* (1) Blows on larynx. (2) Gunshot or cut-throat wounds.
- *Internal* (1) Inhalation of steam or irritating fumes. (2) Foreign bodies. (3) Swallowing of corrosives.

Infections

- *Acute laryngotracheobronchitis.*
- *Acute epiglottitis.*
- *Diphtheria.*
- *Ludwig's angina.*

Tumours

Malignant disease of tongue, pharynx, larynx, upper trachea and thyroid gland.

- When in advanced stage.
- If oedema from radiotherapy embarrasses respiration.
- As adjunct to surgery.

Miscellaneous causes of glottic obstruction

- Haemophilia, angioneurotic oedema.

Bilateral laryngeal nerve palsies

- After thyroidectomy.
- With bulbar palsies.

Cord fixation

Due to rheumatoid arthritis.

2. *Protection of tracheobronchial tree.* In conditions leading to:
- *Inhalation of saliva, food, gastric contents or blood.*
- *Stagnation of bronchial secretions.*
  Aspiration can be done easily, and a cuffed tube is used if necessary.
Conditions include:
- *Bulbar poliomyelitis.*
- *Polyneuritis.*
- *Tetanus.*
- *Myasthenia gravis.*
- *Coma due to many causes (including head injuries, drug overdose and cardiac arrest).*
- *Cervical cord lesions and injuries.*
- *Burns of face and neck.*
- *Multiple fractures of mandible.*

3. *Treatment of conditions leading to respiratory insufficiency.* Any of the conditions in (1) and (2) may cause respiratory insufficiency. It may also result from:

Pulmonary disease

- *Chronic bronchitis and emphysema.* Many patients are elderly and often debilitated. Sedation may inhibit coughing and precipitate respiratory insufficiency.
- *Postoperative pneumonia.*

Severe chest injuries ('flail chest')

Neuromuscular incoordination, causing conditions:

- Leading to (2) above.
- Needing artificial or intermittent positive-pressure respiration (IPPR).
  Tracheostomy aids respiration by:

1. Reducing the 'dead space' (lips to tracheostome) by about 50%.
2. By-passing resistance to airflow in nose, mouth and glottis.

3. Allowing easy 'toilet' of bronchi.
4. Use of mechanically assisted respiration.

Criteria for emergency or elective operations

Fewer emergency operations are necessary now, as a small intratracheal tube can often be passed by a skilled anaesthetist, cyanosis is relieved, and a general anaesthetic administered. With Portex nasotracheal tubes up to 3 weeks can be tolerated by children, and a tracheostomy may be avoided.

Patients needing IPPR should never have an emergency operation; the anaesthetist of the respiratory unit should pass a peroral endotracheal tube, which can be used for 24 h or perhaps longer, when an elective tracheostomy is performed.

Criteria for IPPR:

1. With paralysing disease and normal lungs. If the vital capacity falls to a quarter of normal or if, with deep breath, the patient can count only to 20 and not to 60.
2. With pulmonary disease. If patient loses consciousness or PCO_2 exceeds 70 mmHg.
3. With crushed chest. Clinical judgement is usually sufficient, but PCO_2 measurement is valuable.

In an emergency, with stridor, recession of the suprasternal notch and intercostal spaces, and with anxious, pale, sweating facies, operation must not be delayed. Cyanosis indicates a late and grave stage.

In real urgency, and without proper facilities and training, a *laryngotomy* must be performed.

Emergency operation

1. Anaesthesia

Preferably with intubation and general anaesthetic. Otherwise infiltration with lignocaine 0.5%

2. Position

Head extended over a small sandbag under the neck, and held exactly in the sagittal plane.

3. Incision

Midline vertical, from lower border of thyroid cartilage to manubrium sterni. Cricoid cartilage is the guide and is felt with the finger. Large dilated veins must be avoided or clamped (this includes rarely highly placed innominate vessels), when the incision is deepened to cut through deep cervical fascia.

4. Midline separation of 'ribbon' muscles

With scissors.

5. Thyroid isthmus

Divided usually and ligated, but may be retracted upwards or downwards.

6. Trachea exposed and opened

Circular disc cut out of wall at level of third ring; sometimes also second or fourth rings. The first ring must never be divided. In children a vertical incision is used and no cartilage is removed.

7. Insertion of tube

After aspiration of the trachea a suitable tube is inserted and firmly secured by tapes properly knotted with head in the intended nursing position.

8. Choice of tube

The best type is a cuffed plastic (Portex) tube, but a silver tube may be preferred. The size and shape of the curve are very important, as the anterior and posterior walls must not be traumatized, for fear of ulceration and fatal haemorrhage. A hole or vent on the top of the convexity of the tube is helpful to aid phonation. For assisted respiration, and to avoid aspiration hazards, a low-pressure cuffed plastic tube is needed.

9. Closure of wound

Ligation of bleeding points is essential. The wound is loosely closed, for fear of emphysema, or of making reinsertion of accidentally displaced tube more difficult.

Elective operation

Additional points are:

1. General anaesthetic almost always used.
2. Position: in young patients overextension may lead to the tracheal opening being placed too low.
3. The incision is transverse (or 'collar') about 2 cm below level of cricoid cartilage.
4. Hinged flaps of the tracheal wall are not advisable.
5. Percutaneous techniques are gaining popularity in intensive care units. Hollow needle finds tracheal lumen, instruments and tracheostomy tube are slid over a guide wire. Risk of violating unseen first tracheal ring, leading to perichondritis of cricoid and late stenosis.

Postoperative management

Of the utmost importance.

1. Nursing

Constant attention is essential for the first 24 h at least.

2. Position

The patient must be sitting upright in bed.

3. Suction

Applied regularly, with aseptic technique, passing a sterile catheter into trachea and main bronchi.

4. Humidification

This is essential, using humidifier or moistened gauze over the tracheostomy tube.

5. Prevention of crusting

Aided by use of aerosol preparations. This supplements humidification.

6. Prevention of apnoea

In cases of long-standing obstruction, apnoea may follow restoration of the airway, with lowering of the PCO_2. Carbon dioxide (5–7% in oxygen) is given via flow-meter through the tracheostome if this occurs.

7. Care of tube

The inner tube should project about 0.25 cm beyond the distal end of the outer one, to collect mucus and prevent blockage of the outer tube. The inner tube is taken out and cleaned whenever necessary (hourly at first); the outer tube must be held firmly while withdrawing the inner one. Types having a cut-out portion of inner tube (e.g. Parker) are best avoided, as crusting occurs in the outer tube. Cuffed tubes need firm attachment of the cuff to prevent it overriding the end of the tube: the cuff should be of adequate length and not inflated too much, to avoid pressure necrosis of tracheal mucosa, necessity of periodic deflation of cuff, and the possibility of dilatation of trachea with subsequent disturbance of swallowing. Low-pressure cuffed tubes must always be employed, to minimize the risk of tracheal stenosis.

8. Need for a long tube

With upper tracheal conditions or compression from the oesophagus or thyroid gland, a long Koenig's type or flexible wire tube may be necessary.

9. Speaking valve

After the tissue planes have become sealed off a di Santis valve closing on expiration may be fitted into or incorporated with the inner tube.

10. Decannulation

The tube is removed when the patient is comfortable with it 'corked off'. Difficulty occurs, especially with children, if the tracheostomy has been present for a long time. Gradual reduction in the size of tube, then sealing off, and sometimes a small 'dummy', help readaptation to using normal air passages.

Complications

1. Haemorrhage

May occur if haemostasis is not secured at operation. It can occur from abnormally placed vessels at operation or ulceration by the tip of the tube if of the wrong shape.

2. Displacement of tube

If complete it must be reinserted at once after the wound and tracheal opening are adequately dilated. Replacement is far easier if the lower skin edge is sutured to the lower margin of the tracheal window. Partial dislodgement may pass unobserved for a time, with the tube lying just in front of the tracheal opening. The latter gets easily obstructed. The innominate artery is at risk.

3. Surgical emphysema and pneumothorax

More common in children, and if tracheostomy is too low. Wound must not be closed tightly. Less likely if tissue planes are not dissected too much, and if skin edges can be sutured to tracheal opening (except in young children when this unduly restricts movement). Also less likely if operation is done under general anaesthesia, with intubation.

4. Perichondritis and stenosis

May develop in the subglottic region if the tracheostome is too high. (The first ring must never be molested.) In infants and young children oedema, or even firm granulation tissue, may persist for months. Insertion of a smaller tube, of non-irritating Portex, ensuring no angulation of the tracheal wall above the tube, may help considerably.

Tracheo-oesphageal fistula can result from pressure of an ill-fitting tube against the posterior wall.

A stricture above a well-placed tracheostome may result from trauma by an ill-fitting tube or an opening not large enough. A low tracheal stricture may be a late sequel of prolonged over-inflation of a cuffed tube.

5. Miscellaneous dangers

Occasional tragedies occur from:
- Manipulation of sucker catheter causing syncope with cardiac arrest.
- Oxygen mistakenly administered in catheter down tracheal tube at too high a pressure, causing rupture of lung alveoli and gross fatal emphysema.
- Local sepsis; septicaemia.

Chapter 20

Applied physiology of the trachea and bronchi

FUNCTIONS OF THE TRACHEA AND BRONCHI

Respiratory functions

1. *Conveyance of air.*
2. Patency of airway is maintained by the cartilaginous structure of the tracheobronchial tree which prevents collapse of the tubes during respiration. The cartilages also prevent collapse from the pressure of surrounding structures and allow rotatory and tilting movements of the head and neck on the body.
3. *Diminution of volume of 'dead-space' air* is effected by movements of the trachea and bronchi.
- *During inspiration.* The roots of the lungs move downwards, and the trachea and bronchi increase in length and calibre.
- *During expiration.* The roots of the lungs move upwards and the trachea and bronchi shorten and contract.

Protective functions

1. *Ciliary activity* The ciliated epithelium of the trachea and bronchi is responsible for the trapping and expulsion of small foreign bodies, such as dust and grit. The particles are swept towards the pharynx by a spiral movement of the ciliary escalator and thence swallowed.
2. *Cough reflex* will often expel larger foreign bodies from the lower air passages.
3. *Warming and moistening of inspired air.* The tracheobronchial mucosa helps to bring the temperature of the inspired air to approximately that of the normal body temperature, and provides moisture for humidification.

Phonatory functions

1. *Air column.* The trachea and bronchi provide a column for the passage of air from the 'bellows' (lungs) to the 'reeds' (vocal cords) of the laryngeal wind instrument.
2. *Resonators.* The lower air passages act as resonators during phonation.

Chapter 21

Diseases of the trachea and bronchi

CONGENITAL ABNORMALITIES OF THE TRACHEA AND BRONCHI

Congenital abnormalities of the trachea

Rare.

1. *Stenosis.* May cause few or no symptoms when of slight degree.
2. *Tracheo-oesophageal fistula* is due to a failure of complete formation of the septum between the trachea and oesophagus. This condition is described with diseases of the oesophagus (p. 400).
3. *Abnormal bronchial opening.* The right superior-lobe orifice has been reported to arise directly from the trachea.
4. *Tracheocele.* One type of this rare condition is due to a congenital weakness of part of the tracheal wall.
5. *Tracheomalacia.* The cartilaginous rings are excessively pliable and the lumen 'collapses' during inspiration.

Congenital abnormalities of the bronchi

1. *Abnormal positions of bronchial orifices.* May occur.
2. *Saccular or fusiform bronchiectatic cavities.* May be present.
3. *Stenosis.* Leading to atelectasis.
4. *Compression.* The trachea and bronchi may be compressed by aberrant vessels or grossly deviated by large congenital cysts in the mediastinum.

TRAUMATIC CONDITIONS OF THE TRACHEA AND BRONCHI

Direct injuries

Rare. They are usually associated with laryngeal injuries. The trachea may be injured with cut-throat, stab and gunshot wounds. It may also be ruptured or suffer from partial loss of tissue in crush injuries. It may be torn in operations on the upper end of the oesophagus or on the trachea itself.

Clinical features

1. *Similar to those seen in injuries of the larynx,* including asphyxia.
2. *Surgical emphysema.*
3. *Pneumothorax.*
4. *Mediastinitis.*

Treatment

Tracheostomy is essential and must be followed by bronchial suction.

Surgical repair of the tracheal wall may be possible. Tantalum wire gauze, may be used to replace an excised portion of the wall, or end-to-end anastomosis of normal tracheal wall may be employed, up to 2 cm can be pulled up from the chest. An expanding 'swiss roll' of silicone rubber holds the lumen open while healing occurs. This may be made to bear against a split skin graft if desired and may be removed endoscopically (*tracheoplasty*).

Foreign bodies

Foreign bodies which have passed through the larynx may lodge anywhere in the trachea or bronchial tree, most commonly in the right main bronchus of a child. There may be no history of inhalation, for children may be too frightened to mention it and adults may inhale a foreign body when asleep or drunk. Inhalation may occur during anaesthesia, as for dental extraction. Most accidents occur when a sudden inspiration is taken while an object is in the mouth. The initial symptoms may be slight.

Clinical features

Initial symptoms

1. Cough and dyspnoea occur at the time of the accident.
2. *Bloodstained expectoration* is sometimes present.

There may be a latent period of varying duration before the onset of general symptoms.

General symptoms

Common to all types of foreign bodies, include:

1. *Cough* with or without dyspnoea.
2. *Expectoration.*
3. *'Asthmatoid' wheeze* is common. This is segmental rather than generalized.
Special symptoms depend upon whether the foreign body is of non-vegetable or of vegetable nature.

1. Non-vegetable foreign bodies

A great variety of objects have been recorded. They tend to gravitate into the lower-lobe bronchi, especially on the right side. Their progress depends upon their size and shape. Little or no *inflammatory reaction* occurs in the bronchial mucosa at first. *Granulations* may form later and cause haemoptysis. *Cough,* after its initial presentation, disappears but it returns if the object changes position. *Atelectasis* occurs if the lobe of the lung is completely obstructed, with subsequent danger of infection and the formation of a lung abscess (Figure 21.1a). An obstructive emphysema occurs if a lobe is only partially obstructed (Figure 21.1b), i.e. during expiration (bronchus contracted) but not during inspiration (bronchus dilated). Hard or metallic objects may be present for many months or even years without causing marked or even suspicious symptoms.

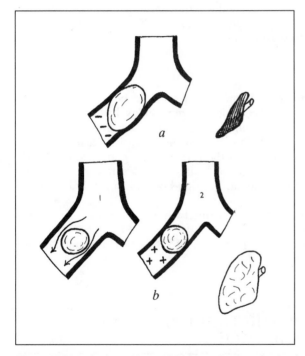

Figure 21.1 Mechanism of bronchial obstruction by a foreign body. a, Complete onstruction (inset – atelectasis); b, valvular obstruction (inset – emphysema). Air enters during inspiration (1) but the bronchus is blocked by contraction on to the foreign body during expiration (2)

2. Vegetable foreign bodies

Include various nuts and pips, fruits, and vegetables. There is always an *intense inflammatory reaction* of the mucosa. This may be a specific allergic reaction to the vegetable oil liberated by the swelling object. Symptoms of acute tracheitis and bronchitis may be present and the patient is obviously ill.

Bronchial obstruction is usually marked. A *valvular emphysema* results when it is partial. *Atelectasis and resulting lung abscess,* or a localized pneumonitis, follow later when it is complete.

Physical signs correspond to the symptomatic changes. At first there may be no signs apart from tracheal or bronchial irritation.

Signs of bronchial obstruction occur later with wheezy rales and evidence of emphysema, atelectasis, acute tracheobronchitis, or lung abscess.

Differential diagnosis

From pulmonary tuberculosis; acute tracheobronchitis; pneumonia and other causes of bronchiectasis and lung abscess; neoplasm; and other mediastinal diseases.

Radiographic examination is essential.

1. *Opaque objects* can be visualized in anteroposterior and lateral views.
2. *Translucent objects* are suspected when the film shows atelectasis, obstructive emphysema, mediastinal shift, consolidation of the lung and abnormal position or movement of the diaphragm.

Treatment

Removal through a bronchoscope. Bronchoscopy should be done as soon as possible, particularly with vegetable objects where delay brings pulmonary complications. Correct instruments are essential. Various grasping forceps and suction tubes are usually sufficient but on rare occasions a magnet has been useful. More space is available for the forceps during inspiration. Small quantities of topical 5% cocaine solution will sometimes release a foreign body gripped by inflammatory oedema. Foreign bodies can rarely be recovered by the flexible fibrescope.

Removal by thoracotomy must be performed when the object is small and has descended into a small lower-lobe bronchus.

Tracheostomy may be necessary if oedema of the larynx develops, either before or after bronchoscopy.

INFLAMMATIONS OF THE TRACHEA AND TRACHEOBRONCHIAL TREE

Inflammations of the trachea

Acute simple tracheitis

Frequently accompanies either a laryngitis or a bronchitis. (When in infants *see below.*) The condition occurs with simple upper respiratory infections and also with influenza and the exanthemas. It may follow instrumentation. Oedema due to an allergic reaction or inhalation of corrosive fumes may occur.

Clinical features

Cough and retrosternal pain are the common symptoms.
  Expectoration of secretions is usually scanty but may be copious.
  Dyspnoea may occur, especially in children.
  Constitutional symptoms are mild unless the causal illness is severe or accompanied by bronchopulmonary infection.

Treatment

Rest in bed.
  Inhalations of Tinct. Benzoin Co. or oil of pine.
  Linctus.
  Systemic antibiotics in severe cases.

Acute laryngotracheobronchitis

Occurs in infants and young children up to age of 4 years. It is described on p. 456.

Acute diphtheritic tracheitis

The tracheal mucosa is usually involved as an extension of the laryngeal inflammation but may be primary. Sloughing occurs with *membrane* formation. Systemic penicillin and antitoxic serum are both essential.

Chronic simple tracheitis

Occurs commonly in association with chronic upper respiratory infections, chronic bronchitis, and bronchiectasis.

Clinical features

Cough is dry and irritating.
Dull retrosternal pain aggravated by coughing.

Treatment

Entails attention to causes in the nose, throat and bronchi.

Tracheitis sicca

A form of chronic tracheitis almost always associated with atrophic rhinitis and/or laryngitis sicca. A severe form is sometimes encountered after laryngectomy. *Dry crusts* on the tracheal wall are very irritating. Treatment is aimed at making the secretions more moist, especially by the use of a humidifier and soda-bicarbonate spray. Obstructing crusts may require frequent removal after laryngectomy. This postoperative condition usually resolves in 2–3 weeks.

Carcinoma of the bronchus

Aetiology

The increase in incidence of bronchial carcinomas has called for inquiry into any factors that might be responsible.
Suspected factors. Include:

1. *Carcinogenic hydrocarbons.* Present in tobacco smoke (particularly in cigarettes), coal smoke (particularly the partially combusted particles from domestic fires) and motor-car exhaust fumes.
2. *Radioactive substances.* Encountered by uranium and cobalt miners and laboratory workers.
3. *Arsenic, chromates and nickel*
4. *Pneumoconiosis*
5. *Chronic bronchitis.* There is evidence that this is an aetiological factor.

Incidence

Sex. Approximately 80% are in the male.
   Age. Approximately 90% occur between 40 and 70 years of age.

Pathology

Three histological types of carcinoma originate from the undifferentiated basal cells of the bronchial mucosa.

1. *Anaplastic carcinoma.*   The commonest type. It includes the 'oat-celled' and 'spheroidal-celled' forms. It metastasizes early.
2. *Adenocarcinoma.* Includes the papillary and 'signet ring' forms. In this type male and female incidence are nearly equal.
3. *Squamous-cell carcinoma.* Usually regarded as the least common type. It often occurs near the hilum and grows slowly.

   NB. Frequently two or more types are found combined in the same tumour if enough sections are made.

Distribution

The primary, secondary and tertiary bronchi are the site of origin in 75% or more of the cases. Clinically these form the 'hilar' group. The upper-lobe bronchi are those most often affected. It is doubtful if primary lung cancer begins in the alveoli. The peripheral group of carcinomas probably arise from the smaller bronchi and spread peripherally.

Spread

Direct spread in the lung is by:

1. *Massive local extension* of the growth.
2. *Peribronchial infiltration.*
3. *Submucosal spread* in the bronchus in both directions. Direct invasion of the mediastinum, the pleura, and the great veins is frequent.

Lymphatic spread. To the hilar nodes is usual and often early. The cervical and other nodes outside the thorax may be affected occasionally and may even appear as the first sign of the disease.

Haematogenous spread. Blood-borne metastases are common, especially in the liver, bones and brain. Not infrequently metastases may cause death in the absence of pulmonary symptoms.

Clinical features

The early manifestations of bronchial carcinoma are often so slight and insidious that valuable months are lost before the diagnosis is made.

1. *Cough.* Persistent and unproductive at first but later yielding a purulent bloodstained sputum.
2. *Sense of discomfort and constriction* in the chest due to endobronchial obstruction.
3. *Pain* follows as pneumonitis and pleurisy supervene.
4. *'Atypical' pneumonia* may be the first indication of the presence of a carcinoma.
5. *Haemoptysis* is occasionally an early sign. With the increase in obstruction and the advent of secondary infection the symptoms increase to those of the later stages.
6. *Dyspnoea* is usually a late sign but paroxysmal wheezing may occur early. Breathlessness is aggravated if either phrenic nerve is involved by mediastinal metastases.
7. *General symptoms* include loss of weight, pyrexia and lowering of the general physical state. Even these have been seen as presenting symptoms.
8. *Bronchial obstruction* may be complete or partial so that atelectasis or emphysema (obstructive and compensatory) can result with corresponding physical signs in the chest. Secondary infection leads to lobar or bronchopneumonia, abscess, or bronchiectasis beyond the tumour. These complications add their own features to the clinical picture. Pleural effusion is frequent and is due to neoplastic involvement of the pleura or to infection spreading from the lung. Aspirated fluid is characteristically bloodstained.
9. *Shoulder pain, paralysis of the hand and Horner's syndrome* may result from invasion of the brachial plexus and sympathetic chain in carcinoma of the apices (Pancoast tumours).
10. *Voice change* follows if the apical tumour invades the recurrent laryngeal nerve. Hilar lymph nodes involve only the left recurrent laryngeal nerve, but either nerve can be involved by the primary growth or by cervical nodes.
11. *Clubbing* of the fingers.
12. *Polyneuritis.*

Radiography

Of the chest is the most valuable single diagnostic measure. The changes most often observed are:

1. *Hilar shadow.*
2. *Atelectasis:* massive or segmental.
3. *Infiltration of the lung:* central or peripheral.

4. *Obstructive emphysema* occasionally, due to 'check-valve' obstruction, in early cases.

5. *Pleural effusion and abscess cavities* are seen late. Peripheral tumours tend to undergo rapid necrosis to give circumscribed shadows, which may lead to a mistaken diagnosis of lung abscess.

CT scan

Gives essential information in some cases.

Cytology of sputum

Or of bronchial aspirate or pleural fluid.

Bronchography

Can demonstrate bronchial obstruction in the segmental bronchi, including those of the upper lobe. Oily or aqueous contrast media may be used.

Bronchoscopy

May demonstrate the lesion. The fibreoptic bronchoscope has greatly increased the diagnostic accuracy and safety of this procedure. It may also permit forceps biopsy, and the collection of secretions for the detection of malignant cells. It may also afford the assessment of operability. Bronchoscopy rarely demonstrates tumours in the absence of radiological evidence but small lesions in the larger bronchi (e.g. carcinoma-in-situ) have been thus detected. Biopsy is positive in about 40–50% of cases subsequently confirmed. It is often difficult to obtain material from the superior-lobe bronchi, in which 50% of tumours originate.

Bronchoscopic appearances of the tumour are varied. Often a red mass, less often a white friable one, occupies the bronchus. Some tumours are nodular, others polypoid or plaque-like with or without ulceration. Peripheral tumours infiltrate to cause stenosis of the bronchus but such areas may yield a positive biopsy. Occasionally a carcinoma-in-situ will obliterate the normal longitudinal folds of a larger bronchus to produce a nodular and stenosed appearance.

Alterations from the normal colour and movements of the bronchi, fixation of the tree, and distortion of its form are points to be looked for. Thickening of the carina and interbronchial spurs may be presumptive evidence of a tumour or its glandular metastases.

Needle biopsy

Through the chest wall, for peripheral tumours.

Exploratory thoracotomy

Desirable whenever radiographic suspicion is present even though bronchoscopic and cytological examinations are negative.

Treatment

1. *Lobectomy or pneumonectomy* with complete removal of the related mediastinal lymph nodes.
2. *Radiotherapy* may be a useful palliative measure for relieving the bronchial obstruction or superior mediastinal venous obstruction by lymph node metastases. Also of value as an adjunct to surgery if mediastinal involvement is found at operation. High-dosage modern therapy is surprisingly effective in Pancoast tumours.
3. *Cytotoxic drugs.* Systemically, can be of some value in oat-cell carcinoma.

STENOSIS OF THE TRACHEA

Aetiology

The causes of stenosis of the trachea include:

Intrinsic causes

From conditions in the lumen or walls.

1. *Congenital narrowing.* Very rarely.
2. *Post-traumatic scar tissue.* From foreign bodies or operations. The upper end of the trachea is endangered after a tracheostomy. At a lower level stenosis may follow the prolonged use of an over-inflated cuffed tube.
3. *Post-inflammatory scar tissue.* From infections of simple or specific nature, the latter including syphilis, tuberculosis, scleroma and leprosy. Postirradiation fibrosis also occurs.
4. *Neoplasms.* Benign or malignant.
5. *Infiltration.* Of the walls by tuberculous caseating lymph nodes or by malignant growths of thyroid, oesophagus, or lungs.

Extrinsic causes

From conditions in the neck or thorax compressing the trachea.
The structures concerned are:

1. *Thyroid gland.* Various types of goitre. This is the commonest cause of compression. It leads to a 'scabbard' trachea.
2. *Lymph nodes.* Tuberculous, neoplastic, or Hodgkin's, in the neck or mediastinum.
3. *Oesophagus.* Impacted foreign bodies or neoplasms.
4. *Mediastinum.* Dermoid cysts, emphysema or abscess following injury and neoplasms.
5. *Aorta.* Aneurysms.
6. *Thymus gland.* Enlargement or abscess.
7. *Pericardium.* Effusion.
8. *Sternum or vertebrae.* Bone diseases.

Clinical features

1. *Dyspnoea* of an increasing degree, is the main symptom. With a slow stenosis, a marked degree of narrowing can occur before symptoms become obvious.
2. *Stridor* occurs in the more severe cases. It is more marked during inspiration. The head position is said to be characteristic in cases of tracheal stridor. It is held forward with the chin down. The upright position is preferred.
3. *Weak voice* may be present but there is no hoarseness. Cough may be negligible or absent.

Treatment

Endoscopic removal of scar tissue may sometimes relieve stenosis from intrinsic causes. Laser resection of scar tissue is of value. After a laser resection repeated endoscopies are often necessary to remove granulations that form on any raw areas.

Dilatation must be considered in mild cases.

External operations may be done to open the trachea, remove the scar tissue, and maintain the lumen during healing with an indwelling Teflon roll. Resection, with mobilization of the lower trachea, and end-to-end anastomosis may be indicated. Tracheoplastic techniques are used to widen the stenosed lumen in infants.

A stainless steel spring wire stent may be inserted in compressed form to expand against the wall of the trachea at the narrow point. The technique has been developed for radiologists to perform while screening the trachea. Good early results are reported.

Tracheostomy may be necessary as a temporary or palliative measure. A long (Koenig's) tube may be essential.

Removal of extrinsic causes of compression will give relief in operable cases.

PART VII
Neurology of the ear, nose and throat

Chapter 22

Anatomy and physiology of the nervous system

THE CEREBRUM

The cerebrum is composed of two symmetrical hemispheres.

Sulci. The surface is thrown into a large number of folds. Each infolding is called a sulcus.

Gyri are the eminences between the sulci.

Longitudinal fissure separates the two cerebral hemispheres from one another, save where the centrally situated corpus callosum joins them together and forms the floor of the fissure.

Corpus callosum consists of a mass of white fibres, functionally connecting the various parts of each hemisphere one with the other.

Falx cerebri is a sickle-shaped fold of dura mater projected into the longitudinal fissure from the skull vault.

Tentorium cerebelli is a broad, tent-shaped fold of dura separating the occipital lobes of the cerebrum from the underlying cerebellum, i.e. separating the posterior fossa from the supratentorial compartment.

Frontal lobe

Composes roughly the anterior half of each hemisphere.

Central sulcus (of Rolando) separates it posteriorly from the parietal lobe.

Lateral sulcus at its anterior end, separates the frontal from the temporal lobe.

Precentral gyrus forms the anterior lip of the central sulcus. It contains 'Betz' cells, the cells of origin of the pyramidal tract on each side.

Voluntary movements of the opposite half of the body are performed by the cells of the motor cortex, activating various parts of the body which are represented in an inverted fashion along the anterior lip of the central sulcus.

'Silent area'. The most anterior part of the frontal lobe is one of the 'silent' areas of the brain; silent because damage to it, particularly if unilateral and gradual, may be undramatic and obscure in symptomatology. This part of the brain is responsible for our foresight, imagination, initiative and planning capacity and for the emotional colouring of these activities. Since there are wide differences between one normal person and another in respect of these faculties, a change in them may not be striking to someone meeting for the

first time a patient with a frontal lobe lesion. When such a lesion is suspected, a careful history from a very close relative or friend is therefore essential.

Broca's area is situated in the lower, posterior part of the frontal lobe of the dominant hemisphere (usually the left). It is that part of the motor cortex directly responsible for the voluntary movements of all the articulatory muscles when used in speech.

Relations

Frontal sinus lies in close relationship to the frontal lobe anteriorly.

Olfactory nerve and its filaments running through the cribriform plate are important inferior relations.

Roof of the orbit and the optic nerves also lie below the frontal lobe.

Circle of Willis in its anterior part, is situated inferiorly to the posterior part of the lobe. So also is the first part of the middle cerebral artery on each side.

Anterior cerebral arteries with their anterior communicating artery, are important relations of its anterior and medial surfaces.

Parietal lobe

Bounded superiorly by the superomedial border of the hemisphere.

Central sulcus forms its anterior boundary.

Horizontal part of the lateral sulcus separates it from the temporal lobe inferiorly.

Posterior boundary is formed by the parieto-occipital sulcus.

Postcentral gyrus lies behind the central sulcus. The parietal lobe cortex, and particularly that of the postcentral gyrus, is responsible for the fullest discrimination of all common sensations, i.e. from skin, joints and the like.

Optic radiations run partly within the deeper substance of each parietal lobe. They travel as a diverging bundle from the lower visual centres to the occipital lobe cortex. A deep lesion may therefore cause a hemianopic visual field defect.

Temporal lobe

Separated from the frontal and parietal lobes respectively by the anterior and posterior parts of the lateral sulcus. The boundary between it and the occipital lobe is ill defined and artificial.

Broca's area. In the frontal lobe, is closely related to the most anterior part of the temporal lobe.

Petrous temporal bone forms the posterior part of the middle fossa and contains the middle and inner ears. This inferior relation of the temporal lobe is of great practical importance to the otologist, for it explains the most common situation of an otogenic brain abscess.

Circular opening in the tentorium cerebelli allows the brainstem to be connected with the cerebral hemispheres and lies close by the inferomedial border of the temporal lobe. A swollen and shifted cerebrum may cause one or other of the temporal lobes to become impacted in this tentorial gap and so thrust the midbrain against its sharp free edge. This not only causes damage to the midbrain but also interferes with the flow of cerebrospinal fluid on its way up to the supratentorial compartment. This *tentorial herniation* is a much-feared complication of raised intracranial pressure and the cause of many otherwise unnecessary deaths.

Auditory area is situated in the superior temporal gyrus.

Uncinate gyrus is situated over the anteromedial part of the temporal lobe and is concerned with the senses of smell and taste. Lesions of this part are liable to give highly distinctive symptoms, the so-called *'uncinate attacks'*, which are of importance in the diagnosis of temporal lobe abscess.

Optic radiations. A part of these radiations traverses the temporal lobe. The radiations may therefore be involved in lesions of the lobe, including otogenic abscess. Hence the visual fields may be of great importance in the diagnosis of such an abscess. The temporal lobe, especially of the non-dominant hemisphere, is a relatively 'silent' area.

Occipital lobe

Rests upon the smooth, sloping upper surface of the tentorium cerebelli which separates it from the underlying cerebellum and brainstem contained in the posterior cranial fossa.

Visual cortex. Specially adapted to the appreciation of visual images.

'Psychic' areas

In the 'no man's land' lying between the temporal, parietal and occipital lobes there are areas of the cortex whose function is of higher appreciation where the results of stimulation of the eye, the ear, and the skin are perceived not as mere sensations but as meaningful happenings, in relation to one another and in the light of past experience. These have been called the 'psychic' areas, the prefix 'psycho-' being attached to the words 'visual', 'auditory', and 'sensory', to distinguish what seem to be three different but anatomically and functionally related parts. At least in respect of the major (or dominant) hemisphere, these areas have an important part in the learning and subsequent function of speech. These areas concerned with 'receptive' speech are closely linked with the more anteriorly placed 'executive' speech areas of the frontal lobe. A lesion involving these inter-connections may therefore disintegrate speech function just as readily as disease of the areas themselves.

THE BRAINSTEM AND THE CRANIAL NERVES

Brainstem

The brainstem, phylogenetically older than the cerebral hemisphere is contained in the posterior cranial fossa.

Optic nerve passes backwards through the optic foramen to become intracranial. Within the skull it runs backwards and medially.

Optic chiasm is formed by the partial decussation of the nerves of the two sides (Figure 22.1). There is a redistribution of the fibres of each optic nerve in the chiasm to form an incomplete decussation, so that the fibres from the nasal halves of each retina cross to the opposite side and those from the temporal halves of each retina remain ipsilateral.

Relations of the optic chiasm

Frontal lobe. Above.
Pituitary gland and sphenoid sinus. Below.
Internal carotid artery and ophthalmic artery, laterally.
Anterior communicating artery joining the two anterior cerebral arteries, may cross it.

Optic tract is formed by the newly constituted part of the visual pathway posterior to the chiasm. Each tract contains fibres that have originated in both retinae. The left optic tract, for instance, is made up of fibres from the left halves of each retina and, since it is these two halves that subserve vision over the right vertical half of the visual field, a lesion of it will produce blindness in the right field, viz. a right homonymous hemianopia. The optic tract runs backwards around the cerebral peduncle of the midbrain and comes to lie below the temporal lobe, where it may be injured by abscesses or other lesions in that lobe.

Lower visual centres contain cell stations in which the optic tract ends. They are:

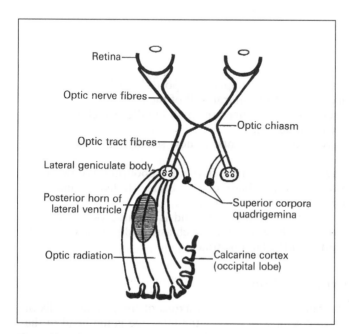

Figure 22.1 Visual pathways

1. *Lateral geniculate body* of the thalamus.
2. *Superior corpus quadrigeminum.*

Optic radiations fan out in the hemisphere as a broad continuous lamina to converge again on to the visual cortex of the occipital lobe. This lamina is so arranged that the uppermost fibres pass almost directly backwards from the internal capsule in the white matter, first of the parietal lobe and then of the occipital lobe. The lowermost fibres take a more circuitous course through the temporal lobe. Between these two extremes there is a continuous sheet of visual fibres but the arrangement is such that, for practical purposes, there are two separate parts of each radiation. The upper and short portion carries stimuli from the upper parts of the retinae, the lower and more circuitous portion carries stimuli from the lower parts of the retinae.

Higher visual centres are situated in the cortical grey matter on the medial surface of each occipital lobe.

Applied anatomy

From the anatomical arrangements described above, the following deductions can be drawn:

1. *Complete lesion of one optic nerve* causes *ipsilateral blindness.*
2. *Complete lesion of one optic tract or one optic radiation* will cause *blindness* of the *vertical half* of the visual field on the opposite side, by blocking stimuli from the homonymous halves of the retinae on the same side as the lesion.
3. *Lesions of the uppermost part of one radiation* will cause *blindness* in the lower half only of the *opposite half-field.*

In the case of a *temporal lobe abscess,* if the damage be confined to that lobe, the field defect will be an *upper quadrantic hemianopia* of the side *opposite* to the abscess. Such a finding is often of inestimable value in the diagnosis of such an abscess, particularly if the lesion be in the non-dominant hemisphere, for speech will then be unaffected, and possibly the only focal evidence of damage will be shown by an examination of the visual fields.

Oculomotor nerves

The IIIrd, IVth and VIth pair of cranial nerves are collectively known as oculomotor.

Third cranial nerve

Nucleus, situated in the midbrain, consists of a group of nuclei on each side, with a centrally situated single one. *The central nucleus* probably innervates the medial rectus muscle of each eye for the purpose of convergence alone. *The paired nuclei* innervate all the muscles moving the eyeball, save for the external rectus (supplied by the VIth nerve) and the superior oblique (supplied by the IVth nerve). In addition, the IIIrd nerve nucleus supplies the levator of the upper lid. A part of the paired nucleus gives origin to fibres travelling within the IIIrd nerve and destined to innervate the involuntary sphincter pupillae and the ciliary muscles which alter the shape of the crystalline lens.

Fibres. Run directly from the nuclei through the substance of the midbrain and come into close contact with the cerebral peduncles carrying the downgoing pyramidal fibres.

Fourth cranial nerve

Nucleus. Lies immediately below that of the IIIrd nerve in the midbrain.

Fibres. Emerge from the dorsal surface of the midbrain, having decussated in the posterior part of the brainstem, and have to encircle the cerebral peduncle on either side before they reach the ventral aspect of the brainstem and come to lie in series with their fellow oculomotor nerves.

Sixth cranial nerve

Nucleus. Lies at a lower level in the brainstem, at the posterior aspect of the pons in the floor of the third ventricle. The fibres of the VIIth nerve curl around the nucleus of the VIth in their circuitous intrapontine path from their nucleus in the middle of the pons to their escape on its ventral surface.

Fibres. Run directly forwards from the nucleus through the substance of the pons. The nerve crosses the superior border of the petrous temporal bone under the petro-clinoid ligament, i.e. in Dorello's canal. It passes from the posterior to the middle cranial fossa with the superior petrosal sinus.

Relations of the oculomotor nerves

1. *Medial longitudinal bundle.* A close relation of all three oculomotor nuclei, probably serving as a connection between them and introducing vestibular stimuli to them.
2. *Cavernous sinus.* All three nerves converge at the cavernous sinus and they all come to lie in its lateral wall, together with the first two divisions of the Vth cranial nerve.
3. *Internal carotid artery.* A part of this artery lies within the substance of the cavernous sinus and is therefore a close medial relation of all these nerves.
4. *Superior orbital fissure.* Gives passage to all three oculomotor nerves as they enter the bony orbit.

Trigeminal nerve

Largely a sensory nerve with a small motor root.

Sensory ganglion (Gasserian ganglion; semilunar ganglion)

Lies in a fold of dura mater on the anterosuperior aspect of the medial end of the petrous temporal bone.

Divisions

Three sensory divisions arise from the anterior end of the Gasserian ganglion.

1. *First division.* Passes forwards in the lateral wall of the *cavernous sinus,* with the second division and all three oculomotor nerves. It therefore lies close to the intracavernous part of the *internal carotid artery.* It passes into the orbit through the *superior orbital fissure* and is finally distributed to the *skin of the front of the head* as far back as a somewhat variable point close to the lambdoid suture, to the *side and tip of the nose,* to the *upper eyelid,* to the *conjunctivae and corneae,* to the *frontal sinus,* and it shares the supply of the *nasal mucosa* with the second division. The first division also supplies the *ethmoidal and sphenoidal sinuses.*
2. *Second division.* Also lies in the lateral wall of the *cavernous sinus,* but leaves the cranial cavity through the *foramen rotundum,* before crossing the *pterygopalatine fossa* to enter the orbit through the *inferior orbital fissure.* Its distribution includes part of the *skin of the temple,* the *cheek,* the *upper lip,* the *mucosa of the cheek,* and the whole of the *upper alveolus with its teeth.* It also takes part in the mucosal supply of the *nasal cavity.*
3. *Third division.* With which travels the whole of the small *motor root,* leaves the skull cavity by way of the *foramen ovale.* It supplies the *skin over the temple* and sometimes the *concha,* the *anterior part of the external auditory canal* and the *tympanic membrane,* and the skin of the *lower face.* It supplies the *inside of the mouth,* the *lower alveolus and teeth,* and common sensation to the *anterior two-thirds of the tongue.* The *motor root* supplies all the *muscles derived from the first branchial arch,* namely the pterygoids, tensor tympani, tensor palati, the masseter, the temporal muscles, the mylohyoid and anterior belly of the digastric.

Main sensory root

Runs backwards from the posterior limit of the Gasserian ganglion to the anterolateral aspect of the *pons,* which it enters. In this extra-cerebral part of its course it is crossed by the superior petrosal sinus and lies in the cerebellopontine angle, together with the VIIth and VIIIth cranial nerves. Within the pons there is a redistribution of fibres, so that those subserving the sense of *touch* end in the *main sensory nucleus,* at the level of entry of the nerve trunk into the pons; those carrying *pain and thermal* sensations travel downwards as the spinal tract, to end at varying levels in the long *nucleus of the spinal tract* which descends to the level of the upper cervical cord. The pain fibres from the first division travel most caudally before entering the lower reaches of the nucleus, those from the third division enter the highest part of the nucleus, the second division fibres ending intermediately. It is therefore possible to have a topographically discriminate sensory loss over the face from a central lesion as well as from peripheral damage to one or other divisions of the nerves. Likewise it is possible that a central lesion in the brainstem substance may produce a dissociated sensory loss over the face; for instance, a loss of pain sense with intact light touch. The nucleus of the small motor component of the Vth nerve lies posteromedial to the main sensory nucleus in the pons.

Facial nerve

Nucleus. Lies deeply within the substance of the *pons*. In that situation, it is closely related on its lateral side to the upper part of the descending tract and nucleus of the Vth cranial nerve and anteromedially to the medial sensory lemniscus.

Fibres. Travel a circuitous route, at first backwards to encircle the VIth nerve nucleus in the floor of the fourth ventricle and then forwards through the pons, to emerge on its anterior surface. After leaving the surface of the pons it runs anterolaterally to enter the *petrous temporal bone.*

Within the cranial cavity. It is closely related to the *VIIIth cranial nerve,* being separated from it by the small sensory root, the *nervus intermedius* of Wrisberg. Here, too, it is near the *Vth cranial nerve.*

In the intrapetrous part. The facial nerve and its sensory root accompany the *VIIIth cranial nerve* into the *internal auditory canal, carrying a common meningeal sheath. Here it has anastomotic connections with the vestibular nerve. At the bottom of this canal it enters the* facial canal which at first runs *laterally* above the vestibule of the labyrinth until it turns *backwards* through a *right angle* on the medial wall above the promontory and the fenestra vestibuli. *At the medial wall of the aditus,* it curves *downwards* to emerge on the inferior surface of the temporal bone at the *stylomastoid foramen.*

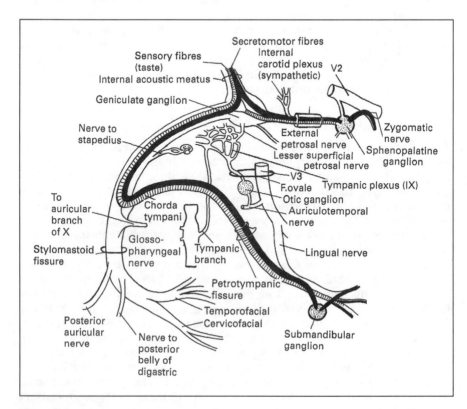

Figure 22.2

In the extracranial part. Once free of the skull, it runs forwards within the *parotid salivary gland.*

Facial (geniculate) ganglion

Situated at the point where the nerve takes a U-turn backwards.

Nervus intermedius

Carries:

1. *Autonomic fibres.* Destined for the supply of the lacrimal, submaxillary and sublingual glands, together with glands of the nasal and oral cavities. These fibres are secretomotor and vasodilator.
2. *Sensory fibres.* Which have their cell stations in the geniculate ganglion.
- Some of these fibres come from the nasal mucosa via the Vidian and greater superficial petrosal nerves. They pass through the sphenopalatine ganglion without relay.
- Other sensory fibres in this nerve travel with the motor branches of the VIIth nerve to the muscles of facial expression and these are thought to carry *proprioceptive* impulses from these muscles.
- Still other sensory fibres, from *skin,* are thought to originate from the region of the concha and other parts behind the auricle. It is thought that the sensory fibres of the VIIth cranial nerve, other than those of taste, end in the descending nucleus of the trigeminal.
- Those fibres forming the *chorda tympani* subserve the special sense of *taste.* These fibres start in the mucosa of the anterior two-thirds of the tongue and travel proximally with the lingual nerve, which they leave to join the facial nerve in the Fallopian canal, a few millimetres above the stylomastoid foramen. The chorda tympani ends in the geniculate ganglion whence the central fibres form one part of the nervous inter-medius.

Motor fibres

Give branches to the stapedius muscle, the posterior belly of the digastric, to a part of the occipitofrontalis, the stylohyoid, the muscles of the pinna, the platysma and to all the mimetic muscles of the face. These are all muscles derived from the second branchial arch.

Sense of taste and its pathways

There is a triple nervous pathway for taste (Figure 22.3).

1. From the anterior two-thirds of the tongue via the *chorda tympani,* travel-ling at first with the lingual nerve, later with the facial nerve in the Fallopian canal. The cell station is in the geniculate ganglion and from there the impulses are transmitted via the nervus intermedius to the pons.
2. *From the palate* via the palatine nerves, nerve of the pterygoid canal (Vidian), geniculate ganglion and nervus intermedius.

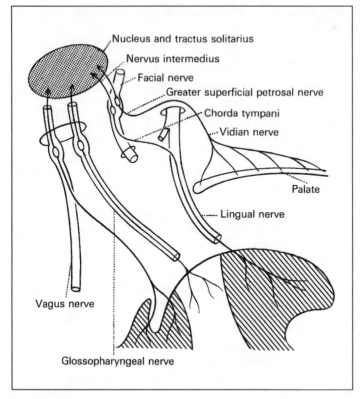

Figure 22.3 Nervous pathways of taste

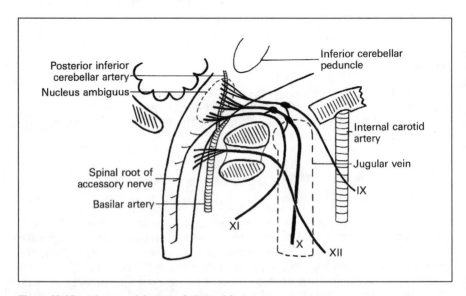

Figure 22.4 Last four cranial nerves (schematic)

3. *From the posterior one-third of the tongue* via the *IXth cranial nerve* and so to the medulla.

4. *From the epiglottis and fauces* via the *Xth cranial nerve* and so to the medulla. No matter by what channel the taste impulses travel to the brainstem, the incoming fibres form the *tractus solitarius* and its surrounding nucleus. This tract and nucleus have a considerable vertical extent, from the pons above and throughout the length of the medulla. From this nucleus the nervous pathway to consciousness is not certainly known but is thought to be by way of the *medial lemniscus of the opposite side.*

Auditory nerve

Described in the Anatomy of the Ear.

Glossopharyngeal, vagus and accessory nerves

Functionally the IXth and Xth cranial nerves have much in common, and this is true to a less extent for the XIth nerve. These nerves are therefore better discussed together (Figure 22.4).

Central connections of the IXth, Xth, and XIth cranial nerves

Efferent connections

1. *Nucleus ambiguus.* Gives origin to special visceral efferent fibres, for the motor supply of the *striated muscles of the pharynx and larynx.* The nucleus stretches throughout the medulla. Outgoing fibres run anterolaterally and leave the medulla on its lateral surface, and are given to the IXth, Xth, and XIth nerves. Those going to the last-named are finally distributed entirely to the Xth nerve at the jugular foramen. This cranial part of the XIth nerve shares the supply of the laryngeal muscles with the vagus.

2. *Dorsal nucleus of the vagus.* An autonomic nucleus serving only a general visceral efferent function. It is a major portion of the cranial *parasympathetic* outflow, the remainder travelling with the IIIrd and VIIth cranial nerves from similar nuclei at a higher level of the brainstem. These outgoing fibres are therefore *preganglionic,* their ganglia being situated at or near the organ affected. The nucleus is situated in the posterior part of the medulla, in the floor of the fourth ventricle. Outgoing fibres run anterolaterally and are joined by those of the nucleus ambiguus before coming to the lateral surface of the medulla as a series of rootlets. These fibres all go to form a part of the Xth nerve trunk, none to the XIth. They supply *smooth muscle and glands* of the *trachea and bronchi, oesophagus, heart and abdominal viscera. Inferior salivary nucleus* is a separate body at upper end of the dorsal nucleus; its outgoing preganglionic fibres are distributed to the IXth nerve trunk, and thence to the *parotid gland.*

3. *Spinal portion of the XIth nerve.* Has its central connections in cells in the lateral part of the *anterior horns* of the *first five segments of the spinal cord.* The fibres emerge from the lateral aspect of the cord as a series of rootlets which ascend to join the cranial portion of the nerve by passing through the *foramen magnum.* The fibres originating from the cord run downwards in the

neck to supply the *sternomastoid* and upper fibres of the *trapezius* muscles. They are therefore functionally somatic efferent nerves and have nothing in common with the cranial portion except for their anatomical contiguity.

Afferent connections

1. *Solitary tract and its nucleus.* Form a vertical mass from the pons above to the lower reaches of the medulla below. It is situated deeply in the medulla. The solitary tract consists of incoming *sensory* fibres derived from the *VIIth, IXth, and Xth cranial nerves.* They subserve *taste* from the anterior two-thirds of the tongue (VIIth), the posterior one-third of the tongue (IXth) and from other taste buds in the pharynx (Xth). The tractus solitarius and its nucleus are also concerned in *visceral sensation* from the *pharynx and larynx* as well as from the remainder of the respiratory and alimentary tracts. The pathway for the upward projection of these sensations to consciousness may be via the medial lemniscus of the opposite side.

2. *Auricular branch of the vagus* (Arnold's nerve; 'Alderman's nerve'). Is the only somatic afferent part of this cranial nerve triad. The fibres end in the *descending nucleus of the Vth nerve.*

Peripheral courses of the IXth, Xth, and XIth cranial nerves

The IXth and Xth cranial nerve trunks are formed from vertically serial rootlets on the lateral surface of the *medulla,* the rootlets being both efferent and afferent. The XIth nerve trunk is formed from a set of cranial fibres, in series with those for the IXth and Xth nerves, and from rootlets which emerge from the lateral aspect of the *spinal cord.* These spinal rootlets run upwards through the foramen magnum to join the cranial ones. The three nerves so formed run forwards in the posterior cranial fossa towards the jugular foramen by which they all leave the skull. As it passes through this foramen the IXth nerve is invested with its own dural sheath, separating it from a similar sheath common to the other two. They share the foramen with the internal jugular vein.

IXth nerve

1. *Motor fibres.* Pass uninterrupted through the jugular foramen and descend between the internal jugular vein and the internal carotid artery. Before passing over the interval between the superior and middle constrictors, they are crossed by the styloid process with its attached muscle. A branch goes to supply the *stylopharyngeus* muscle.

2. *Secretomotor fibres.* Are autonomic fibres derived from the inferior salivary nucleus. They leave the rest of the nerve at the inferior (petrous) ganglion at the jugular foramen and reach the tympanic plexus in the tympanic cavity via the tympanic nerve (nerve of Jacobsen). From that plexus it runs, as the *lesser superficial petrosal* nerve, in its own canal through the temporal bone and so to the *otic ganglion,* by way of the foramen ovale. New fibres arise in the otic ganglion and are finally distributed in the parotid *salivary gland.*

3. *Sensory fibres.* Subserve *common sensation from the* posterior one-third of the tongue, the *posterior faucial pillar,* the *tonsil,* and the *soft palate.* They also subserve *taste* from the *posterior one-third of the tongue.* These fibres are interrupted in the superior ganglion. In some cases the IXth nerve may carry somatic afferent fibres from the skin of the concha.

Xth nerve
Passing through the jugular foramen with the IXth and XIth nerves, descends in the neck. At first the trunk lies between the internal jugular vein posteriorly and the internal carotid artery anteriorly. Lower down these vessels come to lie in the same plane, the artery medial and the nerve between them. Still lower down, the nerve maintains the same relationship with the common carotid artery and the vein in the carotid sheath. Before entering the thorax the nerve crosses the first part of the subclavian artery.

On the right side, in the thorax, the nerve runs down posteromedial to the superior vena cava, then behind the root of the lung, and so on to the posterior aspect of the oesophagus, where it lies until it enters the abdominal cavity through the diaphragm, when it joins its fellow.

On the left side, it passes behind the brachiocephalic vein, medial to the left subclavian and lateral to the left common carotid artery. It runs anterior to the arch of the aorta, crossed by the left phrenic nerve, and so behind the root of the lung and on to the anterior aspect of the oesophagus.

1. *Motor fibres.* Pass in the following branches:
- Pharyngeal. From just below the inferior ganglion, passing between the two carotid arteries to the *side of the pharynx.*
- Superior laryngeal. Also from the inferior ganglion, carrying motor fibres to the *inferior constrictor and cricothyroid* muscles via the external laryngeal nerve, and possibly to the upper sphincter of the larynx.
- Recurrent laryngeal. Supplying all the intrinsic muscles of the larynx except the cricothyroid and the upper laryngeal sphincter. At the inferior ganglion the Xth nerve receives all the cranial portion of the XIth nerve, via the internal ramus of the accessory.

2. *Visceral sensory fibres.* Have the same peripheral course as the motor fibres. Some taste fibres (special visceral afferent) arise from the epiglottis and travel via the internal laryngeal nerve. All of these fibres synapse in the inferior ganglion.

3. *Somatic afferent fibres.* Constituting the auricular branch of the vagus, run via the tympanomastoid fissure and the substance of the temporal bone to the superior (jugular) ganglion, where a synapse takes place. It frequently communicates with the IXth cranial nerve.

XIth nerve
Leaves skull via jugular foramen and in same dural sheath as the vagus.

1. *Internal ramus.* Composed solely of fibres that have originated from the nucleus ambiguus and it passes to the Xth nerve at its inferior ganglion. Its fibres are distributed with those of the vagus to the striated *muscles of the pharynx and larynx.*

2. External ramus. Enters the substance of the *sternomastoid* muscle at the junction of its upper and middle thirds and, after crossing the posterior triangle of the neck, ends in a plexus beneath the upper fibres of the *trapezius* muscle. This ramus is formed solely of fibres having their origin in the *anterior horn cells* of the *upper five cervical* cord segments.

Hypoglossal nerve

Nucleus. Lies close to the midline of the *medulla* in the floor of the fourth ventricle.

Fibres. Emerge on the anterolateral aspect of the medulla, anterior to those of the IXth, Xth, and XIth nerves. The extracerebral fibres run forwards in the posterior fossa, to leave the skull via the anterior condylar foramen in the occipital bone. Immediately beneath the skull the nerve comes into close relationship with the IXth, Xth, and XIth nerves. It lies between the internal jugular vein and the internal carotid artery. At the lower border of the posterior belly of the digastric muscle, it bends forwards and medially and crosses successively the internal carotid, the occipital, the external carotid, and the lingual arteries. As it crosses the lingual artery, it is crossed by the common facial vein. It passes deep to the stylohyoid muscle and enters the substance of the base of the tongue, where it is distributed to the *intrinsic muscles* of the same side. It is a purely motor nerve.

THE CEREBELLUM

Relations of the cerebellum

The cerebellum occupies the *posterior cranial fossa.*

Pons and medulla are separated from it anteriorly by the fourth ventricle.

Petrous temporal bone with its contained internal auditory meatus, lies anterolaterally.

Tentorium cerebelli separates it from the occipital lobes of the cerebrum and the *straight venous sinus.*

Cerebellopontine angle is a potential space lying between the petrous temporal bone anterolaterally, the cerebellar lobe posterolaterally, and the pons medially. The Vth, VIIth, and VIIIth cranial nerves cross this space, and it is here that an acoustic neurofibroma may grow on the VIIIth nerve at the porus of the internal auditory meatus.

Cerebellar peduncles

There are three cerebellar peduncles on either side, supporting the cerebellum and attaching it to the brainstem. All three comprise fibres carrying stimuli to and from the cerebellum.

Superior peduncle arises from the lower part of the *midbrain.*

Middle peduncle arises from the lateral aspect of the *pons.*

Inferior peduncle is formed from the upper part of the *medulla.*

Structure of the cerebellum

The cerebellum consists of a small median lobe, the *vermis,* and two large *lateral lobes.* The inferior part of the vermis (the *nodule)* and the lower parts of each lateral lobe (the *flocculus)* are together the most primitive and (functionally) closely linked parts of the cerebellum. They are together known as the *flocculonodular lobe* and their connections are entirely with the *vestibular system.* The remainder of the cerebellum is called the *corpus cerebelli,* which includes the remainder of the vermis and the two lateral lobes. Phylogenetically the oldest parts of the corpus have connections with the vestibular and the spinocerebellar tracts, while the newer and larger part is connected mainly with the cerebral cortex through the pons.

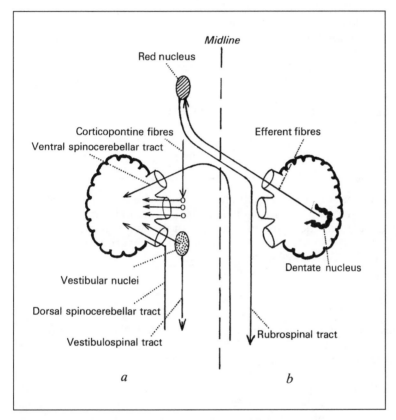

Figure 22.5 Connections of the cerebellum. a, Afferent connections; b, efferent connections

Connections of the cerebellum (Figure 22.5)

Afferent connections

1. *Vestibular fibres.* Enter the cerebellum by way of the inferior peduncle, both directly from the vestibular nerve and indirectly from the vestibular nuclei. These vestibular fibres end chiefly in the flocculonodular lobe.

2. *Spinal fibres.* Originating in the proprioceptors of muscles, tendons and joints, travel up the cord in two distinct pathways, the dorsal and ventral spinocerebellar tracts. The former enters the cerebellum via the inferior peduncle, the latter runs upwards to the midbrain before turning down into the superior peduncle. Both tracts end throughout the cerebellar cortex.

3. *Cortical fibres.* Reach the phylogenetically newer parts of the cerebellum, starting as the corticopontine tracts and relaying in the pontine nuclei, using the middle peduncle.

Efferent connections

The most important efferent pathway from the cerebellum originates from the nuclei, chiefly the *dentate nucleus.* The pathway is projected through the superior peduncle, decussates in the midbrain with those from the other side, and ends in the *opposite red nucleus.* The *rubrospinal tract,* carrying a new set of fibres from the nucleus, crosses the midline and courses downwards through the brainstem, to play upon the *anterior horn cells* of the spinal cord on the same side as the origin of the efferents from the cerebellum. This is probably the most important path used to connect the cerebellar hemisphere with the limb muscles of the same side of the body.

THE MENINGES

The meninges consist of three membranes — from without inwards the dura mater, arachnoid mater and pia mater. They invest the brain and spinal cord, separating them from the cranium and vertebral column respectively. All three layers blend into the connective-tissue coats covering the emerging cranial and spinal nerves.

Dura mater

The toughest and thickest of the three, consists of relatively avascular fibrous tissue. Its outer endosteal layer is attached everywhere to the inner layer of the cranial bones and is accurately moulded over them. Except where the venous sinuses intervene and where the inner layer forms the dural septa the two parts of the dura mater are intimately related. The external layer blends with the periosteum at the foramen magnum and is not directly continuous with the spinal dura which forms a continuous closed sheath within the interrupted bony vertebral column. The lowermost limit of the theca is at the level of the second sacral vertebra.

Dural folds

These are formed from the inner meningeal layer of the dura.

Falx cerebri

A sickle-shaped fold of dura whose attached border encloses the *superior longitudinal sinus.* The free border dips between the two opposing media aspects of the cerebral hemispheres and carries the *inferior longitudinal sinus.* The free edge is attached anteriorly to the crista galli and posteriorly to the upper border of the tentorium cerebelli.

Tentorium cerebelli

A crescentic fold of dura separating the under-surface of the cerebral hemispheres above from the cerebellar lobes below, i.e. separating the supratentorial compartment of the skull from the posterior fossa. The peripheral fixed border is attached from behind forwards on each side to the internal occipital protuberance, the lips of the bony groove for the *transverse sinus,* the superior border of the petrous temporal bone where it encloses the *superior petrosal sinus* and the posterior clinoid process. The free border forms a roughly rounded aperture for the passage of the midbrain and is attached anteriorly to the anterior clinoid process on each side. Its superior surface in the midline is attached to the posterior part of the falx cerebri and at this junction runs the *straight sinus.*

Falx cerebelli

Projects between the two cerebellar lobes in much the same way as the much larger falx cerebri intervenes between the two cerebral hemispheres. Its fixed edge is attached to the inferior surface of the tentorium and to the internal occipital crest, where it encloses the *occipital sinus.*

Subdural space

Only a potential space in health. It separates the cerebral and spinal dura from the underlying arachnoid and contains a little serous fluid.

Arachnoid mater

This is intimately applied to the inner surface of the dura, being separated only by the potential subdural space. It bridges across the sulci and does not dip into them.

Subarachnoid space

This holds the cerebrospinal fluid between the arachnoid and pia mater. There are therefore small pools of CSF in each of the sulci. Larger ones form the *subarachnoid cisterns* where the arachnoid bridges across the wider irregularities between one part of the brain and another, e.g. the cisterna magna between the medulla and the under-surfaces of the two cerebellar lobes. The subarachnoid space communicates with the ventricular system by way of median and lateral apertures in the roof of the fourth ventricle. Each optic nerve is surrounded by a sleeve of subarachnoid space. This ends blindly where the arachnoid blends with the orbit. The cerebral and spinal subarachnoid spaces are continuous with one another at the foramen magnum.

Arachnoid granulations

These are formed by invaginations of the arachnoid into the larger intracranial venous sinuses, particularly the superior sagittal sinus. They are thought to be the pathway whereby the CSF is reabsorbed into the bloodstream.

Pia mater

A much more delicate structure than either of the other two layers, it is intimately applied to the surface of the brain and spinal cord, following its irregularities with precision. The arachnoid and pia are bound together by trabeculae except at the basal cisterns. A perivascular sheath of pia–arachnoid surrounds every artery that enters the brain down to the terminal branches, thus carrying an extension of the subarachnoid space into the brain substance. Below the conus medullaris, the lowermost part of the spinal cord, the pia is continued downwards as the filum terminale, to be attached to the coccyx.

THE CEREBROSPINAL FLUID

The CSF is a clear, colourless fluid occupying the four ventricles of the brain and the cranial and spinal parts of the subarachnoid space.

Secretion

Secretion of the CSF is by the choroid plexuses in all four ventricles. It circulates from the two lateral ventricles to the unpaired third by way of the two foramina of Munro; from the third to the fourth by the narrow aqueduct of the midbrain; and from the fourth ventricle to the subarachnoid space via the apertures in the roof. In the subarachnoid space it flows both upwards and downwards over all the surfaces of the brain and spinal cord.

Absorption

The CSF is reabsorbed into the venous blood stream by way of the arachnoid granulations which project into the larger intracranial venous sinuses especially the superior sagittal sinus. Whether or not this is the only method of egress from the skull is not yet known. The perivascular sheaths surrounding the small vessels which penetrate the cortex bring the CSF into intimate contact with the nerve cells.

Functions

The functions of the CSF are probably twofold at least.
1. *Medium for nutrient and waste-product exchange.* With the nerve cells.
2. *Cushioning water-bed.* For the brain and spinal cord.

Pressure

The pressure by lumbar puncture in the lateral position, the patient being relaxed and breathing easily, and the knees not too tightly flexed towards the chest, lies between 60 and 180 mm of CSF.

Constituents

The more important constituents of the normal fluid, as withdrawn from the lumbar theca, are:

Cells Up to 5 lymphocytes per μl
Protein 0.1–0.4 g/l.
Chlorides 123–135 mmol/l.
Glucose 2.5–3.9 mmol/l.

THE ARTERIAL BLOOD SUPPLY OF THE BRAIN AND MENINGES

The brain is supplied by two pairs of arteries, the internal carotids and the vertebrals. The meninges are largely supplied by the external carotid arteries.

Internal carotid artery

This arises as one of the two terminal branches of the common carotid artery, at the upper border of the thyroid cartilage. It enters the skull through the somewhat sinuous *carotid canal* in the petrous temporal bone. In this canal, where it gives off tympanic branches, it is separated from the anterior aspect of the tympanic cavity and the cochlea only by a thin plate of bone. After entering the cranial cavity it runs forwards through the *cavernous sinus* before turning upwards to pierce the dura mater, medial to the anterior clinoid process. In the cavernous sinus it is related medially to the pituitary body and laterally to the three oculomotor nerves and the first two divisions of the trigeminal nerve.

Branches

After becoming intradural, the artery ends in a suprasellar position by dividing into two terminal branches:

1. *Anterior cerebral artery* which runs forwards above the optic nerve, to gain the anterior end of the superior longitudinal fissure, between the two cerebral hemispheres. In this fissure it runs upwards and then backwards above the corpus callosum and close to its fellow of the opposite side, to which it is joined soon after its formation by the *anterior communicating artery*. The anterior cerebral artery supplies the whole of the medial surfaces of the frontal and parietal lobes and the adjoining parts of the superolateral surfaces.
2. *Middle cerebral artery* which runs laterally between the frontal and temporal lobes of the brain to gain the lateral cerebral fissure, in which it runs to its termination. It supplies the greater part of the lateral surface of the cerebral hemisphere.

Vertebral arteries

These arise from the first part of the *subclavian artery*. After passing upwards through the foramina of the transverse processes of the upper six

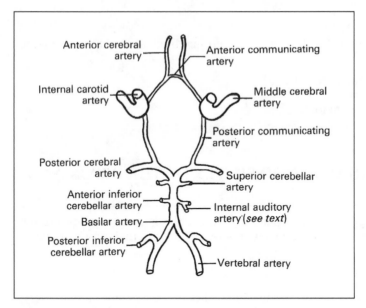

Figure 22.6 Arteries at the base of the brain (circle of Willis)

cervical vertebrae, each artery enters the skull through the *foramen magnum* and joins with its fellow to form the midline unpaired *basilar artery,* at the junction of the ventral surfaces of the pons and medulla. At the upper border of the pons the basilar artery ends by dividing into the two *posterior cerebral arteries.* Among other branches which supply the brainstem and cerebellum, the basilar artery may give rise to the internal auditory artery, though this vessel more commonly arises from the anterior inferior cerebellar, the superior cerebellar, or (rarely) the posterior inferior cerebellar artery.

Circle of Willis (Figure 22.6)

This is an anastomotic circle of arteries situated at the base of the brain and formed anterolaterally by the termination of the two internal carotids, the two anterior cerebral arteries, and the single short anterior communicating artery. Laterally the circle consists of the posterior communicating artery, which is a branch of the terminal part of the internal carotid. Posteriorly the circle is completed with the two posterior cerebral arteries. The circle of Willis is the only place where an adequate anastomosis exists between the various cerebral arteries, which are end-arteries.

THE VENOUS DRAINAGE OF THE BRAIN AND OTHER CRANIAL CONTENTS

The intracranial structures are drained by a system of thin-walled veins without valves, situated within the subarachnoid space and themselves passing their blood to the various venous sinuses. Pain fibres are situated close to venous sinuses. Hence coughing, sneezing or straining at stool increase intracranial pain.

Venous sinuses (Figure 22.7)

These are placed within the two layers of the tough dura mater, many of them close to the skull bones and all of them finally draining into the two *internal jugular veins.* There are, however, numerous emissary veins which pierce the skull bones and serve to connect this intracranial venous system with the veins outside the skull.

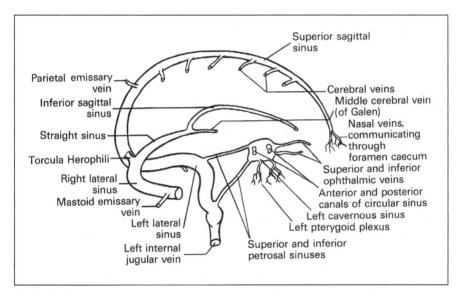

Figure 22.7 Intracranial venous sinuses

Superior sagittal (longitudinal) sinus

Lies between the two layers of the dura mater at the *attached border of the falx cerebri.* It begins anteriorly at the crista galli where it receives radicles from the nasal system, gathers blood from the superior cerebral veins from both sides as it passes backwards, and ends by becoming one or other *transverse sinus* or by flowing into the *confluence of the sinuses (torcular herophili).*

Inferior sagittal sinus

Runs in the *lower free border of the falx cerebri.* Its flow is also backwards, to the point where it ends in the *straight sinus.*

Straight sinus

Lies at the junction of the falx cerebri with the tentorium cerebri. It receives the inferior sagittal sinus and the great cerebral vein of Galen, and ends in

3. In association with disease of the brain and spinal cord

Meningitis may complicate a brain abscess. An initial meningeal reaction is the rule in anterior poliomyelitis.

Bacteriology

Varies with the source of infection. The *meningococcus* is found in epidemic and sporadic cerebrospinal meningitis. The *pneumococcus* may also be the cause of such a 'primary' meningitis but is more often secondary to infection in the lung, nose, or ear. *Other pyogenic invaders* from the nose and ear are *Haemophilus influenzae* and, less often, *staphylococcus.* Anaerobic organisms also may cause infection by direct spread from middle ear or frontal sinus. The *tubercle bacillus* may come from the ear but more commonly from the lung, frequently as part of a miliary bloodstream dissemination. The *virus infections* of the meninges are of less importance to the otologist.

Pathology

Whatever the source of infection, the pathology of acute diffuse pyogenic meningitis is the same.

Intense inflammatory response occurs in the pia and arachnoid. The space between them becomes filled with polymorph leucocytes.

Green or yellow pus may entirely cover the surface of the brain or cord, or it may be confined to the larger subarachnoid spaces, such as the sulci.

Flattening of the gyri is accompanied by some inflammatory reaction in the cortex.

Hydrocephalus may result from obstruction to the flow of CSF by the thick pus and adhesions. This mechanical complication is a much feared danger in tuberculous meningitis, for it may lead to a further increase of intracranial pressure and prevent access of streptomycin to parts of the infection.

Arterial and venous thrombosis may cause signs and symptoms of gross involvement of the brain, most commonly in fulminating meningococcal meningitis. A local and confined meningitis is frequent in the immediate vicinity of a brain abscess or an osteitis, the infection not necessarily becoming disseminated into a diffuse meningitis.

Clinical features

General symptoms are those common to many acute infective diseases.

Fever usually present, the degree depending on the acuteness and extent of the meningeal involvement in all cases, and on the mode of attack of the particular organism in some cases.

Rigors with a high swinging temperature, may result from pyaemia. The clinical picture of meningitis following on ear or sinus infections may merge with that of the original disease, especially after operation, so that difficulties in diagnosis may arise.

Local caused by the irritation of the meninges of the brain and spinal cord, with or without involvement of the underlying nervous tissue. These are much less dramatic in onset when the cause is tubercle bacillus and may follow several weeks of general illness.

Headache is usually generalized, intense and progressively severe. It spreads to the back of the neck and often the whole spine. The pain may travel into the legs.

Neck stiffness may increase to neck retraction. Rigidity is demonstrated by first establishing no resistance in side-to-side neck movement, and then attempting a gentle bimanual flexion of the head, when a spasm of the neck extensors may be felt.

Kernig's sign. Extension at the knee, with the hip joint flexed at a right angle, is painful and limited on both sides.

Altered state of consciousness is frequently present and progressive. It begins as mere drowsiness. Then the patient becomes confused. The next stage is stupor, when the patient responds only to simple commands, followed by semicoma when the only response is to pain. The sequence ends in coma when there is no response even to painful stimuli.

Mental irritability and photophobia are common early signs.

Fits may happen in the early hours of infection, particularly in children.

Cranial nerve palsies sometimes.

Vomiting frequently.

Papilloedema usually late. It forms no essential part of the clinical picture.

Cerebrospinal fluid is always under *increased pressure.* The fluid is usually turbid. *Cells are increased,* sometimes to many thousands per ml. With bacterial, as opposed to viral, infections the majority are polymorphonuclear but a few may be mononuclear. *Protein content is raised,* sometimes very markedly. *Glucose content is reduced,* except in very early cases. *Organisms* may be seen on suitably stained films or may only be identified on culture. *Counterimmune electrophoresis* is helpful for rapid detection of the common pathogens, e.g. pneumococcus, meningococcus, *H. influenzae.*

Differential diagnosis

From:

1. *Brain abscess.*
2. *Intracranial thrombophlebitis.*
3. *Acute general infections:*
- *Typhoid fever.*
- *Pneumonia.*
- *Acute rheumatic fever.*
- *Specific fevers* all of which may produce meningism.
4. *Other diseases producing meningeal irritation* and therefore the signs of meningitis.
- *Poliomyelitis.* The meningeal stage of acute poliomyelitis may precede the paralysis or, indeed, may form the only clinical picture in abortive cases. Evidence of brainstem involvement, cranial nerve palsies, and lower motor neurone paralysis are rare in the early stages of meningitis but are common in the early days of poliomyelitis. The CSF pleocytosis, often mixed polymorphonuclear/mononuclear at first, later becomes chiefly or wholly mononuclear: the glucose and chloride contents are normal.
- *Viral meningitis and meningo-encephalitis* may complicate the specific fevers, especially mumps, or may arise as an acute infection. Due to

various viruses, e.g. mumps, Coxsackie, ECHO, lymphocytic choriomenin-gitis, various arboviruses and herpes simplex. Usually benign. CSF shows moderate rise in white cells, mostly lymphocytes, slight rise in protein, but no fall in glucose.

- *Subarachnoid haemorrhage* in which the onset is sudden, as if 'hit by a hammer'; frank blood is found on lumbar puncture. It is essential to take several separate specimens following a bloody tap to distinguish spontaneous bleeding from needle trauma, and to look for xanthochromia in the supernatant.
- *Neurosyphilitic disease* in which an acute or subacute meningitis occasion-ally occurs at the secondary or tertiary stage. The cells in the CSF are usually all mononuclear. The serological tests for syphilis are positive.

Treatment

Antibiotics. In all cases a lumbar puncture should be performed and the fluid examined chemically and by direct microscopy. It will often then be possible to make a provisional bacteriological diagnosis. If CSF has the characteristics of pyogenic infection antibiotic treatment should be commenced immedi-ately. Otologists are advised to consult bacteriological colleagues about local antibiotic resistance problems in treatment of meningitis of *unknown origin*. If in doubt high dose, i.e. ampicillin (minimum 150 mg/kg/day), or penicillin, plus parenteral chloramphenicol 75 mg/kg/day (adult dose) is a suitable *initial* treatment. In severe cases penicillin 10 000–20 000 units (for adults – children should receive a smaller dose) may be given intrathecally in addition. Any larger intrathecal dose is very dangerous and can prove fatal.

Subsequent treatment will depend on the organism found and its sensitivity to the various antibacterial agents. Treatment must be continued for at least 3 days after the temperature has returned to normal.

Sedatives or hypnotics are sometimes necessary for restlessness or mania.

Ample fluid intake.

Analgesics may successfully control the lesser degrees of restlessness.

Surgery of aural or nasal foci should take second place to the treatment of the meningitis and should await the immediate and dramatic response to specific drugs.

Tuberculous meningitis

Aetiology

Tuberculous meningitis usually results from bloodstream dissemination from the lung but may complicate the rare tuberculous infections of the ear.

Clinical features

Onset is insidious. The patient usually has a prolonged prodrome of general and progressive malaise lasting several weeks before meningeal irritation is obvious.

1. *Headache* is progressive.
2. *Irritability and mental apathy* accompany it in the prodomal stage.

3. *Vomiting and anorexia.*
4. Signs of meningeal irritation may be few and unobtrusive, even when CSF changes are gross.
5. *Pleocytosis* is predominantly mononuclear.
6. *Reduction of sugar content in CSF* is always marked.
7. *Reduction of chloride content in CSF* is probably proportional to the amount and duration of the vomiting. It may be severely reduced.
8. *Acid-fast bacilli in the CSF* is the only certain proof of the infection though the radiological finding of a lung lesion may give great help. In otitic cases the organisms may be found in the ear discharge.

Treatment

Chemotherapy with antituberculous drugs has revolutionized treatment and prognosis. Combinations of first line drugs are used – streptomycin, rifampicin, isoniazid and pyrazinamide. In moribund or stuporose patients streptomycin is sometimes given intrathecally, for an initial short period. Early treatment is obligatory for best results. Tuberculous meningitis is best managed by specialized teams.

Prognosis

Depends almost entirely on the stage at which specific treatment begins.

Arachnoiditis

The arachnoid mater may be involved in an inflammation of either the dura mater (pachymeningitis) or the pia mater (leptomeningitis), when the clinical picture is of one of those two conditions. A localized involvement of the arachnoid may, however, occur primarily.

Aetiology

1. *Chronic middle ear infection* may occasionally give rise to a localized area of arachnoidal thickening and adhesions to surrounding parts.
2. *Trauma* may play a part.

Clinical features

1. *Gradually increasing intracranial pressure* produces headache (particularly occipital), vomiting, papilloedema and visual deterioration.
2. *Involvement of the Vth, VIIth, and VIIIth cranial nerves* is common.
3. *Involvement of the cerebellum* may occur. The symptoms and signs are those of a cerebellopontine angle or cerebellar tumour. This diagnosis is usually suggested by CT scan and the true state of affairs is not revealed until operation is undertaken. A *retention cyst* of the CSF is then usually found, enclosed within the meshes of a thickened and opaque arachnoid. An *internal hydrocephalus* may result from arachnoidal involvement of the openings in the roof of the fourth ventricle.

Extradural abscess

Aetiology

An extradural abscess is usually caused by a direct extension of infection from subjacent osteitis and is most commonly secondary to a mastoiditis. It occurs with both acute and chronic infections of the middle ear cleft and paranasal sinuses.

Pathology

The collection of pus is usually well encapsulated but on occasion it may spread widely, stripping the dura from the bone.

Clinical features

Sometimes indeterminate and the finding of such an abscess is usually made by chance at operation. However, an extradural abscess over the surface of a part of the brain may exactly mimic an abscess within the brain and diagnosis may be difficult. A CT scan will clearly differentiate an intracerebral abscess from an extradural collection, but will less readily distinguish extradural from subdural abscess. This may only be possible at operation.

Treatment

Along the same lines as for a brain abscess (p. 551). Drainage is preferably done through the primary focus, but if spread is extensive craniotomy may be required.

Subdural abscess (empyema)

Aetiology

A subdural abscess may result from:

1. *Open head injury.*
2. *Extension of infection from the paranasal sinuses or mastoid air cells.*

Trauma not infrequently plays a part in those secondary to nose or ear infection.

Clinical features

As a rule the symptoms and signs differ in no way from those of an *abscess in the brain substance* at the same site. Collections of pus in this situation may occasionally travel widely over the surface of the brain and give little evidence of their presence save for intractable headache, fever and a progressively severe malaise. The diagnosis may be one of the most difficult in neurology and is often made by chance in the investigation of severe headache without brain damage and fever of unknown cause. CT scan may be crucial to the diagnosis.

Treatment

Similar to that of extradural abscess. Evacuation of pus through a burr hole or a craniotomy is necessary.

Brain abscess

Definition

A circumscribed collection of inflammatory products within the substance of the cerebrum, brainstem, or cerebellum.

Aetiology

1. *Infections of the ears or paranasal sinuses.* Account for approximately one-half of all brain abscesses. Three-quarters of these are otogenic. Rather more than one-half of the otogenic abscesses are found in the ipsilateral temporal lobe, the remainder in the ipsilateral cerebellar hemisphere. Those secondary to frontal sinusitis are all in the anterior pole of the frontal lobe of the same side. The commonest organisms found are the streptococcus, pneumococcus and *Staphylococcus aureus*. There tend to be mixed flora in otogenic and rhinogenic infections and gram-negative bacilli, moulds and fungi are common.
2. *Infections of the lungs, skin, bone and cardiac valves.*

Routes of infection

1. *Direct track of infection* leading to the abscess cavity.
2. *Septic thrombus* in which there has been a short 'jump' across normal tissue by way of the blood vessels.
3. *Bloodstream infection* from the lung or other distant focus, in which the 'jump' has been a longer one. There is a tendency in these latter cases for the infected thrombus to be seeded at the junction of the white and grey matter.

Pathology

Once within the brain, the organisms multiply.

Purulent cerebritis results from focal necrosis and liquefaction with a surrounding area of intense oedema.

True abscess is formed only when the natural process of demarcation succeeds. The rate of formation of the capsule varies considerably. It is usually definable within a week or so but it may be several weeks before a tough membrane forms to safeguard the surrounding brain.

Meningitis may develop to some degree over the abscess, depending on its distance from the surface. As the abscess wall grows thicker and tougher the surrounding brain oedema lessens and may disappear.

Clinical features

1. General symptoms and signs

Onset may be acute and fulminating, or slow and insidious, especially when the events are happening under cover of antibacterial drugs. Particularly when the infection has spread gradually through the bone from the ear or the frontal sinus, the onset is apt to be slow and unremarkable.

- *Progressive malaise.* The patient looks ill.
- *Fever,* usually irregular and moderate in degree.
- *Anorexia.*
- *Shivering or rigors* may be included in a more acute onset.
- *Delirium* is a frequent symptom and more often seen with an abscess than with any other intracranial 'tumour'.

2. Symptoms and signs due to raised intracranial pressure

- Headache, which is constant, progressively severe, and generalized. The maximum pain may be related to the site of infection, particularly with otogenic and rhinogenic infections. Headache may be worse in the early morning or related to change of posture.
- *Nausea and vomiting* occur sooner or later.
- *Deterioration in level of consciousness.* Coma may ensue.
- *Papilloedema* is the inevitable result of progressive pressure, but is a late and not essential sign of brain abscess. Diagnosis must not await its appearance.

Epilepsy

Generalized (grand mal) or focal seizures are particularly common, especially in children. Pattern of focal seizures depends on the site of abscess, e.g. posterior *frontal lobe* (motor cortex) lesions may present with twitching in the contralateral arm, leg or face. From the *parietal lobe* (sensory cortex) bouts of paraesthesiae may occur in the contralateral limbs. Seizures from *temporal lobe* lesions have a variety of forms: a short-lived hallucination of smell or taste, a momentary feeling of remarkable familiarity with the environment *(déjà vu)* or involuntary smacking movements of the lips and tongue. Auditory and visual hallucinations may also occur: the former are unsystematized; the latter tend to be recurrent formed images, momentary and vivid, carrying a strong nostalgic content, though the detail is poorly described.

Focal seizures are of value in lesion localization. They may progress to a full grand mal attack with tonic/clonic movements of the limbs and loss of consciousness. Tongue biting and incontinence are common.

4. Focal symptoms and signs

These are caused by the brain damage due to infection or by the surrounding area of oedema, and are dependent upon the area involved.

- *Frontal lobe abscess* is notoriously difficult to locate by clinical means alone, particularly in the most anterior part of the lobe. The most suggestive symptom is apathy; failure to grasp the significance of events; lack of desire to do so; lack of concentration when being examined or questioned; euphoria; inappropriate behaviour; and failure to respond normally to incontinence and personal uncleanliness. Slight changes in personality are not apparent to the stranger, and all of these failings are likely to be more apparent to relatives. Signs of a progressive upper motor neurone lesion of the opposite side of the body will develop if the lesion extends backwards into the motor cortex, with weakness or clumsiness of the appropriate limbs, increased tendon reflexes and an extensor plantar response. Dysphasia may be caused by involvement of the postero-inferior aspect of the dominant frontal lobe.

● *Temporal lobe abscess* may also be relatively 'silent', but:

(a) Upper quadrantic hemianopia in the opposite field of vision is a frequent finding, and

(b) Dysphasia is liable to result when the dominant hemisphere is involved. An abscess posteriorly placed in this lobe will tend to produce a disorder of understanding of the spoken word (receptive dysphasia). More anteriorly placed lesions will produce expressive dysphasia.

● *Cerebellar abscess* of otitic origin, is always situated in the ipsilateral cerebellar hemisphere usually the most anterior part of it where it is closest to the petrous temporal bone. Symptoms and signs are therefore those of a unilateral lesion.

(a) Clumsiness or weakness of limb movements on same side. A fault in the leg is often complained of as an unsteadiness of gait, sometimes as a staggering towards the side of the lesion. This unsteadiness may be described as 'giddiness' or 'dizziness'.

(b) Vertigo when severe or prolonged, probably indicates an associated lesion of some part of the vestibular system outside the cerebellum.

(c) Neck stiffness may be produced by adjacent meningeal reaction.

(d) Nystagmus is coarse and slow and towards the side of the lesion, and is maximal when the eyes look in that direction.

(e) Loss of cerebellar control of a limb results in failure to maintain a steady posture of the limb away from its rest position; and slowness and irregularity of rapid repetitive movements *(dysdiadokokinesis);* inability to perform a movement with accuracy and economy; inability to walk or even stand with normal balance. The finger–nose test may reveal an *intention tremor.*

(f) Large cerebellar abscesses may cause fourth ventricular obstruction and hydrocephalus.

5. CSF cell count

This is usually moderately raised (about 100 per μl). Whether polymorphs or lymphocytes predominate depends on the acuteness of the lesion. Protein content is disproportionately raised.

If an abscess is suspected lumbar puncture is contraindicated as it may cause cerebellar herniation (coning) and death. A CT scan can be diagnostic, and collaboration with a neurosurgeon is mandatory.

Investigation

CT scan will confirm the nature of the lesion and demonstrate its exact site. The abscess appears characteristically as a lesion surrounded by a ring that enhances markedly with intravenous contrast medium. In early stages, this relates to increased vascular permeability; in late stages to the formation of the capsule.

Treatment

1. *Antibiotics* are given intravenously in combination:
- Penicillin – for aerobic and anaerobic streptococci.
- Chloramphenicol – broad spectrum.
- Metronidazole for anaerobic gram-negative bacilli.

These antibiotics may be modified when the sensitivities of the organism have been determined. Consultation with the microbiologist is essential.

2. *Burr hole aspiration* through a blunt brain cannula. Reaccumulation of pus frequently occurs and is detected by regular CT scanning. Aspiration may be required three or four times before the abscess cavity is completely obliterated.

3. *Primary excision* by craniotomy is an alternative. This ensures removal of the necrotic bacterial centre, but carries an increased risk of producing or increasing a neurological deficit.

4. *Treatment of the primary source of infection* (e.g. otitis media, sinusitis) is essential within a few days of the primary procedure, otherwise further bacterial spread will occur. *5. Conservative (non-surgical) management* only may be possible if abscesses are multiple or surgically inaccessible.

Complications

1. *Acute infection* may overwhelm the natural resistance of the brain, fail to form an abscess, and spread fatally. Unskilled abscess tapping may seed infection into healthy brain.

2. *Rupture into a ventricle* may occur spontaneously, or from diagnostic or therapeutic manoeuvres.

3. *Pressure cone* may result from impaction of the temporal lobes into the tentorial opening or impaction of the cerebellar tonsils into the foramen magnum.

Intracranial venous thrombosis

Venous sinus thrombosis is a natural defence (venous isolation) against the dissemination of organisms into the bloodstream from otogenic or rhinogenic infection. Subsequent infection of the clot increases the danger of dissemination. In the pre-antibiotic era, the incidence of sinus thrombosis complicating suppurative otitis media was stated to be 1–200 cases, but this is now much reduced.

Aetiological factors

Sinus thrombosis may result from:

1. Purulent infection

Close to one or other of the venous sinuses.

2. Trauma

Involving the venous channel, less often.

3. Distant focus

Rarely, as a complication of infected venous thrombosis within the pelvis, when the metastatic infection may reach the venous sinuses by way of the vertebral system of veins. The free communication between the venous sinuses and the veins of the head and neck allows not only direct and continuous spread but also spread by short or long metastatic 'jumps'.

4. Unknown aetiology

Thrombosis may arise spontaneously. Severe inanition and dehydration, especially in the infant, predisposes. Congenital variants of the intracranial venous channels may play an important part, e.g. if one sigmoid sinus is vestigial or absent (not uncommon), a blockage of the other is liable to be more devastating.

Pathological considerations

The clot may be uninfected or infected, partially or completely obstructive. The areas of the brain drained by the sinus may be congested or softened. Recanalization of the clot commonly occurs. An individual vein draining from a discrete area of the brain may be affected alone. Alternatively, a major sinus, or more than one, may be blocked. A combination of blocked veins and sinuses may happen. The effects of sinus blockage, especially one containing many arachnoidal villi such as the superior sagittal, are likely to be more drastic than a small venous thrombosis.

Clinical features

In addition to the symptoms of the infected focus, these features depend upon:

1. *Symptoms of septicaemia* such as malaise, headache, swinging temperature, and possibly rigors and sweating.
2. *Focal symptoms of neurological dysfunction.*
3. *Symptoms of raised intracranial pressure* in some cases.

Cavernous sinus thrombosis

Aetiology

1. *Infective lesions of the upper face* via the facial and ophthalmic veins.
2. *Infections in the ear* via the superior and inferior petrosal sinuses.
3. *Infections in the pharynx and upper jaw* via the veins of the pterygoid plexus.
4. *Sphenoidal sinusitis* by direct spread.
5. *Frontal sinusitis* via the frontal diploic, supraorbital, or ophthalmic veins.

Clinical features

The signs may be unilateral or bilateral depending on whether or not there is spread from one sinus to the other via the small intercommunicating channels.

1. *Engorgement and oedema* of the upper part of the face, eyelids, and conjunctiva, come with dramatic suddenness.
2. *Proptosis of the globe* occurs without pulsation behind the swollen and closed lids.
3. *Congestion of the retinal veins.*
4. *Papilloedema* may be caused by congestion of the ophthalmic vein.
5. *Complete external and internal ophthalmoplegia* are produced by paralysis of the IIIrd, IVth, and VIth cranial nerves.
6. *Impaired sensation* over the bridge of the nose and forehead, from involvement of the first division of the Vth cranial nerve. These signs all disappear on subsidence of the pressure from the clot.

Sigmoid sinus thrombosis

Aetiology

Thrombosis secondary to suppurative otitis media occurs as the result of:

1. *Phlebitis* due to contact of the sinus with a perisinus abscess or infected bone. This may be associated either with acute or with chronic mastoiditis.
2. *Progressive thrombophlebitis* less frequently. This starts in the venous tributaries from the bony mastoid, the labyrinth, or the tympanic cavity.
3. *Surgical trauma* to the sinus, rarely.

Pathology

Thrombosis secondary to a perisinus abscess or to contact with septic bone occurs in the following stages:

1. *Periphlebitis,* i.e. a localized pachymeningitis of the dural wall of the sinus where it is in contact with the perisinus abscess or diseased bone, usually at the upper bend.
2. *Endophlebitis* with deposition of a mural clot which may spread proximally and distally.
3. *Occlusion of the sinus lumen* by increased thickness of the clot and by clotting of the stagnant blood on either side of the point of occlusion.
4. *Infection of the clot* which causes it to extend further proximally and distally. The ends are sterile though the central part may become an intrasinus abscess.
5. *Softening of the ends of the clot* by infection, with release of organisms and infected fragments into the bloodstream, causing septicaemia.

Thrombosis is usually associated with a virulent acute infection by haemolytic streptococci. In children a primary thrombosis of the jugular bulb may occur directly from the tympanic cavity.

Clinical features

Occlusion of the sigmoid sinus by a thrombosis will cause no symptoms unless organisms reach the bloodstream in sufficient quantities to cause a septicaemia.

Such a thrombosis may be found unexpectedly at operation. The sinus then presents as a hard ridge with or without dural granulations on it.

1. *Rigors* are caused by the escape of organisms. They are followed by sweating. The temperature is hectic, being 39.4°C (103°F) or more during the rigor and then falling. Between the rigors the patient may feel surprisingly well.

2. *Papilloedema and engorgement of the retinal veins* do not usually occur. When present these signs suggest further septic intracranial complications or an extension of the clot into the superior longitudinal or cavernous sinuses.

3. *Positive blood culture* is sometimes obtained if the sample is taken during a rigor.

4. *Polymorphonuclear leucocytosis* is usual. The content and pressure of the CSF are unchanged in the absence of other intracranial complications.

Diagnosis

Rigors in the presence of suppurative otitis media always suggest sigmoid sinus thrombosis. Difficulty may be encountered when otitis media is associated with other diseases causing rigors, e.g. pneumonia, pyelitis, malaria and typhoid fever. In cases of doubt the sinus must be explored.

Complications

Due to:

1. *Extension of the aseptic clot.* The clot usually occupies the sinus lumen from the entrance of the superior petrosal sinus to the jugular bulb.
- *Spread into the sagittal sinus* via the torcula, may cause 'otitic hydrocephalus'.
- *Spread to the superior petrosal sinus* may cause venous infarction of the lowest part of the motor cortex to give an *upper motor neurone facial weakness* perhaps involving the arm and even leg. When thrombosis of the superior petrosal sinus is present, however, it is usually primary. Later it may spread to the sigmoid and sometimes to the cavernous sinus.
- *Spread to the jugular bulb and internal jugular vein* may produce *pain in the neck* and resentment to neck rotation but not to flexion. This may closely simulate the neck rigidity of diffuse meningitis unless care be taken. The clot may be felt as a tender cord in the neck. The IXth, Xth, and XIth cranial nerves are occasionally paralysed by the pressure of a clot in the jugular bulb.
- *Spread to the inferior petrosal sinus* may produce a *Gradenigo's syndrome*, as the VIth cranial nerve lies close to the sinus near the petrous tip.
- *Spread to the mastoid emissary vein* causes tenderness and *oedema of the scalp* over its foramen.
- *Retrograde spread to the cortical veins* to produce focal symptoms.

early cases it is rare to have evidence of focal brain damage but there may be cranial nerve palsies (due to thick inflammatory exudate) especially of the VIth nerve. This has no localizing value in the presence of raised intracranial pressure. Papilloedema is late and slight. The CSF contains a large increase in cells (the majority being polymorphs) raised protein, reduced sugar and reduced chlorides. The pressure is always greatly raised, and organisms are usually found.

Brain abscess

Often has a subacute or insidious onset. Fever is less obvious than with meningitis. Commonly there is an extracranial source of infection (e.g. ear, frontal sinus or lung). Focal evidence of brain damage is usually present. Signs of meningeal irritation are uncommon, though there may be neck stiffness and rigidity with abscesses in the posterior fossa. There are then, however, usually signs of cerebellar incoordination in one set of limbs to suggest an abscess in one cerebellar lobe. The CSF may have normal constituents or there may be a slight pleocytosis, with a relatively greater increase of protein. Organisms are usually absent.

Intracranial thrombophlebitis

May have a sudden or subacute onset. The general symptoms are frequently much less florid than with meningitis or abscess, and in particular the patient is commonly alert and fit-looking. There is often no evidence of focal brain damage and there is no meningeal irritation. Papilloedema is early and severe in thrombosis of the longitudinal sinus. The CSF contents are usually normal, though there may be slight pleocytosis.

Whenever there is doubt, CT scan to exclude an intracranial mass or abscess must be done before the risk of lumbar puncture is taken.

LESIONS OF THE CRANIAL NERVES

Lesions of the cranial nerves and their connections may cause symptoms referable to the ears, nose and throat; while disease arising in these structures may involve certain cranial nerves.

Olfactory nerve lesions

Anosmia is discussed under Physiology of the nose.

Optic nerve lesions

Though the complications of ear, nose and throat disease rarely affect the IInd cranial nerve, it is important to understand the following conditions.

Papilloedema

Oedema of the papilla (optic nerve head as seen with the ophthalmoscope) may be caused by a general rise of intracranial pressure when it is nearly always bilateral. When unilateral it may be caused by:

1. Retinal vein thrombosis.
2. Ophthalmic vein thrombosis.
3. Cavernous sinus thrombosis.
4. Compression of the ophthalmic vein, e.g. by orbital tumours.
5. As part of the oedema of a lesion within the substance of the anterior part of the optic nerve, i.e. a retrobulbar neuritis.

Papilloedema due to a general rise of intracranial pressure results from the raised pressure within the sleeve of subarachnoid space compressing the ophthalmic vein as it crosses that space. Such a state has to be rapidly progressive or long uncontrolled before it will cause a diminution of central visual acuity, though this may occur in severe and unrelieved high pressure accompanying, for instance, intracranial thrombophlebitis, and must be watched for.

Retrobulbar neuritis

Refers to a lesion within the substance of the optic nerve. The commonest cause is a plaque of disseminated sclerosis; only a few causes are truly inflammatory. Retrobulbar neuritis is usually unilateral and subacute in onset and inevitably causes very marked diminution of central vision, frequently blindness. If the lesion is sufficiently far forward its surrounding oedema may be visible over the optic disc. Such papilloedema of retrobulbar neuritis is traditionally called 'papillitis', but its optic appearance alone cannot distinguish it from other causes of disc swelling.

Optic atrophy

Refers to the abnormal pallor of an optic disc whose component fibres have been degenerate for at least a few weeks. The degeneration may follow:

1. Retrobulbar neuritis from any cause.
2. Compression, damage or ischaemia of the optic nerve.
3. Continued papilloedema from any cause of raised intracranial pressure.

Diminution of visual fields and acuity

The importance of the peripheral fields of vision to the otologist has been discussed under the section on Anatomy. Bedside testing of the peripheral field is easily and accurately done by confrontation. Central vision, whose acuity is much greater, depends on the integrity of the retinal macula and the fibres from it proceeding to form the major and central part of the optic nerve. It is for this reason that a lesion within its substance (retrobulbar neuritis) causes a central scotoma and great loss of visual activity. A scotoma also may be demonstrated by confrontation using a small white-headed pin. Visual acuity should be tested and charted by using Snellen's test type at 6 metres from the patient. Such testing is required regularly in the management of intracranial thrombophlebitis (thrombotic hydrocephalus).

Oculomotor nerve lesions

Total lesion of the IIIrd cranial nerve

Causes

1. Complete ptosis of the upper lid which cannot be lifted voluntarily.
2. *Dilated and paralysed pupil.* The eyeball is at rest in a slightly abducted and depressed position owing to the unopposed action of the external rectus and superior oblique muscles. These active muscles can fully abduct and slightly depress the globe and there is *diplopia,* masked by the ptosis.

Lesion of the VIth cranial nerve alone

Causes partial or complete inability to abduct the affected eye, together with an appropriate diplopia.

Isolated paralysis of the IVth cranial nerve

Not easy to detect, except by analysing the diplopia.

Combined lesion of the IIIrd, IVth and VIth cranial nerves

Causes an immobile eyeball and pupil (external and internal ophthalmoplegia).

Light and convergence reflexes

Anatomy

The pupil is constricted by the IIIrd nerve (parasympathetic) and dilated by the sympathetic system, which reaches the iris via the carotid sympathetic plexus, having originated from the lateral grey matter of the lower cervical cord. These cells are under hypothalamic control. The sympathetic system concerning the eye therefore traverses both limbs of the U-shaped pathway; one within the brainstem, the other in the neck, so that the anatomy of a Horner syndrome may extend over a wide area, within or without the CNS.

Light reflex

Afferent impulses, as a result of light shone into one eye, traverse that optic nerve and play upon both IIIrd nerve nuclei so as to produce bilateral pupillary constriction. The consensual light reflex is one way of determining whether a unilateral pupillary paralysis is the result of a IInd or a IIIrd nerve lesion.

Convergence reflex

When the eyes converge or the lens accommodates for near vision, there is a pupillary constriction. This reflex is dependent upon the integrity of a different part of the IIIrd nerve nucleus from that which innervates the external muscles. This anatomical dissociation may be responsible for the Argyll Robertson pupil in which pupillary constriction to light may be lost while it is retained to convergence.

Diplopia

May be due to a disorder of one or more oculomotor nuclei or nerves; of the neuromuscular physiology; of the muscle itself; or of the lens or retina. Supranuclear lesions of the oculomotor nerves cause palsies of conjugate eye movements and therefore no diplopia.

Causes of diplopia

1. *Lesions of the oculomotor nerves* due to:
● *Raised intracranial pressure* or dislocation of the cranial contents from any cause. The VIth cranial nerve (and less often the others) is liable to damage from displacement of the brain by a tumour, e.g. an acoustic neuroma.
● *Brainstem lesions*
(a) Vascular accidents, e.g. posterior inferior cerebellar artery thrombosis.
(b) Disseminated sclerosis.
(c) Neurosyphilis.
(d) Encephalitis lethargica.
(e) Primary or secondary tumours.
● *Extracerebral lesions*
(a) Aneurysms of or near the circle of Willis. Such cases are liable to be confused with frontal sinusitis.
(b) Pyogenic or syphilitic meningitis.
(c) Complications of intracranial thrombophlebitis, particularly Gradenigo's syndrome.
(d) Nasopharyngeal carcinoma via the basal foramina.
(e) Trauma.
2. *Neuromuscular lesions.* Myasthenia gravis often presents with diplopia.
3. *Orbital lesions* such as neoplasms, abscess and other infective or traumatic conditions, which result in diplopia by displacing the globe or interfering with the action of the oculomotor nerves or muscles.
4. Ocular diplopia due to fatigue or alcohol. Here, objects overlap (as in a bad mirror or on a television screen). They are not separated by daylight.

Trigeminal nerve lesions

Sensory symptoms

Include *numbness, 'pins and needles' and pain.*

Unilateral motor paralysis

Produces slight, if any, symptoms. The masseter and temporal muscles of the two sides may be seen and felt to be unequal when the jaw is closed tightly. The opposite pterygoid muscles tend to push the jaw to the paralysed side when the mouth is opened.

Examination

Made by:

1. *Pin prick,* examining each of the three divisions separately.
2. *Light touch,* using the pulp of the finger.
3. *Corneal reflex,* using cotton wool and warning the patient that the eye reflexes are going to be tested. Absence is a sign of trigeminal nerve involvement in acoustic 'neurofibroma'. Corneal anaesthesia may lead to progressive ulceration.

Lesions of the trigeminal nerve

Include:

1. *Tic douloureux* and other facial neuralgias (q.v.).
2. *Lesions within the brainstem:*
- Disseminated sclerosis, which causes pain and/or sensory loss.
- Thrombosis of brainstem arteries.
- Syringobulbia.
3. *Extracerebral lesions.*
- Cerebellopontine angle lesions, causing compression.
- Meningitis, pyogenic or syphilitic.
- Aneurysm or tumours in the region of the cavernous sinus.
- Nasopharyngeal tumour with intracranial spread.
- Apical petrositis ('Gradenigo's syndrome').
- Glioma of the cerebellar hemisphere will occasionally involve the Vth and VIIIth cranial nerves, to simulate an acoustic neurofibroma.
4. *Extracranial lesions* are rare except for trauma and neoplasms of the nasopharynx and upper jaw.

Facial nerve lesions

Supranuclear lesions

Facial weakness of upper motor neurone origin varies greatly in degree. Severe and sudden lesions cause very obvious but always incomplete weakness, the lower parts of the face suffering most. After a variable interval there is return of function, usually quicker and more complete than in the accompanying paralysis of the limbs on the same side. There is a tendency for there to be a dissociation (in either way) between emotional and voluntary movement paralysis. Recovery is usually greater and quicker in the upper than in the lower part of the face.

Lower motor neurone lesions

The weakness is usually equally distributed between upper and lower parts of the face. Complete paralysis causes asymmetry of the face at rest. The lower lid and angle of the mouth sag on the affected side. Wrinkles are smoothed out and the mouth is pulled to the active side on smiling. Tears overflow and saliva may dribble out on the paralysed side. The paralysed buccinator allows food to collect in the cheek. The platysma fails to move the skin of the neck.

Level of lesion

This determines the exact clinical picture.

1. *In the pons.* Other cranial nerve nuclei and the long motor and sensory tracts are usually involved if the cause be vascular blockage or an expanding lesion. Taste and lacrimation are unaffected. Poliomyelitis, vascular accidents and tumours act at this level.

2. *Before entering the internal auditory meatus.* Meningitis and cerebellopontine angle tumours may involve the Vth and VIIIth cranial nerves with the facial. Taste and lacrimation are unaffected unless the nervus intermedius is also involved.

3. *After entering the internal auditory meatus.* The cochlear and vestibular divisions of the VIIIth cranial nerve may be involved with it, by trauma or by tumours. The nervus intermedius may also be involved.

4. *In the Fallopian canal.* It usually suffers alone, most commonly as the result of Bell's palsy. Lesions between the union of the motor fibres with the chorda tympani and the geniculate ganglion cause loss of taste over the anterior two-thirds of the tongue. Lesions above the point at which the nerve to the stapedius leaves it may be associated with hyperacusis (phonophobia). Tests for taste (by traditional methods or by electrogustometry), stapedius reflex action (acoustic impedance tests), salivation and lacrimation (Schirmer's test), if carefully done, permit a fair degree of accuracy in locating the upper extent of a discrete lesion. In diffuse lesions affecting much of, or the whole nerve, these tests can help to indicate the severity of a 'neuritic' process, as some functions are preserved and others lost.

5. *Below the stylomastoid foramen.* Motor paralysis only is found; taste, stapedius function and lacrimation are all unaffected.

Pathology of facial paralysis

The nerve may be affected by inflammation, compression, contusion, ischaemia, stretching, section, application of excessive heat (e.g. electrocautery), cold, ultrasonic energy and local anaesthetics.

Neuropraxia (reversible conduction block) results from minor degrees of injury.

Wallerian degeneration occurs in more severe lesions. The axons disappear distal to the lesion. Recovery is by *regeneration* of fibres and depends on: (1) resolution (or removal) of the cause of nerve injury; and (2) physical conditions which permit sprouting axons to grow down inside the neurilemma tubes and reinnervate motor end-plates. At least 3 months must elapse before reinnervation becomes evident in facial paralysis due to a lesion in the temporal bone. Final result is often marred by *residual weakness, associated movements or synkinesis* (from misdirection of regenerating fibres), fixed *contracture* of facial muscles, and sometimes *crocodile tearing* (watering of the eye during eating).

Electrodiagnosis

Essential to determine whether neurapraxia or denervation is present. May also permit conclusions regarding the gross continuity of the nerve trunk, and the progress of recovery during reinnervation.

Minimal nerve excitability (NE) test

Measures threshold (in milliamps) of the nerve trunk below stylomastoid foramen to percutaneous stimulation with an electrical pulse of 1-ms duration. Complete loss of excitability denotes severe or total denervation. Raised threshold (compared with normal side a difference of more than 4 or 5 mA is probably significant) means a substantial number of fibres is degenerate. This test is useful at any time after the first 3 days of the paralysis.

Electroneuronography

Measures the amplitude of the evoked muscle-action potential. It is claimed to give a higher degree of accuracy in prognosis than the older techniques.

Electromyography (EMG)

Needle electrode inserted in paralysed muscle detects electrical activity at rest, during attempts to move the face (both voluntary and involuntary) and (in nerve conduction-time tests) during percutaneous stimulation of the nerve trunk.

Fibrillation potentials appear any time after 7 days and indicate denervation (not quantitatively).

Motor unit potentials during attempts to move face indicate functioning nerve fibres and imply nerve trunk is in gross physical continuity even though paralysis is clinically complete.

Polyphasic (recovery) potentials occur during reinnervation, and are a good prognostic sign even before any return of movement is visible.

General management of facial paralysis

At the onset the nature and prognosis of the paralysis must be explained to the patient, with appropriate reassurance, and when early recovery is expected (i.e. in cases of simple neurapraxia) nothing more may be necessary.

In severe or complete paralysis, and in all cases with denervation:

1. *Care of the eye* involves prevention (or treatment) of corneal abrasion by protecting the eye from dust. If lacrimation is impaired methyl cellulose eye

drops at frequent intervals will prevent the consequences of a 'dry eye'. Lateral tarsorrhaphy may be necessary.

2. *Support* for the sagging cheek and corner of mouth may be provided by a 'plumping bar' which fills the upper buccal sulcus.

3. *Self-massage* of the paralysed muscles, and *galvanic stimulation* have probably only placebo value.

When recovery has begun, *active exercises* are useful. Persistence of crocodile tears after final but incomplete recovery of the face may be treated by *tympanic neurectomy*. Total failure to recover can be treated by plastic surgery (tendon transplants, fascial slings and muscle transplants) or by faciohypoglossal anastomosis. These procedures are only indicated if there is no hope of spontaneous recovery and direct surgical repair of the facial nerve has failed or cannot be attempted.

Causes of peripheral facial paralysis

Intracranial

Brainstem lesions such as tumours, vascular accident, poliomyelitis and multiple sclerosis. Cerebellopontine angle lesions include acoustic neuroma, arachnoidal cysts, primary cholesteatoma and meningitis.

Intratemporal

Otitis media (acute or chronic), trauma (surgical or accidental), herpes oticus (Ramsay Hunt syndrome, 'geniculate herpes'), idiopathic (Bell's palsy) and tumours.

Infratemporal

Parotid tumours and trauma (surgical or accidental).

Miscellaneous

Including sarcoidosis, Melkersson–Rosenthal syndrome, polyneuritis, glandular fever and leukaemia.

Facial paralysis in acute otitis media

Usually incomplete and occurs if nerve sheath (exposed by congenital dehiscence or adjacent mastoid air cell) becomes inflamed.

Treatment

Antibiotics. Early myringotomy if not improving. Cortical mastoidectomy if clinical mastoiditis is present. Exploration of nerve not necessary. Recovery almost always is early and complete.

Facial paralysis in chronic otitis media

Occurs if nerve is compressed, later destroyed, by cholesteatoma. Rarely it occurs in 'glue ear'.

Treatment

In cases of neurapraxia *immediate* operation to remove cholesteatoma and decompress nerve sheath is mandatory. Sheath should not be opened. Satisfactory recovery is to be expected.

In cases of severe or complete denervation operation must include full exposure of nerve from stylomastoid foramen to geniculate ganglion. Sheath must be opened and nerve excision and grafting performed if nerve trunk continuity is lost.

In tuberculous otitis media treatment with systemic antituberculous drugs should lead to resolution of the paralysis. Direct surgical treatment of the nerve should be reserved for cases showing no recovery after the disease has been cured.

Postoperative facial paralysis

Predisposing factors are congenital abnormality of intratemporal course of the nerve (rare) or lack of surgical landmarks within the ear. Landmarks may be unidentifiable from advanced disease or previous surgical intervention. Nerve may be exposed (congenitally or by disease) and therefore abnormally vulnerable.

Severe paralysis of immediate onset results from severe injury to nerve, e.g. transection or transfixion. Spontaneous recovery is not likely. Immediate exploration of nerve is necessary to define site and nature of lesion, and repair damage. A free nerve graft (from lateral cutaneous nerve of thigh) may be necessary. Recovery is by reinnervation, and marred to greater or lesser extent by residual weakness and synkinesis.

Incomplete paralysis of delayed onset results from minor trauma, usually pressure of packing in ear. Pack must be promptly removed. Significant denervation is usually thus avoided, recovery should be early and complete in most cases. Systemic steroids (e.g. Dexamethasone) in high dosage may lessen the intraneural oedema and reduce the likelihood or severity of denervation.

Rarely, paralysis subsequently worsens and denervation dominates EMG findings. Immediately this position is established, the nerve should be explored with the object of examining the lesion and establishing optimum conditions for regeneration.

Facial paralysis due to head injury

May be unnoticed in comatose patients, or those with severe facial injuries. Sometimes associated with evidence of damage to labyrinth, middle ear, tympanic membrane or meatal walls.

Minor contusions of the nerve and sheath cause neurapraxia. Paralysis is often incomplete and *delayed in onset*. Recovery is early and complete. No treatment of the nerve is indicated.

Severe nerve injuries, such as laceration or complete disruption, cause complete paralysis of *immediate onset.* Recovery by regeneration is often incomplete and may fail altogether. In all such cases the nerve must be explored and repaired as soon as the general condition of the patient allows. In some cases the lesion is at or above the geniculate ganglion and the middle cranial fossa approach may be necessary.

Facial paralysis in herpes oticus

Pathology

Caused by the virus of herpes zoster. Nerve trunk shows inflammatory changes, with round-cell infiltration. Geniculate ganglion bears no special brunt of the disease. Other cranial nerves often affected – V, VIII, IX, X, XI.

Vesicular rash occurs in ear, sometimes on face, scalp and in mouth or throat. Exudate contains the virus.

Symptoms and signs

Pain, often severe, may precede vesication and facial paralysis by hours or days.

Deafness and giddiness, with nystagmus, often occur.

Facial paralysis develops suddenly, but may increase relatively slowly during first 7–14 days. Usually becomes severe, often complete. A high proportion of fibres usually degenerate, so that recovery is slow to begin, and final result imperfect.

Taste, lacrimation and stapedius function are almost always affected from the onset. Taste recovers fairly quickly. Crocodile tears are a common late sequel.

Treatment

Acyclovir is effective if used early.

As for the 'General management of facial paralysis' (see p. 566). There is no evidence that decompression of the nerve, or vasodilator therapy, have any useful effect. Steroids in high dosage may be justified in severe cases.

Idiopathic facial paralysis (Bell's palsy)

Pathology

Cause is not known. *Virus infection* suspected. Some cases may be due to zoster virus without vesication.

In decompression operations marked swelling of the nerve has been noted just above the stylomastoid foramen when the sheath is opened. Recently, swelling has also been observed in the supragenicular part as exposed by middle fossa approach. For obvious reasons there are no histopathological data relating to the nerve itself, though biopsies of sheath and chorda tympani have been reported.

Primary *ischaemia* (due to constriction of vasa nervorum) followed by tissue damage and consequent secondary ischaemia due to swelling of contents of Fallopian canal form the basis of one popular theory of causation of Bells palsy. Evidence for this is circumstantial and direct proof is lacking.

Symptoms and signs

Paralysis is sudden in onset. *Pain* is variable, often absent, and may appear before paralysis begins. *Impairment of taste* also may be noticed before the paralysis. *Hyperacusis* due to stapedius paralysis is common. *Epiphora* is usually due to weakness of the eyelids. Diminished lacrimation is uncommon.

Examination shows the severity of paralysis. Tests for taste, stapedius function, salivation and lacrimation indicate probable severity of the lesion. Ears and other cranial nerves are clinically normal. In cases with marked pain around the ear, deep tenderness on pressure is often severe between mastoid and ramus of mandible.

Prognosis

Incomplete paralysis almost invariably is followed by complete recovery within 2–4 weeks.

Complete paralysis may be followed by full and early recovery if nerve excitability remains unimpaired after first 3–5 days (i .e. neurapraxia). Very few such cases go on to late degeneration.

If *nerve excitability* is lost, denervation occurs. Recovery begins only after 3–4 months and final result will be imperfect. (Some 10–15% of all cases of Bell's palsy.)

In *mixed* cases final quality of recovery depends on ratio of neurapraxic to degenerated fibres. EMG is a useful guide to prognosis.

Treatment

As for the 'General management of facial paralysis' (see p. 566). No specific treatment to prevent denervation or promote regeneration is known. The following have their advocates:

1. *Vasodilator therapy.* Nicotinic acid by mouth, stellate ganglion block, intravenous infusion of histamine, etc., could be justified only if given in the first few hours of the illness. No convincing benefit has been shown in published literature.

2. *Prednisolone.* In large dosage (60–80 mg/day for 4 days, tapering to withdrawal at 9 days) is claimed to reduce denervation if commenced during the first 6 days. As this regimen is potentially hazardous, it is only appropriate for cases (about 10% of all Bell's palsies) who have a poor prognosis untreated. The place of steroid therapy is still disputed, no conclusive evidence having been produced that recovery is favourably influenced.

General contraindications to steroid therapy must be carefully excluded before a decision is made to treat any case.

Selection of Bell's palsies for steroid therapy:
- The paralysis must be total.
- The paralysis must be of recent onset – less than 7 days, preferably only one or two.

- Slight pain only is not relevant, but *severe* pain has ominous prognostic significance.
- Electrogustrometric threshold more than 100 A above that of the healthy side of the tongue is unfavourable.

Immediate referral to an otologist is essential for diagnosis, and evaluation of need or otherwise for steroid therapy. These activities must be completed on the day of presentation and daily review thereafter is necessary.

3. *Surgical decompression of the nerve.* The general opinion is that surgery should not be undertaken. It does not prevent denervation, even if performed immediately nerve excitability is lost. To operate even earlier would be to operate unnecessarily in all those cases which would have recovered completely without treatment. Similarly there is no convincing evidence that late decompression (e.g. after 3, 4 or 6 weeks) promotes regeneration of nerve fibres. Despite these objections the operation in various forms is still practised in some countries and the reported indications for surgery are very diverse.

Facial paralysis due to tumours within the temporal bone

Rare. May be due to:

1. *Acoustic neuroma.*
2. *Glomus tumour* (chemodectoma).
3. *Carcinoma* (of external or middle ear).
4. *Metastasis* (e.g. from tumours of breast, bronchus, prostate, etc.).

In all such cases *treatment* is that of the neoplasm. If paralysis persists after apparent cure of the growth plastic surgery may minimize the cosmetic defect, or Dott's nerve grafting operation, by-passing the temporal bone, may be considered. 'Cross-face' nerve grafting techniques are currently under trial.

5. *Primary tumours of facial nerve.* Neurofibroma and fibrosarcoma are rare. Slowly increasing facial paralysis is followed by deafness, and sometimes otoscopic and radiographic abnormalities. *Treatment* is excision and repair of the nerve by a free graft.

Facial paralysis due to infratemporal lesions

Malignant tumours of parotid gland require excision and immediate repair of the nerve. Auriculotemporal nerve can be used as a free graft, its branches being anastomosed to the cut peripheral ends of the facial, and its trunk to the proximal stump just below stylomastoid foramen, or even within the temporal bone.

Injuries, either surgical or accidental, require prompt exploration and nerve repair (end-to-end suture or free graft).

Neonatal facial paralysis is usually incomplete, transitory, and due to pressure of obstetrical forceps over stylomastoid foramen. Severe cases are more likely to be due to fractured skull or brain injury.

Miscellaneous causes of facial paralysis

Agenesis of facial nerve

Extremely rare. Varies in severity. Only treatment is plastic surgery if severity of paralysis justifies it.

Primary cholesteatoma

(Retrolabyrinthine, 'congenital').

Melkersson–Rosenthal syndrome

Recurring attacks of facial paralysis and swelling of lips. Congenital furrowing of tongue. Cause unknown. Paralysis is similar to Bell's palsy and recovery is usual.

Sarcoidosis

Can cause paralyses of cranial nerves. The facial may be affected, either alone, or in conjunction with parotid gland enlargement. Recovery is usual, though some fibre degeneration is common.

Recurrences are common on either the same or the opposite side. Any patient who has had 'Bell's palsy' more than once should be thoroughly investigated for evidence of sarcoidosis.

Acute polyneuritis (Guillain–Barré syndrome).

Involvement of other nerves, paraesthesiae, systemic illness, and CSF changes indicate an infective polyneuritis. In such cases absence of sensory disturbances suggests *poliomyelitis.*

Glandular fever and leukaemia

Unusual causes of facial paralysis, which generally recovers, while the systemic disease may remain undetected. Blood examination is essential.

Facial hemispasm

Attacks of violent involuntary hemifacial muscular contractions. Rare, and affects mainly older patients. Cause not known. The twitchings are almost incessant and no treatment is permanently effective. Direct surgery may be tried in expert hands – 'needling' of the horizontal part of the nerve (by per-meatal tympanotomy), intraparotid selective division of individual branches, and posterior fossa craniotomy to eliminate suspected compression by a vascular loop at the porus acousticus all have been advocated. Nerve section and facio-hypoglossal anastomosis may rarely be justified.

Eighth nerve lesions

The cochlear and vestibular portions may be affected separately or together. Conditions arising in the end organs of the nerve are discussed under the appropriate otological sections. Acoustic 'neurofibroma' is an important lesion of the trunk, usually arising from the vestibular portion.

Acoustic neurufibroma

Pathology

This tumour grows from the sheath of Schwann (neurilemma). It is non-invasive and appears as a firm, nodular, yellow tumour with the nerve splayed out on its surface. It usually begins at the point of emergence of the nerve from the internal auditory meatus. Histologically it consists of packed sheaves of connective-tissue cells whose nuclei are arranged in palisades. Central softening may follow ischaemic degeneration.

Clinical features

The tumour occurs equally in both sexes, with a wide age incidence, usually between 30 and 60 years. Bilateral cases may occur and are then often associated with general neurofibromatosis. This association is less often found in the commoner unilateral cases. Symptoms usually appear in the following chronological order:

1. *Acoustic symptoms*
- *Deafness:* Sensorineural in type, not uncommonly overlooked.
- *Tinnitus.*
- *Vertigo* – less commonly.
2. *Trigeminal symptoms*
- *Pain, tingling and numbness* occur in any or all divisions of the trigeminal nerve but the pain is rarely of the quality of tic douloureux.
- *Diminished corneal sensation and reflex.*
- *Motor paralysis* is less easy to detect than sensory signs.
3. *Headache.* This presents at first as a dull ache behind the ear, probably from dural irritation by the enlarging growth. It appears before a rise in the intracranial pressure is apparent. Eventually pressure on the aqueduct and fourth ventricle causes dilatation of the upper three ventricles, to give rise to generalized headache, nausea, vomiting, and papilloedema.
4. *Cerebellar symptoms* follow when the tumour affects the ipsilateral cerebellar lobe. Unsteadiness (often called giddiness by the patient) is common when the cerebellum is involved.
- *Staggering* towards the side of the growth when trying to walk in a straight line.
- *Clumsiness* in the finer movements of the ipsilateral hand, arm, or leg.
- *Nystagmus,* usually a fine rapid one of first degree to the side opposite to the lesion, with a coarser slower one (also of the first degree) to the side of the tumour.
5. *Diplopia.* This is usually a result of raised intracranial pressure, i.e. a late and false localizing sign.
6. *Facial paralysis.*
7. Terminal symptoms.
- *Blindness* from papilloedema.
- *Coma.*

Diagnosis

The VIIIth nerve tumour is much the commonest lesion of the cerebellopontine angle. Posterior fossa meningioma, Vth nerve neuroma, cerebellar tumour, primary cholesteatoma, aneurysm and arachnoiditis all give similar clinical pictures but are far less common. Tests of cochlear and labyrinthine function reveal a sensorineural (usually non-recruiting) deafness and usually a canal paresis. Auditory evoked brainstem electrical responses and electrocochleography can give great help at this stage. Radiographs show erosion of the internal auditory meatus in many cases. Most recently, CT scanning with high definition and enhancement techniques has greatly improved diagnostic accuracy, though intrathecal air or myodil contrast radiography may still be necessary.

Treatment

Partial or complete removal. By craniotomy the mortality and morbidity are still formidable when the growth is large. However, surgical risks are justified when sight and life are both threatened by the tumour.

Small tumours can be removed with far greater safety by translabyrinthine approach. The otologist's microsurgical techniques result in preservation of facial nerve function in a high proportion of cases but close cooperation with a neurosurgeon is mandatory.

Glossopharyngeal, vagus and accessory nerve lesions

Glossopharyngeal nerve paralysis

Paralysis of the stylopharyngeus muscle is symptomless. Loss of sensation over a variable portion of the tonsil and fauces occurs and taste is lost over the posterior one-third of the tongue. Glossopharyngeal neuralgia is discussed under Facial pain.

Vagus nerve paralysis

1. Soft palate

Bilateral paralysis causes a nasal intonation with nasal escape and regurgitation of fluids through the nose. Unilateral paralysis is usually symptomless but the palate is drawn to the opposite side. Minor asymmetry is seen in normal persons.

2. Pharynx

Bilateral paralysis produces profound *dysphagia*. Unilateral paralysis causes a varying degree of dysphagia and the posterior wall moves to the opposite side.

3. Larynx

The symptoms and signs of the various laryngeal paralyses have been described in the section on the Larynx.

Accessory nerve paralysis

That part of the nerve which arises from the cervical cord supplies the sternomastoid and upper part of the trapezius muscles. The former rotates the head to the opposite side. Paralysis of the latter causes a flattening and weakness of elevation of the shoulder and often some slight winging of the scapula at rest.

Hypoglossal nerve lesions

Bilateral paralysis

Causes severe *dysarthria* and difficulty with the performance of the first part of deglutition. *Atrophy of the tongue muscles* and the formation of broad wrinkles in the mucosa and a coarse fasciculation follow. There is partial or complete *inability to protrude the tongue.*

Unilateral paralysis

Causes these symptoms to a much less degree and the *tongue protrudes to the weakened side.*

Pathology of lesions of the lower cranial nerves

General considerations

The IXth, Xth and XIth cranial nerves are frequently involved together for the following reasons: they share their origin in the nucleus ambiguus; they are closely related within the skull; they have a common exit from the skull. The XIIth cranial nerve although having a separate exit from the skull is in close relationship to these nerves centrally, intracranially, and below the base of the skull.

Combined lesions

May be either unilateral or bilateral. Commoner causes include:

Lesions within the medulla

1. *Arterial lesions,* e.g. lateral medullary syndrome.
2. *Syringobulbia.*
3. *Tumours,* either primary (glioma) or secondary.
4. *Motor neurone disease* (progressive bulbar palsy).
5. *Acute anterior poliomyelitis.* Bulbar.

Lesions within, or at the exit from, the skull

1. Posterior fossa tumours, e.g. acoustic 'neurofibroma'.
2. *Basal meningitis.* Acute and chronic (syphilitic and tuberculous).

3. *Basal fractures and new growths* involving the jugular foramen. This includes nasopharyngeal carcinoma.

Lesions high in the neck

Any combination of the four nerves may be involved in traumatic, inflammatory, or neoplastic disorders, particularly by carcinoma of nearby tissues and by the reticuloses.

Special examples of combined lesions

Combined paralysis of the last four cranial nerves is not of serious consequence *per se* when it is unilateral, but it is of the utmost gravity when it is bilateral. The paralysis may be either of lower or upper motor neurone or a mixture of the two. The commonest example of lower motor neurone involvement is in motor neurone disease which is also the common cause of the mixed (upper and lower motor neurone) kind. When motor neurone disease affects wholly or maximally the motor nuclei of the medulla (bulb) the disease is called 'progressive bulbar palsy'. When the upper motor neurone is predominantly or purely affected the clinical picture is called 'pseudobulbar palsy', meaning that the patient looks like an example of progressive bulbar palsy. Progressive bulbar palsy and pseudobulbar palsy present similar clinical pictures. Ironically, bilateral paralysis of the bulbar muscles, though more disabling, is less easily recognizable than unilateral ones which cause conspicuous asymmetry.

Motor neurone disease (progressive bulbar palsy)

A progressive degeneration of unknown aetiology affecting both the lower and the upper motor neurones of the brain and cord. *Lower motor neurone degeneration* usually begins in the cord, to give a gradual *weakness* with *wasting* and *fasciculation* in the limbs, most often the hands. An accompanying upper motor neurone lesion is usually detectable, if only by the extensor plantar response. *Lower motor neurone degeneration* in the *bulb* (progressive bulbar palsy) affects the *lower cranial nerves,* causing *dysarthria, dysphonia,* and eventually inability to cough or to swallow. Inanition and pneumonia lead to death.

Pseudobulbar palsy

A spastic paralysis which selectively involves the bulbar motor nuclei. *Arteriosclerosis,* less often disseminated sclerosis, are the common causes of the degeneration of the pyramidal fibres high in the brainstem. Motor neurone disease is less common. Owing to the rich bilateral innervation of the cranial nerve nuclei by the upper motor neurones from each cerebral hemisphere, a unilateral lesion of the pyramidal tract causes few and transitory signs within the cranial nerve territory. The facial muscles are an exception. With a bilateral lesion, there is *weakness* (or near-complete paralysis) *of the muscles used in chewing, swallowing and speaking,* with effects similar to those of bulbar palsy but without wasting or fasciculation. The tongue is slow-moving and pursed. Speech is slurred and monotonous. The face tends to be immobile and expressionless like that of parkinsonism. The facial emotional reactions tend to be excessive, uncontrollable, and often inappropriate to the mood. The jaw jerk is increased. The gait is tottery and shuffling, corners are turned by 'marking time'. Death usually results from inhalation pneumonia, though the dangers are not so great as in bulbar palsy.

Treatment

Although there is no curative treatment for these conditions, *in selected cases* surgery to protect the lower respiratory tract from inhalation can be of palliative value. Cricopharyngeus myotomy, epiglottopexy and even laryngectomy have a restricted but useful role in management.

Lesions of the recurrent laryngeal nerves

1. Low in the neck

Either recurrent branch of the vagus may suffer as the result of several conditions, many of which can produce a bilateral paralysis.
- *Diseases of the lymph nodes* including lymphadenitis; primary or secondary malignant disease; and lymphoma.
- *Carcinoma of the cervical oesophagus.*
- *Diseases of the thyroid gland* including benign and malignant goitres and operations on the gland.

2. Lesions special to the right recurrent laryngeal nerve

- *Aneurysms* of the subclavian and innominate arteries.
- *Carcinoma* of the apex of the right lung.
- *Tuberculous disease* of the right cervical pleura.

3. Lesions special to the left recurrent laryngeal nerve

- *Aortic aneurysm.*
- *Carcinoma* of the thoracic oesophagus and of the left lung and their mediastinal metastases.
- *Tuberculous disease* of the left pleura.
- *Enlargement of the left auricle* in mitral stenosis.
- *Other intrathoracic masses,* e.g. lymphoma.

4. Idiopathic

Some 30% of cases have no identifiable cause. Many recover spontaneously in weeks or months. A virus aetiology seems probable.

Zoster

Definition

An acute viral inflammation of the first sensory neurone and the areas of skin and mucosa supplied by it.

Aetiology

The varicella virus (identical with chickenpox) has been isolated. Zoster may give rise to varicella in contacts or vice versa. The incubation period seems to be about 2 weeks.

It is widely held that the virus is dormant in the spinal and cranial nerve ganglia and may be activated by local trauma or alteration in general immunological status.

Pathology

Acute inflammation of the ganglia occurs in the posterior root ganglia or in the sensory cranial nerve analogue. Haemorrhage and nerve-cell degeneration may be seen.

Perivascular cuffing with mononuclear cells and to a less extent with polymorphs, occurs in related portions of the spinal cord or brainstem. Similar changes are found throughout the peripheral nerves affected.

Inflammation of neighbouring meninges. Commonly.

Vesicle formation in skin results from inflammatory infiltration of the epidermis and dermis.

Clinical features

Although occurring at any age, it is distinctly more common in the latter half of life. The two forms of greatest importance to the otologist are:

1. *Trigeminal zoster*
- *Prodrome* of a few days is frequent. This consists in vague ill-health, a slight *fever,* and *pain* which can be very severe in the part that will subsequently show the rash.
- *Rash* then appears, usually over one only of the three divisions on one side. It presents as a series of *papules* (later *vesicles),* set on an irregular erythematous base. The pain is greatly intensified as the rash comes out and remains severe until fading begins, after a few days. The erythema fades and the vesicles crust and fall off, to leave small, permanent depressed scars in the skin. These areas are found to be variably but permanently anaesthetic.
- *Superficial ulceration of the cornea* may occur when the ophthalmic division is involved. The healing of these ulcers may lead to permanent scars and so to loss of vision.
- *Intractable neuralgia* may result from zoster but is not inevitable, some patients having no sequelae.
2. *Facial nerve zoster* (geniculate herpes) in which the geniculate ganglion and the nerve trunk are involved in the zoster infection.
- *Facial paralysis* appears suddenly.
- *Vesicular rash and pain* precede or accompany the paralysis. These symptoms involve the skin over the mastoid process or external meatus, or the mucous membrane of the anterior faucial pillar.
- *Loss of taste* occurs over the anterior two-thirds of the tongue on the affected side.

- *Cochlear and vestibular disturbances* (Ramsay Hunt syndrome) are explained as a spread of infection to the eighth cranial nerve.
- *Hoarseness and dysphagia* may result from involvement of the vagus.

Diagnosis

Trigeminal zoster is obvious except in the prodrome.

Facial nerve zoster. The diagnosis depends on the finding of a facial paralysis associated with the typical rash. If the rash is missed the diagnosis of Bell's palsy may be wrongly made.

Treatment

Antiviral agents (systemically and topically) such as acyclovir are becoming available and must be used in the early stages to be effective. Steroids in large dosage are advocated by some to reduce oedema, especially if the eighth nerve as well as the seventh is involved.

Prognosis

1. Facial paralysis – recovery is commonly long-delayed and incomplete with defects of coordination and mass movements.
2. Sensorineural hearing loss is often severe. Spontaneous improvement is unusual but it can occur.
3. Post-herpetic neuralgia is unusual in facial nerve zoster. When it follows trigeminal zoster, analgesics or carbamezapine can help.

HEADACHE

Headache is one of the commonest symptoms in medical practice. Not all of the structures forming the head are pain-sensitive, nor do all the sensitive ones respond to all the stimuli that would invoke pain in the skin. The following structures are capable of appreciating certain painful stimuli:

1. *Tissues covering the cranium,* including the arterial walls which respond to stretching. The periosteum is also pain-sensitive but not the underlying cranium.
2. *Dura mater* covering the base of the skull, and the tentorium cerebelli. Here it is sensitive chiefly to traction or dislocation. Other parts of the dura mater, including the falx cerebri, are not.
3. *Blood vessels,* including the meningeal arteries, the larger cerebral arteries, and the intracranial venous sinuses elicit pain on traction.
4. *Certain parts of the leptomeninges* are painful when dragged upon or inflamed.

It has been found experimentally that stimulation of pain-sensitive structures in the supratentorial compartment or the tentorium itself causes pain referred to the front of the head. From the posterior fossa pain is referred to the occiput. Many of the causes of headache have been discussed in other sections of this book, but some general principles will be enumerated and certain conditions important in the differential diagnosis of headache will be described in some detail.

Aetiology

1. Raised intracranial pressure

May result from:
- *Expanding lesion* within the unyielding bony skull, e.g. tumours, abscesses, or collections of extravasated blood. Expanding lesions raise the pressure not by their size alone but also by virtue of the surrounding oedema, particularly with brain abscesses, and their capacity for interfering with the normal flow of CSF. A posterior fossa tumour, for instance, is apt to distort the fourth ventricle or the aqueduct, to cause a subsequent dilatation of the other ventricles.
- *Inflammation of the brain and its meninges*
- *Block to the outflow of venous blood* from the skull; or the prevention of absorption of the CSF into the bloodstream.
- *Arterial hypertension* in its severer forms.

Nature of the headache in raised intracranial pressure: in terms of severity and situation, the headache bears no relation to the precise pathology. The headache is usually of recent origin and does not date back for years. At first intermittent, it tends to remit less often as time passes and to become increasingly severe. It is usually at its worst on waking in the morning and is exaggerated by exertion or by postures in which the head is low. Nearly always frontal, it may involve any other part also. In due time it is associated with nausea and vomiting. There is nothing characteristic about the vomiting due to increased intracranial pressure.

2. Meningitis

- *Acute diffuse purulent meningitis.* The headache is usually generalized but it is particularly prominent over the back of the head. There is also neck pain and often pain over the entire spine. The mechanism of the positive Kernig's sign is that flexion at the hip joint of the straight leg causes a pull on the inflamed lumbosacral nerve roots by way of the sciatic nerve. The consequent muscle contraction, to prevent further hip flexion, is akin to the abdominal muscle guarding over peritonitis.
- *Chronic meningeal irritation,* e.g. tuberculous meningitis. The headache is slower in onset, but in the end it attains the same severity.

3. Intracranial aneurysms

Cause extravasation of blood into the subarachnoid space when they rupture. The pain of a subarachnoid haemorrhage is similar in cause and effect to that of an acute diffuse infective meningitis, but it is more acute in onset like a hammer-blow to the head. The majority of aneurysms are thought to be congenital and most occur on or near the circle of Willis. At the time that they give rise to symptoms, associated vascular hypertension may play an important part in the aetiology of the following complications:

- *Rupture* is the commonest cause of spontaneous subarachnoid haemorrhage. The physical signs may be identical with those of an acute fulminating meningitis, but the history of sudden onset is likely to be sufficient to distinguish them.
- *Pressure effects* of an unruptured aneurysm on the adjacent structures may cause confusion with a frontal sinusitis. These effects may be sudden or slow, transient, or recurring. When caused by aneurysm on the anterior end of the circle of Willis, there is a sudden onset of intense pain within (or around) one eye. This may last for hours, days, or weeks and is constant or fluctuating in intensity. It is likely to go undiagnosed unless the pain is accompanied by evidence of compression of a cranial nerve or of the visual pathway, or unless it is complicated by rupture. Paralysis of one or more of the oculomotor nerves may, however, occur suddenly, often at the onset or soon after an attack has begun. Cranial nerve symptoms should not be taken lightly and without investigation as being due to a sinus infection; they are very uncommonly so.

4. Migraine

A paroxysmal disorder, attacks lasting a portion of, or a whole day, rarely 2–3 days with total freedom between episodes. *Each attack is characterized by headache plus nausea, vomiting and/or photophobia.* The head pain may be unilateral or bilateral. An aura preceding the headache is unnecessary for the diagnosis.

Aetiology

- *A congenital predisposition,* often *genetic,* is the underlying cause.
- *An initiating process,* head injury, meningitis, an emotional crisis, hormonal changes (puberty, pregnancy or the contraceptive pill) in women can start attacks.
- *Triggering factors, hunger, certain foods* – cheese, chocolate, alcohol, citrus fruits, *sleep* – too much or too little, *hormonal variations* in women, *changes in the environment* – heat, cold, excess light or noise, *local head pains* – sinusitis, upper respiratory infection, pain from neck or eyes, *exercise, travel* and *emotional stimuli,* particularly after a period of *stress,* can all trigger individual attacks.

Pathology

Migraine is an organically determined functional disorder without permanent structural fault (compare Raynaud's phenomenon).

It is disputed whether the primary disturbance is in the nervous system, secondarily stimulating blood vessels, or vice versa. The site of the vascular reaction is also under discussion – meningeal, cerebral or extracranial: in severe attacks all may be involved.

Clinical features

Infrequently migraine begins in childhood when boys and girls are equally affected. With the hormonal changes of puberty, females have an increased incidence, women being more affected than men (1.5:1). Migraine headaches commonly begin in the 'teens, twenties or thirties. Onset after the age of 40 is unusual and a neurological opinion is advisable.

If attacks begin with a headache and no aura then the patient has *common migraine;* an initial neurological aura followed by headache makes it *classic migraine* (10–15%).

- *Earliest warning symptoms* – prodromata: several hours before the headache, patients or relatives may be aware of undue tiredness, yawning, craving for food (often carbohydrates) mood changes – elation or depression, or change in bowel frequency.
- *Aura.* A neurological disturbance lasting 10–60 min after which the headache and accompanying symptoms slowly begin.

  Visual aura is the most common, presenting as a scotomatous or hemianopic field defect, or moving or stationary white or coloured lights. Diplopia or blurred vision also occur, lasting 10–60 min before headache begins.

  Paraesthesiae of the hand or circumoral region.

  Weakness of one or both arms and/or legs.

  Dysphasia and mild mental confusion.
- *Headache,* unilateral or bilateral, may be frontal, occipital, or generalized and of any severity. The pain is usually described as aching, boring or throbbing. Often accompanied by nausea and vomiting, the headache may be sufficiently disabling to cause the patient to seek a darkened room and lie still until sleep brings relief.

The aura and the headache may occur singly or together, but headache alone is common. Anxiety can increase attacks.

Diagnosis

Is made on the history alone, and there must be no abnormal physical signs on examination. The classic example can hardly be mistaken but fragments of an aura, or admixture of aura and headache make recognition more difficult. Frontal and/or facial pain are more frequently migrainous than they are due to paranasal sinus disease. Swelling of, or watery discharge from, nasal mucosa, especially if unilateral, suggests migrainous neuralgia. Overt migraine commonly follows a history of childhood vomiting which probably has a similar vascular mechanism. Migraine must be differentiated from *tension headache* – a continuous 'pressure', 'awareness', on top of the head or in a band distribution 'like a hat'. The temporalis, frontalis or occipital muscles can also give rise to headache (*see below*).

Treatment

- *Explanation and reassurance.* At present there is no cure but we can reduce the frequency and severity of attacks, prevent many and abort others. Many patients harbour unnecessary fears.
- *Prevention* is by avoiding precipitating factors (listed above) that need to be pointed out to the sufferer.

- *Aborting attacks.* Appropriate medication must be taken as early as possible.

Ergotamine tartrate 1–2 mg by mouth is highly effective in some patients who must be free from systemic and cerebral arterial disease.

Metoclopramide 10 mg to counteract the nausea, and analgesic (aspirin 900 mg or paracetamol 1000 mg) is highly effective taken early in the headache phase.

Prochlorperazine ('Stemetil') suppositories may be required if the nausea has advanced beyond oral therapy.

'*Migraleve*', a proprietary preparation containing paracetamol and an antihistamine is effective in some.

- *Speeding resolution.* Patients have different means of ending attacks: sleep, a hot meal or vomiting.
- *Interval therapy.* Patients with more than 2 attacks a month can be helped by clonidine (in smaller dosage than for hypertension), propranolol or pizotifen.
- *Complications.* When anxiety or depression complicate migraine, treatment along psychiatric lines is indicated.

5. Pains from head and neck muscles

Pain from the *temporalis muscle(s)* can arise from grinding teeth at night (bruxism), impacted wisdom teeth, a 'high bite', temporomandibular joint dysfunction, or an anxiety state when the patient clenches the jaws too tightly. Treatment: refer to an interested dental surgeon.

Pain from *upper neck muscles* can radiate over the head or the pain may be referred to the forehead. Treatment is by a physiotherapist or a rheumatologist.

Pain from the *frontalis muscle* is usually due to bad posture at work or while driving. Treatment: the mechanism of muscle pain, experienced by all after unusual exercise, needs to be explained to the patient who can often correct the posture. Physiotherapy also helps.

6. Cervical spondylosis

May give referred pain from irritation of the uppermost posterior nerve roots. It radiates upwards from the neck to the occiput and even over the vertex to the front of the head. It may be associated with prolapse of one or more of the cervical intervertebral discs. Painful stiffness of the neck recurs, with pains radiating over one or both shoulders and perhaps into the arms. *Neurological evidence of a root lesion* may be present, affecting one or both arms. *Radiological changes* are evident in the *cervical spine*.

7. Temporal arteritis (giant-cell arteritis)

A cause of mistaken diagnosis but is rare. There is an acute inflammation of the arteries of the head and elsewhere.

Aetiology. The cause is unknown. It occurs in men and women over the age of 55. The natural history, symptoms, signs and pathology are consistent with an inflammatory process.

Pathology. Characteristic lesions have been found in the temporal, occipital, carotid, retinal, mesenteric, coronary, and renal arteries.

Inflammation of the adventitia and media of middle-sized arteries is the essential lesion. Small areas of necrosis may be seen in the media, perhaps due to thrombosis of the vasa vasorum. The elastic laminae are fragmented. The intima is frequently thickened but only occasionally inflamed.

Organized thrombosis of the affected artery is common. Lymphocytes, plasma cells and large mononuclears infiltrate the lesion and typically giant cells are present.

Clinical features. Before the typical symptoms appear, there may be a *prodrome* of weeks or months, consisting of a mild general malaise, lassitude, weakness and aching pains of mild severity in the limbs. Symptoms then appear suddenly or insidiously.

- *Pain in the head* may be chiefly over the temples and frontal region, or the occiput or both. The head begins to ache intolerably and constantly. The pain is an intense, boring ache, often with a well-marked throbbing quality and occasionally superimposed with short, lancinating pains darting over the scalp.
- *Exquisite tenderness over the scalp* is typically present in the areas where the pain is worst. The patient may be unable to put his head on the softest pillows in certain positions. Classically, the patient cannot comb or brush the hair.
- *Swelling and redness* of the overlying skin, may be seen in the course of a temporal (or other superficial) artery uncovered by hair. Such an artery may be unduly prominent and may be followed by a light finger touch as a hard, hot, tender cord for a part of its length.
- *General manifestations:* the sufferer is a characteristic picture of intense misery, in severe pain, hardly daring to move his head, lacking sleep, anorectic, often wasted, with a mild fever, and perhaps sweating. This state of affairs usually lasts acutely for at least a fortnight, often longer, before the inflammation subsides and the pain and tenderness ease.
- *Ocular complications* occur in a considerable number of cases. Partial or complete loss of vision is the most serious and is due to involvement of the ophthalmic artery on one or both sides. The papilloedema which often accompanies such an arteritis may lead to a mistaken diagnosis of increased intracranial pressure.

Laboratory findings. An elevated erythrocyte sedimentation rate, 60 or more, helps to confirm the clinical diagnosis, but is often unnecessary. Some false negative results are obtained

Treatment is directed to the relief of pain and the prevention of blindness.

- *Prednisone* 60 mg initially, followed by 40 mg 8-hourly, and then gradually reduced. The condition is a medical emergency because sight is always at risk. The subjective and objective responses to treatment are dramatic, the pain resolving within 24 hours. Duration of treatment, and dosage after the acute phase are dictated by the clinical condition and the ESR.
- *Analgesics.*

Prognosis. The disease seldom kills directly but thrombosis of a coronary or mesenteric artery is an occasional cause of death at the height of the disorder. Loss of vision is usually permanent, as may be the other neurological symptoms

8. Psychologically determined headache (tension headache)

Often has a history going back many years. It is conspicuously less remitting than that of organic origin. Simple descriptive words which suffice for the patient with organic headache are not enough for the neurotic or hysteric. Anxiety symptoms or obvious depression usually accompany the headache.

FACIAL PAIN

Functional neuralgias

These are the neuralgias in which there is no demonstrable pathology.

So-called 'typical' neuralgias

1. Trigeminal neuralgia (tic douloureux)

Definition

A specific clinical syndrome in which there is recurring paroxysmal pain of brief duration (a matter of seconds), within the territory of the trigeminal nerve. It has been called tic douloureux to distinguish it from other painful conditions of the face.

Aetiology

The cause is *unknown,* except in the examples which complicate a gross disease of the nervous system, such as a tumour or disseminated sclerosis. It has recently been suggested (Janetta) that an arterial loop pressing on the sensory root in the posterior fossa is responsible. Females are more commonly affected than males, in the ratio of about 3:2. It occurs mostly over the age of 50.

Clinical features

Severe pain may last initially for days, weeks or months. Within such a bout there are oft-recurring, short-lived attacks of very severe pain of varying frequency. Each attack is described as jabbing, stabbing, burning, cutting or like an electric shock. The pain usually begins in a well-localized area at a point over the cheek, or near one nostril, or in the upper or lower alveolus, or on one side of the tongue. It often spreads from the initial point to a wider area within the affected division of the nerve. Attacks occur spontaneously or are initiated by chewing, talking, touching the affected side of the face (as in washing or shaving), or cold winds blowing on the face. Remissions are common but attacks can worsen in frequency and intensity, the remissions tending to shorten and finally to cease altogether.

Diagnosis

Certain strict criteria must be observed.

Pain is unilateral: although both sides may very rarely become affected, the paroxysms of pain never affect both sides at the same time.

Pain is trigeminal i.e. must be within the territory of the Vth cranial nerve alone.

Pain is severe: agonizingly intense while it lasts.

Pain is paroxysmal: each attack within a bout lasting only *seconds* up to one minute at the longest.

Pain is precipitated: Some attacks must be precipitated. 'Trigger' zones are usually present, where the slightest stimulus will provoke an attack. Such zones are over the lower end of the nasolabial fold and over the gum of either jaw.

There are no abnormal signs relevant to the trigemina or any other cranial nerve. A little hyperalgesia may be present over the affected side of the face soon after an attack.

Treatment

Frequent spontaneous remission, at least in the early stages of the natural history, allow of spurious claims for a host of remedies.

1. Carbamazepine (Tegretol) is effective, beginning with a small dose – 100 mg b.d. then t.d.s. then 200 mg b.d. and then t.d.s. Not uncommonly, in severe cases, it produces a striking initial benefit, which after some months wears off, so that radical treatment becomes necessary.

2. Radical treatment is necessary for the severely affected. The sensory neurone at the ganglion can be destroyed by thermocoagulation or electrolysis. The sensory root can be divided surgically, or a muscle graft may be interposed between the root and the artery compressing it (Janetta procedure).

2. Glossopharyngeal neuralgia

Definition

A rare form of neuralgia confirmed to the limits of the IXth cranial nerve and behaving like trigeminal neuralgia.

Aetiology

The cause is *unknown.* It occurs equally in the two sexes, at any time during the second half of life. A *long styloid process* or an *ossified stylohyoid ligament* has been associated with the condition, but surgical removal has not been successful in treatment.

Clinical features

Severe pain is felt in sudden bouts in the region of the *tonsil* on one side only and, maybe, deep in the ipsilateral *ear* as well. Aural pain does not happen alone. The pain has the same qualities as that of trigeminal neuralgia. Beginning spontaneously, it may be brought on by swallowing, talking, or other tongue movements. There are no abnormal physical signs, either locally in the tonsillar area or in the nervous system.

Diagnosis

Occasionally an early faucial carcinoma may simulate this type of neuralgia.

Treatment

1. *Conservative treatment* is called for until it is clear that such treatment is of no avail, for there is a somewhat greater tendency for natural cure than in trigeminal neuralgia. Tegretol should be used in the same dosage as in trigeminal neuralgia.
2. *Surgical division of the nerve* is perhaps best performed intracranially, as division peripherally does not give uniformly successful results.

'Atypical facial pain'

There is a group of patients suffering from constant or recurring pains in the face and forehead, not characteristic of either of the two disorders just described, in whom no cause can be found.

1. Atypical facial pain

Clinical features

Pain is variously felt over the cheek, nose, upper lip or lower jaw, or all these places. It frequently transgresses the midline to become bilaterally symmetrical, and just as often radiates widely to the neck on one or both sides. It is described as aching, shooting, or burning and is often accompanied by reddening of the skin and lacrimation, or watering of the nose. It lasts for hours, days or weeks; sometimes, indeed, it is incessant. The main difference from trigeminal neuralgia is that the pain is often bilateral and involves areas outside the trigeminal supply; it is longer and less remitting and is not truly precipitated. Many patients are in a tense, anxious, or depressed state. A psychological factor is an important, if not the sole, cause, and the condition is more common in women than in men.

Treatment

Strong and repeated reassurance is essential.
   Sedation is less harmful than repeated doses of analgesic drugs.
   Surgical division or phenol injection of the trigeminal nerve can give temporary relief although the resultant sensory loss adds to the burden.

2. Migrainous neuralgia (cluster headache)

Occurs more commonly in men than in women (4:1) and is allied to migraine.

Clinical features

Attacks occur in clusters of 4–12 weeks followed by freedom of months, often 1–2 years. During a cluster the patient is woken in the early morning hours by a pain behind one, always the same, eye that becomes injected, red and tears. The eyelids and the ipsilateral nasal mucosa become congested. The pain builds up over a few minutes, becomes very severe, making the patient pace around or press on the affected eye for ½–1 hour and then the attack resolves having lasted a total of ½–2 hours. When the nose is congested it may be blocked or discharge a clear fluid. In some cases the attacks occur by day and a few patients have several attacks in the 24 hours.

Diagnosis

There is no aura. The periodicity, duration, clustering, daily recurrence, the nose and eye on the same side simultaneously affected are characteristic. During a cluster, alcohol often provokes an attack 20–40 min after starting to drink.

Treatment

Ergotamine tartrate by mouth, inhalation or suppository 2 hours or more before an attack is due is effective in 8 out of 10 patients. Prophylactic therapy is used before going to bed in nocturnal attacks and twice daily in diurnal episodes.

Methysergide 1–2 mg t.d.s. is the second line in prophylaxis, Many patients also take analgesics when the pain is incompletely controlled by prophylactic therapy.

Inhaling oxygen at the beginning of the pain can abort attacks.

All treatment is stopped when the cluster is finished.

3. Sluder's neuralgia and Vidian neuralgia

Sluder described an intractable pain in the region of the nose, eye, cheek and (maybe) lower jaw. This he called lower-half faceache, the cause of which (he said) may lie in a lesion of the sphenopalatine ganglion, secondary to infection in the paranasal sinuses. Such a faceache has similarly been ascribed to a lesion of the Vidian nerve within its canal. The evidence is very slight and the results of treatment are far from satisfactory. It seems likely that many of these patients were suffering from trigeminal neuralgia or migrainous neuralgia. The sphenopalatine ganglion is better left untouched.

As stated, much the commonest cause of chronic recurring head/face pain is one where there seems to be a functional disturbance of blood-vessel tone and calibre, while structural disease of the central or peripheral nervous system in this context is rare. As a corollary to this, treatment along purely physical lines is likely to fail unless it acts along psychological pathways. Direct attention to psychological mechanisms is more rewarding.

Symptomatic neuralgias

In the symptomatic neuralgias a number of organic and well-defined lesions cause facial pain by involvement of the trigeminal nerve and its central connections.

Intracranial lesions

1. Central lesions

Occurring in the brainstem and including primary and secondary tumours of the pons and medulla, patches of disseminated sclerosis, thrombotic lesions, and syringobulbia. Secondary carcinomatous deposits, in any of these situations or in the skull base, may also cause facial pain. Occult nasopharyngeal carcinomas may cause facial pain by involving one or other divisions of the Vth nerve. There are usually symptoms other than facial pain, the pain is rarely like that of idiopathic neuralgia in detail; there are none of the true precipitants of trigeminal neuralgia; and there is usually some sensory loss within some part of the trigeminal territory, as well as involvement of adjacent structures.

2. Post-herpetic neuralgia

Herpes zoster may affect the Gasserian ganglion of the trigeminal nerve. The cause is the zoster virus.

Clinical features

- *Vesicular rash* covers one division – commonly the first – of the trigeminal territory.
- *Intense pain* always accompanies the rash during the acute stage and for a few days before it appears. As the rash fades the pain often disappears gradually with it; but the pain may remain, particularly in the elderly, and if it does so for a period longer than 3 or 4 months it rarely disappears. The pain is described as constant, intense, burning, or searing.

Treatment

The pain of long-installed post-herpetic neuralgia is a most intractable condition. It is important to realize that surgical division or alcohol injection of the trigeminal is rarely successful. A careful explanation and reassurance are the first essentials. Anxiolytics, antidepressants and supportive therapy provide the mainstays of treatment.

Extracranial lesions

Infective and neoplastic lesions of the paranasal sinuses are common causes of local pain. There are, however, two other conditions that must be remembered when the cause is not obvious.

1. Dental neuralgia

- *Dental caries* with or without gross infection, may simulate trigeminal neuralgia. Chewing and thermal stimulation are, however, the only precipitants. Careful palpation and percussion of the teeth should be performed in cases of doubt, together with appropriate radiology even in an edentulous patient, to exclude pain from a retained dental fragment.

- *Dental extraction* may be followed by a chronic, recurring, intense pain from the neighbourhood. It is always initiated spontaneously and sometimes also on direct stimulation, by temperature variation or by touch. Paraesthesiae are often present over a small adjoining area of the alveolus. Nothing is found save for a small 'trigger' zone inside the mouth perhaps associated with a lowering of the threshold to pin-prick and to touch over a small adjoining area. The pain may continue for weeks or months before gradually dying away. Possibly damage to a branch of one of the dental nerves is the cause, much like the causalgia from damage to other peripheral nerves.

2. Temporomandibular joint pain

Lesions of the temporomandibular joint give rise to chronic pain in the face. The pain varies from a dull, recurring ache over the affected joint to the most intense, agonizing, short spasm of pain which may radiate to the cheek, temple, lower jaw, ear or mastoid. These sudden sharp pains are related to jaw movements when trismus may result. Additional symptoms may arise in some cases, in the form of slight ipsilateral conductive deafness, tinnitus, or recurring vertigo (Costen's syndrome). The direct cause seems to be a degenerative condition of the joint, and in some cases at least this is caused by persistent overclosure of the lower jaw resulting from loss of teeth, ill-fitting dentures, or tearing of the temporomandibular ligament by yawning or the indelicate use of mouth gags during anaesthesia. It is differentiated from trigeminal neuralgia by its constant association with jaw opening, crepitus over the joint, radiographic changes of degeneration within the joint, and the dramatic temporary relief that comes of procaine deeply injected into the petrotympanic fissure.

Treatment is by a consultant dental surgeon.

VERTIGO

Physiology of balance

Equilibrium

Infers the maintenance of an unfixed but constantly appropriate orientation within our surroundings.

Maintenance of equilibrium

Depends upon:

1. *The vestibalar apparatus* discussed in the section on the Ear.
2. *Other sensory mechanisms*
- *Exteroceptive* includes the special sensation of sight. Stimulation of the skin and deeper structures by outside influences, such as changes of the pressure and texture of the ground under the feet.

● *Proprioceptive* impulses from *joints, muscles* and *tendons.*
3. *Motor mechanisms* include correct and ever-changing involuntary *muscle tone* of trunk and limbs, i.e. proper functioning of the pyramidal and extrapyramidal systems; and the appropriate control by the cerebellum and its connections.

Vertigo

Definition

Vertigo was defined by Gowers as 'any movement or sense of movement, either in the individual himself or in external objects, that involves a defect, real or seeming, in the equilibrium of the body'. 'Rotation' is not a part of this definition. There is no known underlying anatomical or pathological difference between the causes of rotatory and non-rotatory giddiness.

A more modern approach is to see vertigo as a sensation of movement caused by stimulation of the labyrinth or its central connections. We have all experienced this feeling on a round-about or after a boat-ride, and it contrasts with unsteadiness experienced after standing in a hot operating theatre for a long time, or rising from bed in the early morning.

Mechanism

Vertigo may be caused by any abnormal stimulation from outside applied to the sense organs concerned in normal maintenance of balance, or by disease (structural or functional) of these sensory end-organs or their central connections.

Types of vertigo

1. Physiological vertigo

Vertigo not caused by a fault of the body workings but by stimulation of normal and intact sensory structures. Examples are:
● *Giddiness of heights* from visual stimulation.
● *Giddiness after spinning movements* from stimulation of the semicircular canals.
● *Giddiness from sudden change of floor texture* from unexpected stimulation of the skin and deeper tissues of the feet.

2. Pathological vertigo

Vertigo resulting from *disease* which affects any one of the many functions used in balance:
● *Disease of the vestibular end-organs, vestibular nerve or its central connections.*
● *Diplopia.*
● *Sudden blindness.*
● *Loss of sensation from the feet, as in tabes, peripheral neuritis, disseminated sclerosis, or subacute combined degeneration of the spinal cord.*

- *Severe weakness from upper or lower motor neurone disease.*
- *The rigidity and slowness of movement of parkinsonism.*
- *The ataxia of cerebellar disease.*

Nystagmus

Nystagmus may be defined as involuntary, rhythmical, oscillatory movements of the eye. Such movements, when they are pathological, are always due to abnormal maintenance of eye posture.

Postural control of the eyes

Depends upon:

1. *Retinal impulses,* themselves dependent upon adequate visual acuity.
2. *Normal power* of the external ocular muscles.
3. *Labyrinthine impulses* acting through the vestibular nerves, nuclei, and central connections and finally the external ocular muscles.
4. *Proprioceptive impulses* arising from the neck muscles. The posture of the eyes and the balanced maintenance of that posture at any given moment are therefore dependent on an orderly stream of impulses from peripheral sources acting upon these external eye muscles.

Types of nystagmus

Physiological nystagmus

Optokinetic nystagmus is the commonest example, seen in the normal person when focusing on a series of fast-moving objects at a sufficiently close distance, as in 'railway nystagmus'. These involuntary eye movements are exactly the same as those of common pathological nystagmus, except that the quick phase of the oscillation is towards the centre or rest-point. Other examples of physiological nystagmus are found after rotational or caloric stimulation of the labyrinth.

Pathological nystagmus

May result from lesions involving any of the mechanisms responsible for the normal maintenance of eye posture.

1. *Ocular nystagmus* is common in congenital bilateral blindness, particularly when macular vision is affected, but may occur without any defect of vision. This nystagmus is usually coarse and variable from moment to moment; the two phases of the oscillation are of the same speed and amplitude. The nystagmus is therefore, pendular or jelly-like. Miner's nystagmus is a form of the ocular variety. Another form of ocular nystagmus is seen when one or more of the external eye muscles is weak for any reason. This type closely mimics vestibular nystagmus: there is a slow and a fast phase, but is confined to one eye, and only in the direction towards which the weakened muscle moves the eye.

2. *Vestibular nystagmus* has a quick and a slow component, the two phases being in opposite directions. Except in rare instances the quick phase is always directed towards the periphery, i.e. away from the central rest-position of the eyes. This kind of nystagmus is thought always to be due to a lesion somewhere of the vestibular system. The slow drift to the midline is the basically abnormal part of the movement, the quick component being a reflex attempt to maintain a desired posture of the eyes. By tradition, in Britain a nystagmus is named after the direction of its quick phase, e.g. a nystagmus whose quick component is towards the right is called a nystagmus to the right.

3. *Brainstem lesions* produce nystagmus in a vertical direction.

4. *Cerebellar lesions* (or lesions of the cerebellar connections) produce horizontal nystagmus, usually more marked to the side of the lesion.

5. *Toxic nystagmus* is seen when excess of alcohol, sedatives, anticonvulsants, or other drugs, has been taken. The nystagmus is horizontal and seen on lateral gaze.

6. *Rotatory nystagmus* – the eyes swivel round in an arc best observed by looking at conjunctival vessels. It is seen in labyrinthine or brainstem lesions.

7. *Ataxic nystagmus* is seen in lesions of the medial longitudinal bundle. The nystagmus is horizontal, coarser in the abducting than adducting eye when looking sideways. Multiple sclerosis is a common cause.

Degrees of nystagmus

Vestibular nystagmus is divided into three degrees which denote the severity and acuteness of the lesion but not its anatomical site.

First degree – when the nystagmus is present only if the eyes are directed away from the rest point, i.e. peripherally in any direction.

Second degree – when there is nystagmus on gazing straight ahead.

Third degree – there is so violent a nystagmus to one side that deviation of the gaze to the opposite side is insufficient to stop it, and there continues a nystagmus whose quick component is now directed towards the midline.

Direction of nystagmus

Varies with the site of the lesion. A destructive lesion of the vestibular end-organ or the vestibular nerve will produce a transitory, horizontal nystagmus with its quick phase towards the opposite side.

A unilateral cerebellar lesion will produce a nystagmus with its quick phase to the same side. A lesion of the vestibular system within the cerebellum tends to give a slower, coarser and more remarkable nystagmus than that from a lesion of the vestibular nerve or end-organ.

It is thought that the labyrinthine end-organ is the site of rhythmic tonic impulses which are carried by the vestibular nerve to its own nucleus of the same side. The utricle is probably responsible for these impulses.

If the impulses from one labyrinth or from one nucleus should cease suddenly (as with labyrinthine destruction), then the unaffected impulses from the opposite side will be unbalanced and tend to produce slow, drifting, turning movements of the eyes to the side of the damaged ear.

This slow drift will be reflexly corrected in the form of repeated quick jerks in the opposite direction, i.e. there will be a nystagmus with its quick phase to the side away from the damaged labyrinth.

If the damage is confined to the end-organ or vestibular nerve, this nystagmus will gradually cease as the ipsilateral vestibular nucleus begins to initiate new impulses of its own (Bechterew's compensatory mechanism).

When after the passage of time spontaneous nystagmus of this kind can no longer be seen, the remnant of the unbalanced outflow from each utricle may be seen (in an induced caloric nystagmus) as a directional preponderance to the healthy side.

Pathological vertigo

Sudden recurring attacks of giddiness, with normal or near-normal balance between whiles, are usually symptomatic of a vestibular disorder.

Labyrinthitis, Menière's disease and acoustic neurofibroma

Described elsewhere.

Positional vertigo

First described by Bàràny as a disorder of the otolithic part of the vestibular apparatus.

1. Benign paroxysmal positional nystagmus

Defined as recurring paroxysmal, short-lived attacks of vertigo in certain critical positions of the head in space.
Aetiology
- *Head injury* can cause positional vertigo that is reproducible when the patient is examined, and often accompanied by rotatory nystagmus. Surgeons must be aware of the symptoms and signs—all too often the patient is wrongly diagnosed as 'neurotic'.
- *Infective ear disease.*
- The majority happen without apparent cause and without structural disease.
Pathology
The very few cases that have so far come to autopsy show changes in the maculae of the utricle, and to a less extent of the saccule, on one side. These changes were found mainly in the utricular epithelium and subepithelial tissues, and are consistent with either trauma or chronic low-grade inflammation.
Clinical features
Are characteristic and a firm diagnosis can usually be made on the history. In the post-traumatic group, symptoms usually come on within a few days of the injury.
- *Brief attacks of vertigo* of sudden onset are noticed when the patient puts his head in certain positions, most commonly as he lays his head on the pillow. Turning from one side to another in sleep may wake the patient with vertigo. A single attack is not uncommon on getting out of bed in the morning. During the day the attacks are apt to appear on looking upwards.

- *Positional nystagmus* is diagnostic. The patient is sat up on an examination couch in such a way that his head will just project over it when he lies down. The test is explained. He is then instructed to keep his eyes open and to look at the centre of the observer's forehead. His head is held gently with both hands and turned slowly but firmly to one or other side (at an angle of about 45° from the sagittal plane) as he is laid backwards. After a latent period of a few seconds rotatory nystagmus will be seen in positive cases. This is directed towards the *undermost ear*. This lasts several seconds before gradually fading and is associated with a vertigo of the same quality that the patient has been suffering. The nystagmus soon fatigues on repetition of the test. A nystagmus in the reverse direction may occur on sitting the patient up. The evidence suggests that in unilateral disease, the abnormal labyrinth is that of the undermost ear.
- *Cochlear symptoms are absent.*
- *Caloric abnormalities* may or may not be found.

Prognosis

There is a natural tendency for a spontaneous cure which may be delayed for several months; recurrences are common.

Treatment

- *Reassurance and explanation.*
- *Antivertigo drugs* – Avomine, Dramamine, Serc, Stugeron, Stemetil, Vertigon – can be very helpful.
- *Posterior canal denervation.* Described by Gacek. The posterior cingular nerve is approached via the round window niche. There is a high risk of total hearing loss.
- *Posterior canal obstruction.* The posterior canal is 'blue lined' after a cortical mastoidectomy. The canal is carefully opened and obstructed with bone paté.

2. Central type of positional nystagmus

Acute lesions (especially demyelination, metastases, and vascular disorders) of the brainstem are liable to cause attacks of vertigo with a positional factor.

Clinical features

The history is usually shorter and more florid than in the benign type. Lasting nystagmus and perhaps other abnormal neurological signs are found and the positional nystagmus is often superimposed upon a spontaneous one and is directed towards the uppermost ear when the head is held backward and to one side. A typical positional nystagmus may be seen with such central lesions; it continues long or indefinitely and is not fatigable.

Table 23.1 Differentiation between benign peripheral and central causes of positional nystagmus

Peripheral	Central
1. Onset delayed by up to 10 sec	Onset immediate
2. Patient distressed while nystagmus lasts	No distress
3. Nystagmus fatigues in trigger position, and on repetition of the test	Nystagmus does not fatigue

Vestibular neuronitis

Vertigo, usually paroxysmal probably caused by a lesion of the vestibular nerve. The cochlea is not involved.

Aetiology

The sexes are equally affected and the majority of cases occur initially between the ages of 30 and 50. The clinical picture of streptomycin intoxication *(see below)* is identical with the usual form of vestibular neuronitis. The facts that vestibular function is severely upset, that cochlear function is normal, and that there is no evidence of a brainstem lesion have led to the belief that the lesion could be somewhere in the vestibular nerve trunk or in the vestibular nuclei and not in the peripheral end-organ.

Clinical features

The onset of symptoms is frequently preceded a week or 10 days earlier by a sore throat, acute sinusitis, or other upper respiratory infection.

1. *Vertigo* can last several days before a gradual recovery begins. Less often the onset is insidious as an unchanging mild disturbance of balance. Still less often recurrent multiple attacks of vertigo happen against a background of chronic instability.
2. *Nausea and vomiting* are commonly associated.
3. *Hearing is normal.*
4. *Vestibular dysfunction.* In the acute stage, spontaneous nystagmus of the vestibular type may be present. In all cases an abnormality of vestibular function is shown by abnormal caloric responses: canal paresis, (commonly bilateral), directional preponderance, or a mixture of the two.

Treatment

1. *Reassurance and explanation.*
2. *Antivertigo drugs* ('vestibular sedatives').

Prognosis

Vestibular neuronitis has no complication and does not affect life. Recovery is usual in a few weeks, but can take many months.

Other causes of vertigo

1. *Epilepsy* in which vertigo may also form an *aura.* The vertigo is momentary and is most commonly an aura of grand mal. It is not uncommon, however, for an epileptic to suffer occasionally his own particular kind of aura without it being followed by loss of consciousness. Such an aura occurring alone may masquerade as something quite different from the epilepsy when it is in truth merely a subliminal attack. The vertiginous aura of epilepsy arises from the temporal lobe, in the highest vestibular connections.

2. *Multiple (disseminated) sclerosis.* The brainstem is a common site for the plaques of 'demyelination', the underlying pathology of disseminated sclerosis. If vestibular connections are involved vertigo results. The medial longitudinal bundle is frequently involved giving vertigo, nystagmus and sometimes ocular palsy. Vertigo is usually of sudden onset, intense and associated with vomiting; it lasts for hours or days or even longer in diminishing degree. Other abnormal physical signs are usually present in the nervous system.

3. *Vascular accidents.* A thrombosis or embolic block of any of the arteries supplying the vestibular system may cause vertigo. *Thrombosis of the posterior inferior cerebellar artery* is the classic example.

- *Acute vertigo* with repeated vomiting is associated with marked prostration and other symptoms of shock. The severe vertigo will continue unabated for hours or days and will take considerably longer to disappear completely.
- *Paraesthesiae* and loss of pain and thermal sensation on over the same side of the face.
- *Dysphagia* due to ipsilateral paralysis of the palate, pharynx and larynx, caused by damage to the nucleus ambiguus or its outgoing fibres.
- *Nystagmus and incoordination of the ipsilateral limbs* are caused by ischaemia of the cerebellum or its connecting fibres.
- *Sensory loss over the opposite side of the body* may occur with pain and thermal loss due to involvement of the spinal lemniscus, the upward continuation of the spinothalamic tract from the spinal cord into the brainstem.

4. *Basilar (brainstem) ischaemia* is associated with very sudden loss of balance and falling, without warning and usually without loss of consciousness. It occurs in later life, usually from atherosclerotic disease.

5. *Tumours*

- *Acoustic 'neurofibroma'* only rarely causes severe attacks of vertigo.
- *Brainstem and cerebellar tumours* commonly cause severe ataxia of the limbs, trunk, or gait, but rarely cause severe vertigo. The rate of progression of the lesion probably determines the individual symptoms.

6. *Raised intracranial pressure* from any cause, is likely to give mild and short-lived attacks of unsteadiness. It may also cause momentary recurring attacks of complete blindness, commonly related to sudden head movements.

7. *Herpes zoster oticus* has long been assumed to be a cause of acute vertigo. It may occasionally be associated with nystagmus and deafness, facial paralysis and vesication in or about the external ear (Ramsay Hunt syndrome).

8. *Drugs.* Many therapeutic drugs have an unwanted effect on the nervous system, often causing vestibular imbalance, e.g. hypnotics, anticonvulsants, anti-parkinsonism drugs, etc. Others, such as hypotensive drugs, cause unsteadiness or even syncope by affecting the cardiovascular system rather than the nervous system direct.

Streptomycin and other ototoxic antibiotics have a specific effect on the vestibular end-organs especially in large doses, in the elderly or those with reduced renal function, causing ataxia and vertigo which last until the patient accustoms himself to use alternative means of balance and to compensate for a paralysed vestibular system. Rehabilitation is often incomplete.

SPEECH AND ITS DISORDERS

The learning of speech

Reception of speech

1. Hearing, seeing and feeling

The infant sees and feels objects that surround him, and hears the sounds that they emit and the conversation of adults.
- *Occipital lobe.* Visualizes these objects.
- *Parietal lobe.* Perceives the finer or more discriminative feel of them.
- *Temporal lobe.* Receives the sounds that they make or the spoken words concerning them.

2. 'Psychic' areas

As time passes, the infant gains an ever-growing and richer appreciation of the objects that he sees, hears and feels; their meaning, various relationships, value to him and their names as told to him by others. It is thought that this understanding of them is partly a function of areas of cortex that are close to, but not part of, those areas that receive the relatively uncomplicated sensations of sight, touch, and hearing. These association areas have been called 'psychic' areas, each of the three senses mentioned having such an association area at the command of the brain as a whole and of speech function in particular. If the sensory, visual and auditory areas of the cerebral cortex on the surface of the brain are taken to represent roughly an inverted triangle, then the three appropriate 'psychic' areas may be thought of as within that triangle, close to one another, mutually building and storing an understanding of the world about the child. A part of this growing storehouse is given over to the learning of speech. In respect of speech, it is the dominant hemisphere that takes over the task, i.e. the side opposite to the dominant hand.

Execution of speech

Later on, by arduous practice and mimicry the child learns to say these names himself adding other words that conjure up in another's mind what he himself has seen, felt, heard, or thought.

1. Motor speech area

In the motor cortex of the major hemisphere, close to the site that initiates movements of lips, tongue and palate, there is a special area concerned with speech alone, working in close harmony with adjacent sensory areas. This motor speech area, situated at the lower end of the *precentral gyrus,* propagates impulses in a variety of changing patterns, to move the many muscles concerned with articulation. Later, from another specialized area, muscles of the hand are made to comply with the disciplined movements of writing.

2. Upper motor neurone

This neurone transmits the preformed pattern of stimulus to the appropriate muscles. Fibres start in the motor cortex, course through the internal capsule to the *cranial nerve nuclei* in the brainstem concerned with speech; and, in respect of writing, to the anterior horns of grey matter in the cervical portion of the spinal cord.

3. Lower motor neurone

This neurone produces the finely graded muscular contractions and relaxations that are required for utterance. In this task the lower motor neurone calls on the help of the cerebellum and its connections to produce an orderly stream of words, each sufficiently separate from the last but not spaced too far apart.

Disorders of speech

Dysphasia

A disturbance of the internal mechanism of speech that results from a lesion in the cortical speech 'centres' or their connections with one another. There are many degrees of dysphasia, from an aphasia (or virtual speechlessness) on the one hand to the slightest and occasional fault on the other. The quality of the speech disorder is different from that in dysarthria, a disturbance of articulation. The fault in dysphasia is one of misunderstanding the spoken or written word or symbol, or the improper formulation (not the enunciation) of words or groups of words. There are a number of differing types of dysphasia, dependent on whether the responsible lesion involves a large or small part of the cerebral speech areas. A small localized area of damage may cause:

1. Receptive dysphasia

The fault lies in the auditory or visual association areas of the cerebral cortex, or in the subjacent white matter.

Auditory aphasia (word deafness). The patient, with adequate hearing, has an impaired or absolute loss of understanding of the spoken word. He can read normally and he can write normally so long as there is no associated loss of 'internal' speech, i.e. the ability to think in words. In some cases his spoken speech is also grossly affected, maybe to the extent of 'jargon aphasia', for he has lost the power of proper censorship of his own spoken words.

Visual aphasia (word blindness). Despite normal visual acuity, there is an asymbolia for words, letters and often for mathematical or musical signs. Spoken speech may be normal, and indeed writing may be possible but not understood by the patient when he has written it. The close proximity of the auditory and visual association areas and their common blood supply make a combination of word-deafness and word-blindness likely. Both lesions lie close to the visual pathways and may be associated with an homonymous hemianopia if the lesion is deeply situated in the hemisphere.

2. Expressive dysphasia

This may be due to a lesion of the cortical motor speech (Broca's) area or of the connections running in the white matter and linking this area with the receptive centres. There may or may not be an associated disturbance of internal speech, probably depending on which of these two anatomical lesions is present. The retention of intact thought-processes in relation to speech, dependent on this internal speech, is indicated by the patient's ability to indicate (by circuitous means) that he is fully aware of what he wants to say though quite unable to say it. Other patients, aphasic in respect of spoken speech may be able to write fluently; this indicates that internal speech is not in abeyance for it is as necessary to the written word as to the spoken word. Any disease-process affecting the cerebral hemisphere may lead to a disturbance of speech if appropriately situated. *Vascular accidents* and *brain tumours* are the commonest causes.

3. Congenital dysphasias

An acquired lesion in the appropriate part of the dominant cerebral hemisphere of an adult deals a blow to the complex speech function that has been slowly laid down over many years. Recovery depends on a return of function in the injured part. If the lesion is congenital or early acquired, however, and if it is unilateral, there is no resulting dysphasia because either side of the brain may take over the learning of speech in the early months or years. Apart from this ability to compensate more than the adult, the acquired dysphasias are in no way different in the young child. Congenital dysphasias are therefore rare and presumably due to bilateral involvement of the brain.
Aetiology
Primary agenesis or cerebral trauma suffered during birth have for long been invoked as probable factors.
Types
The commonest are those that have a fault on the receptive side of speech.

- *Congenital auditory imperception* or congenital word-deafness. This is not uncommonly familial and may occur in succeeding generations. It is considerably more common in males. Despite normally acute hearing, there is an inborn inability to appreciate the meaning of spoken words and, in some cases too, confusion in the understanding of the meaning of other sounds. The fault is not discovered until the child has passed the age at which it should learn to speak. Although the child responds normally to noises, he pays no attention to spoken words unless it be to the emotional emphasis given to them, and his own speech is confined to grunts and pantomime. The majority of cases are associated with a normal intelligence and mental capacity but not, of course with a normal learning. It is thought that the responsible lesion is in the psycho-auditory cortex and must be bilateral.
- *Congenital dyslexia* or congenital word-blindness. This is commoner than congenital auditory imperception There is a relative or absolute inability to perceive the meaning of written symbols, though visual acuity and the

fields of vision are ¨normal. It may be familial and is said to happen significantly more often in children with a family history of left-handedness or ambidexterity. Mirror writing is a not uncommon symptom, when the child may not only produce such writing but will also read the written word from right to left and mispronounce accordingly. Less florid examples are liable to be overlooked or ascribed to mental defect or 'backwardness'. Recognition is important because many agree that this may be a discrete brain fault causing slowness reading and therefore learning in a child of normal intellect.

Differential diagnosis

From deafness, mental deficiency, or very rarely, autism.

Management

No medical treatment is possible. Such children have special educational needs which must be met.

Dysarthria

Dysarthria is a disorder of articulation resulting from faulty working of appropriate cranial nerve nuclei, their peripheral connections, or the muscles, ligaments or joints upon which they act. In dysarthria there is no fault in understanding of the spoken or written word, and there is no difficulty with the formulation of ideas or choice of words.

1. Supranuclear lesions

The majority of the cranial nerve nuclei receive innervation from both cerebral hemispheres via both pyramidal tracts. Therefore unilateral pyramidal tract lesions do not lead to a paralysis of the muscles of articulation, and dysarthria occurs only with bilateral supranuclear lesions. Bilateral lesions of the pyramidal pathway high enough to involve the corticobulbar tracts cause a distinctive dysarthria, congenitally in a cerebral diplegia, or acquired in degenerative or ischaemic changes. The voluntary muscles used in speech show a weakness and clumsiness combined with an increase of tone, i.e. a spasticity. Speech is slow, sometimes with explosive outbursts, laboured and slurred, and it has a distinctive 'stiff' quality; frequently there is an associated difficulty in swallowing, choking, especially in the early morning, and drooling of saliva. Often there is a poverty of facial expression and a slowness of gait. This condition has been called 'pseudobulbar palsy', to distinguish it from bulbar palsy, in which the nuclei and their nerves are involved rather than the upper motor neurone.

2. Nuclear, infranuclear and muscular lesions

The VIIth, Xth, and XIIth cranial nerves are directly concerned with speech.
● *Facial paralysis,* especially when bilateral, affects the production of labial and dental sounds, making them indistinct and 'woolly'. A bilateral congenital nuclear agenesis is occasionally seen, while pontine tumours, vascular lesions and poliomyelitis all involve the nucleus of this nerve. The nerve is also involved by various lesions in the posterior fossa, middle ear cleft, and outside the skull.

- *Lesions of the vagus nerve* cause a paralysis of the soft palate which, if bilateral, produces 'nasal escape', from inability to shut off the nasopharynx from the mouth cavity. If the responsible lesion be nuclear or in the main trunk of the nerve above its ganglion then *paralysis of the vocal cord* will be associated, e.g. in bulbar poliomyelitis.
- *Lesions of the hypoglossal nerve cause ipsilateral weakness and wasting of the tongue.* If unilateral the dysarthria is slight and soon compensated. A bilateral paralysis is much more disabling to speech. Consonants sound clumsy, slow, and 'thick'. Lesions of this nerve at the nuclear level are most often due to bulbar poliomyelitis, syringobulbia, vascular lesions of the bulb and progressive bulbar palsy.
- *Myasthenia gravis* in which the fault lies at the neuromuscular junction, may cause any of the above types of dysarthria as a result of undue fatigability of one or more muscles. The dysarthria is variable, accentuated by exercise and reversible with anti-cholinesterase drugs.

3. Lesions of the extrapyramidal motor system

Give rise to changes in muscle tone, posture and movement, due to pathology in the basal ganglia. Disease of a part of this system, such as parkinsonism, gives rise to changes in muscle tone, posture and movement. The muscles show an increase of tone in the form of rigidity, slowness of voluntary and associated movement, a tremulousness but no true weakness. The speech is slow, monotonous, indistinct and sometimes high-pitched. Certain congenital lesions of the basal ganglia produce a peculiar writhing restlessness of voluntary movement—athetosis. Speech may be affected with other movements. to produce a jerky. explosive, indistinct enunciation.

4. Lesions of the cerebellum and its connections

The cerebellum and its connections are concerned with graduating and harmonizing voluntary movement. Speech may suffer from divorce from cerebellar control. There are a number of component faults in cerebellar dysarthria, and not all may be present in one patient. Slurring and scanning occur, and there may be an explosiveness of speech. Such defects tend to be more florid when the midline structures of the cerebellum are involved or the disease is bilateral. Tumours of the cerebellum, tumours compressing it from without, degenerative lesions and multiple sclerosis all cause a cerebellar dysarthria.

Stammering

Stammering is a functional disorder of speech without any underlying structural cause. There is no associated dysphasia and no abnormality of the lower motor neurones or muscles concerned with speech. The break in the normal flow of speech, either a complete arrest or a repetition of sounds or syllables, is probably psychological in origin. Its close association with left-handedness or forced right-handedness suggests an anatomico-physiological basis. Its association with neurotic traits is strong. Diagnosis is easy because the patient can sing fluently. Treatment is by speech therapy.

Disorders of voice

Dysphonia

Follows changes in the larynx and has been discussed in the appropriate sections.

Rhinolalia

A change in the tonal character of the voice. There are two types:

1. *Rhinolalia operta* results from incomplete closure of the nasopharyngeal sphincter. It occurs with cleft palate, 'short' palate, and with limitation of palatal movement from mechanical impedance or paralysis.
2. *Rhinolalia clausa* results from obstructive lesions in the nose and nasopharynx. It occurs with the common cold, adenoids, nasal polypi and septal deformities.

Other changes

1. *Weakness of voice* from pulmonary insufficiency.
2. *Changes following impairment of hearing.*

Index

Abducent nerve, 14, 527
Abscess
  apical, 25
  brain, 522, 550, 551, 553, 554, 558, 560
    aetiology, 551
    clinical features, 552
    complications, 554
    differential diagnosis, 560
    investigations, 553
    meningitis with, 551
    pathology, 551
    thrombosis in, 556
  bronchial, 511
  cerebellar, 150, 553, 558
  extradural, 550
  frontal lobe, 552
  intracranial, 198
  laryngeal, 469
  Luc's, 118
  lung, 357, 508, 511
    in carcinoma, 516
    pneumonitis and, 511
  mediastinal, 517
  metastatic, 119
  nasal septum, 215, 217, 220, 345
  nasolacrimal passage, 276
  nasopharynx, 333
  oesophageal, 403, 404, 413
  orbit, 248
  parapharyngeal, 349, 350
  peritonsillar, 346, 349
  petrous bone, 110
  pharyngeal, 118, 346
  postauricular, 118
  retropharyngeal, 351, 352
  in sinusitis, 238
  subdural, 550
  temporal bone, 527
  thymus, 517
  tonsillar, 348
  von Bezold's, 118
  zygomatic, 118
'Abscess-tonsillectomy', 350
Absolute bone conduction test, 52

Accessory auricles, 81
Accessory nerve
  anatomy, 533
  lesions, 575
  paralysis of, 575
  peripheral course, 534
Achalasia of cardia, 441
Acne rosacea, 221
Acoustic impedance, 131
Acoustic nerve
  division in tinnitus, 166
  lesions of, 572
  neurofibroma, 165, 572, 573, 579
  electrocochleography in, 60
  MRI in, 30
  radiology, 29
  in Wegener's granulomatosis, 135
Acoustic neuroma, 156, 277, 536, 571
  recruitment in, 55
  tone decay in, 55
Acoustic trauma, 143
Acquired immune deficiency syndrome, 311, 384
Acromegaly, 257, 388
Actinomycosis, 233, 328, 337, 468
Acyclovir, 91, 326, 337, 338
Adamantinoma, 260
Adenoidectomy, 345, 353
Anodontia, 320
Adenoid facies, 344
Adenoid pad, 294
Adenoids, 111, 119, 244, 267, 343
  diagnosis, 344
  removal of, 111, 309
  symptoms and signs, 344
  treatment of, 345
Adenoma
  ear, 93
  nose, 250
  oral, 358
Aditus ad antrum, 11, 12
Aerocele, 210
Aero-otitis, 104
Aerophagy, 412

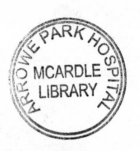